Praise for *Americc*

"Deeply researched and meticulously crafted, *American Breakdown* is at once a damning indictment of the systems shaping our way of life and an engrossing narrative of the lives of two women connected across the centuries. A literary triumph, brimming with righteous anger, empathy, curiosity, and hope."
—Olivia Campbell, *New York Times* bestselling author of *Women in White Coats: How the First Women Doctors Changed the World of Medicine*

"Part medical mystery, part literary excavation, Jennifer Lunden's intimate and intricate debut chronicles her search for the source of her unexplained chronic illness and the parallels she finds in the biography of Alice James. In the end, Lunden arrives at an explanation for her body's mutiny, but her scalpel-like prose also identifies and resects the illness latent in our entire ailing system—personal, political, planetary. . . . This mesmerizing book is an essential story for our time, maybe *the* story."
—Ted Genoways, James Beard Award–winning author of *The Chain: Farm, Factory, and the Fate of Our Food*

"Using herself as an investigative tool, Lunden unspools an incredibly re-searched story not just of her 'mysterious fatigue' but of how a bankrupt healthcare system in a broken country gaslights women about their bodies and minds. A tale that is both enraging and affirming. If you demand answers about *anything*, let Lunden be your guide."
—Kerri Arsenault, winner of the Society of Environmental Journalists' Rachel Carson Environment Book Award and author of *Mill Town*

"Jennifer Lunden has written a wide-ranging, fascinating, and deeply personal account of unexplained illness, showing that behind the all-too-common word 'unexplained' lie decades of medical failings. By tracing lines of medical epis-temology, the impact of research funding, and the proliferation of chemicals in modern life, both in her own life and across historical parallels, she takes on nothing less than the entire Western medical system. Her research is com-prehensive, her writing both rousing and riveting. Anyone who has ever felt abandoned by healthcare will find not only comfort in this crucial book, but inspiration to push for change."
—Alex Marzano-Lesnevich, United States Artists fellow and author of *The Fact of a Body: A Murder and a Memoir*

"Epic in scope and impeccably researched, from wallpaper to junk food to the pharmaceutical industry and art, Lunden unfolds a personal and historical medical mystery, filled with secret poisons and unexpectedly poignant, relatable moments. *American Breakdown* offers a vital message of hope and advocacy for our bodies and future."

—Emily Maloney, author of *Cost of Living*

"Deftly moving between the personal and the political, Jennifer Lunden offers both an intimate, affecting account of two women's illnesses and an eye-opening indictment of how American capitalism is harming us all."

—Maya Dusenbery, author of *Doing Harm: The Truth About How Bad Medicine and Lazy Science Leave Women Dismissed, Misdiagnosed, and Sick*

"More than a medical memoir, Lunden's book is a multifaceted exploration of how runaway capitalism, gender bias, and a broken medical system may lead to the collapse of our society. In the tradition of *Silent Spring*, she lays out a roadmap for revolution."

—Kris Newby, author of *Bitten: The Secret History of Lyme Disease and Biological Weapons*

"An earnest chronicle of the enigma of chronic fatigue syndrome, the byzantine dysfunction of the medical world and the chemicals and pesticides that are making so many of us ill, *American Breakdown* is told in short, accessible, and interwoven fragments that will be familiar and edifying to anyone who has been sick and tried to find an answer to the painful question, *Why?*"

—Caitlin Shetterly, author of the award-winning memoir *Modified: GMOs and the Threat to Our Food, Our Land, Our Future*

"Visionary and exacting, *American Breakdown* is a revolutionary guide for responding to chronic illness in an industrial society."

—Katherine E. Standefer, author of Kirkus Prize Finalist *Lightning Flowers: My Journey to Uncover the Cost of Saving a Life*

"An absolutely beautiful book, and a life story that is all too familiar. How many brilliant books need to be written by patients suffering from these overlooked and undervalued illnesses before the medical community starts to pay attention? If there is any justice in the world, *American Breakdown* will be the tipping point."

—Sarah Ramey, author of *The Lady's Handbook for Her Mysterious Illness*

American Breakdown

Our Ailing Nation, My Body's Revolt, and the Nineteenth-Century Woman Who Brought Me Back to Life

Jennifer Lunden

HARPER

NEW YORK · LONDON · TORONTO · SYDNEY

HARPER

A hardcover edition of this book was published in 2023 by Harper Wave, an imprint of HarperCollins Publishers.

AMERICAN BREAKDOWN. Copyright © 2023 by Jennifer Lunden. All rights reserved. No part of this book may be used or reproduced in any manner whatsoever without written permission except in the case of brief quotations embodied in critical articles and reviews. For information, address HarperCollins Publishers, 195 Broadway, New York, NY 10007.

HarperCollins books may be purchased for educational, business, or sales promotional use. For information, please email the Special Markets Department at SPsales@harpercollins.com.

Parts of this book, often in slightly different form, were previously published in *Creative Nonfiction, Orion, Longreads, The Yale Journal for the Humanities in Medicine*, and in *Charlotte Perkins Gilman: New Texts, New Contexts*, eds. Jennifer S. Tuttle & Carol Farley Kessler (Columbus: Ohio State University Press, 2011).

FIRST HARPER PAPERBACKS EDITION PUBLISHED 2025.

Designed by Nancy Singer

Library of Congress Cataloging-in-Publication Data has been applied for.

ISBN 978-0-06-294139-8 (pbk.)

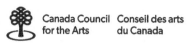

Canada Council   Conseil des arts
for the Arts   du Canada

We acknowledge the support of the Canada Council for the Arts.

Considering how common illness is, how tremendous the spiritual change that it brings, how astonishing, when the lights of health go down, the undiscovered countries that are then disclosed . . . it becomes strange indeed that illness has not taken its place with love and battle and jealousy among the prime themes of literature.

—Virginia Woolf, *On Being Ill*

In threatening to undo or unfix the self . . . illness also holds the potential to reveal the everyday world in a new light.

—David B. Morris, *Illness and Culture in the Postmodern Age*

This book is in part about gender bias in healthcare. Although beyond the purview of the book, it's important to note that patient treatment and outcomes are also impacted by conscious and unconscious bias based on gender identity and presentation, sexual orientation, race, religion, disability, weight, age, and history of mental health diagnosis or substance use disorders. And of course, healthcare providers can themselves be discriminated against within their profession based on these embodied experiences and/or identities.

CONTENTS

PART V Recovery

Bedridden

bedridden: confined (as by illness) to bed

confine: something (as borders or walls) that encloses; *also*: something that restrains <escape from the confines of soot and clutter. —E. S. Muskie.>

archaic: RESTRICTION. obsolete: prison.

—*Merriam-Webster's Collegiate Dictionary, 11th ed.*

CHAPTER 1

Bankruptcy

I imagine her in the summer of 1862, swimming with friends off the coast of Newport, all of them laughing and teasing, splashing around, showing off—the things young people did in the water in the mid-nineteenth century, and still do. They've swum out beyond the surf and the water is calm and warm, and for a moment, perhaps, Alice James feels free.

She is thirteen, on the cusp of young womanhood and all its accompanying constraints. The water sparkles in the sunshine, rippling around her body. Does she swim the breaststroke to protect her hair? Does she float on her back and look up at the vast blue sky? Or does she dive down deep, eyes open, reveling in a world so different from the one above the surface?

Looking back almost thirty years later, Alice wrote in her diary of that vanished girl, lamenting her "blank youthful mind, ignorant of catastrophe."

———

I was twenty-six years old when I first laid eyes on the gold spine of Jean Strouse's *Alice James: A Biography* and pulled it down from the shelf. I'd heard about Alice; we had something in common. We'd both been felled by a mysterious fatigue.

The book is fragile now. Its cover barely holds on to the spine, and some of the pages are falling out, and most of them bear some kinds of markings. The price, two dollars and fifty cents, is still penciled inside the front cover. Someone else had owned the book before me. When I bought it, I took a purple pen to her name, crossed it out and wrote my own and the year: 1994. I'd been sick for five years.

I didn't know then that the book was treasure in my hands. It would become my company, my work, my healing.

At the time, I was the live-in caretaker of a 1789 historic house museum in Maine, its substantial perennial garden laid out in measured decorum inside a white picket fence. When I think now of that garden, I see it bursting in the violent bloom of high summer—stands of white liatris spiking the azure sky; gold rudbeckia, six feet tall and toppling; aphids on the helianthus; mold on the phlox; weeds overwhelming all the back beds. The garden was too much for me.

From the bedroom window on the second floor, I could see the explosion of color, a carnival of red, yellow, purple, and pink. But I rarely looked down upon the garden from the bedroom window. Because what I saw more than anything, even from that vantage, was my failure to keep up.

For me, the garden was something to be contended with. When I should've been weeding it, taming it, saving it from itself, instead I lay in bed in the cool of the oscillating fan reading about my dead bed-comrade, Alice James.

In Alice, I met my Victorian counterpart, my kindred spirit. And somehow, reading about her—bright, witty, proud, and stuck—I began coming unstuck.

Why was Alice sick? Why was I?

From my bed, and with the aid of interlibrary loan and a helpful librarian, I set out on a journey to find some answers. I spent years researching American history, nineteenth-century and contemporary toxicology, biology, medical history, economics, environmental history, sociology, chaos theory, and more, and by the time I finished, things were a whole lot clearer.

———

Ninety-nine years before I was born, Alice collapsed. She was nineteen years old in 1868, two years younger than I would be when illness took me under. Her eldest brother, William, had just given up preparing for a career in medicine and was floundering toward his destiny as the father of American psychology. Henry, who would become one of America's most celebrated authors, had just seen his first story in print. Her brothers Wilkie and Bob were pursuing their own career opportunities three years after surviving Civil War combat.

All her siblings suffered, intermittently, with perplexing pains and debilitations. But Alice, from that point on, spent most of her life in bed with nothing to commend her to posterity but a private diary she didn't even begin to write until many years later.

Alice had fallen victim to a mysterious epidemic that was sweeping the country. Its symptoms were not fatal but left sufferers in a state that sometimes felt closer to death than to life. The hallmark of the illness was an inexplicable, incapacitating fatigue that sent many, like Alice, to their beds. Almost no bodily system was spared. Victims endured headaches, insomnia, digestive problems, chronic pain, anxiety, inability to concentrate, and vertigo. They sank into dark depressions. Physicians were at a loss to produce an effective treatment.

In 1869, esteemed neurologist George Beard gave this diverse set of symptoms a name: neurasthenia. For forty years, the illness wreaked havoc throughout the country. Then, as mysteriously as it arrived, it seemed to drop off the face of the planet.

Or maybe it didn't.

———

As Hemingway once wrote about bankruptcy, it was gradual, and then it was sudden. Something was wrong.

The year was 1989. I had just moved to Portland, Maine, 650 miles from my home in Canada, launching at last into adulthood and everything I believed it would bring. I would build, finally and from the ground up, a life of my own choosing.

I bought the newspaper every day, clipped potential opportunities from the want ads, taped them into a loose-leaf binder, made calls, dressed up for interviews, shook hands firmly, smiled, looked people in the eye. I studied maps. Drove circles around the city, finding my way.

I was excited. I was scared. I was happy.

To tide me over, I signed on at a temp agency. Every morning I got up and called in, asking for work. I was the hired hand in factories and cafeterias. I was the envelope stuffer.

———

I found a studio apartment in a 1920s-era building, a former hotel. The elevator had an iron gate that slid back manually. High ceilings, hardwood floors, pigeons cooing on the ledge. The windows were open the morning I found the place; I could smell the ocean in the air.

One sunshiny day, after I hung the crystals from the windowsills and pinned the Georgia O'Keeffe print over my bed, I stood in the middle of my room and looked around. Everything was in its place. My apartment was clean and bright, and my big orange tabby, Cassie, who'd ridden shotgun all the way from Canada, lay curled up and content on my corduroy patchwork quilt.

I sat down on my bed to revel in my new home. The bedroom was papered in dappled blue wallpaper flecked with gold: I felt like I was immersed in a Monet painting. The light made patterns on the wall, and when it hit the crystals just right, my floor was scattered with rainbows.

But something was happening to my body. I was tired, inexplicably. I kept thinking I would feel better, and then I didn't.

I felt so weak.

But weakness was a shameful thing; it didn't belong to me.

Hadn't I been strong enough to watch my mother drive away when I was eleven and barely shed a tear? To take over the care of my six-year-old brother and cook dinner after school while my father worked? Wasn't I an A student who quit college to teach in a remote village in Belize? Hadn't I worked in a refrigerator tubing factory till I'd saved enough to pack my Toyota and drive across two countries, setting down roots in a city where I knew not a soul?

I was strong.

Wasn't I?

———

The temp agency sent me to a local dairy whose conveyor belt had broken. The foreman, dressed in a thin white coverall, handed buckets to the other two temp workers and me, showing us how to scoop up the cottage cheese and lug it up to the next floor, where we would dump it into another giant vat.

I needed the money. Trembling with exhaustion, I kept scooping and carrying, scooping and carrying.

———

I dragged through my days, and finally, on June 30, 1989, dragged myself three blocks up the street to the walk-in clinic. I wondered, *Is it physical . . . or is it psychological? Is it just the stress of the move? What if it's something worse?*

It felt like something worse.

The doctor listened as I told her about my move to Maine and the mysterious fatigue. She took my blood and said she'd call with the results.

———

I got a job as a residential aide at a group home, but each day at work was like walking through water. My job would not have been considered physically strenuous for any healthy person. I reminded three women with developmental disabilities how to use the washing machine, fold and put away their clothes, take out the trash, and boil the wieners on the menu for that night's dinner. Often I just sat with them in the living room and watched TV. But all of these jobs involved sitting or standing. Every day I was exhausted and every day I was getting worse.

That same year, a syndrome the press dubbed the yuppie flu was entering the public consciousness. Four years earlier, an outbreak in the idyllic skiing community of Incline Village, Nevada, near Lake Tahoe, made national news. Over 160 people in the town of 30,000—most of them women—had been taken down by a mysterious fatigue.

In 1989 George Herbert Walker Bush had just been sworn into office. The *Exxon Valdez* spilled 11 million gallons of crude oil into the pristine waters of Prince William Sound. A crane lowered the now-iconic bronze bull to the sidewalk in front of the New York Stock Exchange. Prozac, the wonder drug, would soon become the most widely prescribed antidepressant in the country. And in China, a lone man in a white shirt stood down a long line of tanks in Tiananmen Square, then disappeared.

Somebody from work brought me an old black-and-white TV and set it up for me at the foot of my bed. I accepted it gratefully, a concession to my illness. I couldn't even hold a book. I lay there and watched *Guiding Light* and *Entertainment Tonight* and *Late Night with*

David Letterman. I stopped getting up to brush my teeth at bedtime. I slept fitfully through the night, sweating inexplicably, waking with headaches. I began taking baths in the morning rather than stand in the shower, but even that sapped the life out of me.

The telephone rang one day in early July. I answered it from my bed. The doctor from the clinic told me I had a mild case of mononucleosis. The good news, she said, was that the test showed I was in the recovery stage. "But you're going to have to take it easy for two or three weeks."

I had a diagnosis, and it would be better soon. What a relief.

"But how did I get it?"

"Who knows? A water fountain at work? No way of knowing, really. You're just going to have to rest up. It's a virus. There's nothing we can do but wait for it to pass."

———

But it didn't pass.

I lay on my bed limp, exhausted. Spent.

But I had to work, shop for groceries, do my laundry. So I kept going, resting when I could, but mostly I kept on going.

On August 8, 1989, I wrote in my journal, handwriting all angled and askew, "I'm so tired I can hardly hold the pen."

That is when I called my mother.

She was studying photography in a small town two hours north of Portland. I told her how sick I was, how full of despair. When she invited me to convalesce at her place for a few days, even promising to come and fetch me, my body slumped with relief.

In the car, Cassie curled up in my lap. I gazed out the window, watching the city disappear, and burst into tears. "I can't do it anymore, Mom. I can't. I'm just so *tired*."

"Oh, Jen," said my mother. "I'm sorry it's so hard right now."

"I'm too tired to be cheery or fun or interesting or intelligent . . . I feel so ugly and unlovable. I'm *nothing*. I'm just a blob." I wiped away tears, but more came. "I'm in this mass of chaos that I can't put back in order. I can't *do* it. There's too much, and I'm too weak. Everything's falling apart."

"Maybe instead of trying to put the chaos in order, you could just simply *observe* it."

"I hate it when you tell me to *just observe*."

"It might relieve you of your suffering."

"I *can't* just observe. I'm *in* it. If I don't hold everything together, who will?"

We sped up the highway. I turned and looked at my mother. "Mom, I've *never* felt lovable." I started to cry again. "I didn't feel like you *loved* me."

"Oh, Jen." She glanced over at me, her expression tender with regret. "I'm sorry . . . I . . . I probably didn't." I could feel myself crumbling inside.

"I was so caught up in my own misery," she continued. "I just didn't have it in me then to love you the way you should have been loved." Outside the window, the city had been replaced by Maine's dense forest. "I'm sorry," she added.

I cried harder. Was it better to be validated? Was it worse to know that my feelings were true?

Alice was twenty-four the year her mother, Mary, died. She would later describe her as "a beautiful illumined memory, the essence of divine maternity." Henry would write: "she was the house, she was the keystone of the arch. She held us together, and without her we are scattered reeds."

What Alice and I shared was as notable as what we did not.

———

A year earlier, in 1988, the disorder had been given its official name, *chronic fatigue syndrome*. With telltale imprecision, the name failed to accurately represent the incapacitating array of co-occurring symptoms. In addition to debilitating fatigue, sufferers also described chronic pain in joints and muscles, headaches, cognitive dysfunction, depression and anxiety, sleep disturbance (insomnia and/or hypersomnia), digestive problems, fever, vertigo, and more. It was like a wicked flu that never went away.

While two Incline Village doctors tried desperately to determine what was happening to their patients' bodies and other researchers also took up the cause, the syndrome was the butt of jokes at the Centers for Disease Control and Prevention (CDC). When any of the epidemiologists complained of being tired or stressed, their colleagues quipped that they must have contracted the strange condition, which at the time was believed to be associated with the Epstein-Barr virus (EBV). The syndrome's chief investigator, Gary Holmes, had scrawled on a poster of the Statue of Liberty on the wall in his office, "Give me your tired, your weak, your EBV-positive, yearning to be diagnosed."

The derisive skepticism from one of the U.S. government's top health agencies soon trickled down to doctors and the mainstream media. The CDC's preliminary findings about the Incline Village outbreak, published in the widely distributed *Morbidity and Mortality Weekly Report* in May 1986, prompted the Associated Press to report, "Federal health officials said there is not yet sufficient proof that a new disease which supposedly ravaged the Incline Village area last year actually exists." On ABC's *Nightline*, medical correspondent Dr. Timothy Johnson stated bluntly, "The question is whether the cause is biological or emotional." And on a CBS news show, medical expert Dr. Richard Jacobs, an associate clinical professor of infectious disease at the University of California at San Francisco, declared: "This is a trend. It's a real fad."

After my weeklong retreat at my mother's, I returned to my little apartment in the city, and a friend's roommate, who suffered from the illness, sent me a packet of clippings and support-group handouts. I knew she was trying to be helpful, but I hadn't asked for the information and didn't want to be a part of that club.

But what else could it be? Page by page, I read through the packet. Finally I called the doctor. "What if it's chronic fatigue syndrome?"

"If you think that way," she replied, "you'll make it so."

———

In 1988, Stephen Straus, the only National Institutes of Health (NIH) physician with an interest in the illness, declared, "It's clear to me that most of the people there [Lake Tahoe], whatever they had, weren't part of an epidemic. Now, the question is, of those who were there, were they just fatigued and achy and psychoneurotic? Or was this mass hysteria?" Later that day, referring to the belief that the illness primarily struck yuppies, he quipped, "Maybe these are the individuals who, you know, they just don't want to drive their BMW unless they feel up to it, and they need our help to get behind the wheel." He added, without offering any evidence, "There's a large history of psychiatric problems in these patients." Almost a decade later, in 1997, feminist scholar Elaine Showalter listed the syndrome alongside alien abduction and satanic ritual abuse as examples of "hysterical epidemics" in her book *Hystories*.

Meanwhile, tens of thousands of people were falling ill, losing their jobs, and watching the lives they'd built for themselves wither on the vine.

———

I needed a doctor; I couldn't afford a doctor. I had no option but to take an extended leave of absence from work.

I called my father and asked if he and my stepmother would help me out financially. He said they would be willing to lend me the money to get by for the next month, but I could hear the constriction in his throat. My father had worked hard all his life. He rarely sat down, even on weekends. And he was athletic: played tennis in summer and squash in winter. When I was a teenager, if he passed my room and saw me reading in bed, he would pause in my doorway, clear his throat, and ask me to clean the litter box or help my stepmother fold the towels. Now, on the phone, he said, "Maybe you just need to get a clerking job. Something less stressful. At a record store or something."

"Dad. The group home job is actually pretty easy. I like it. A record store would be worse. I'd have to be standing. All day. This isn't an emotional thing. I'm physically *exhausted*."

I had to find a primary care doctor, someone who could see me consistently, someone who could help.

The receptionist behind the plexiglass window handed me an intake form on a clipboard and asked me to fill it out, waving me toward the waiting room. Nondescript chairs lined three of the walls. There was a lonely feel to it, despite attempts at warmth—the maroon area rug edged in vining pink flowers, the dollhouse and wooden bead maze tucked away in the corner.

I looked down at the clipboard and checked off all the boxes that pertained to me, and, finished, picked up a magazine. An ad for DuPont promised better things for better living. A photocopier ad promised built-in automatic anxiety reduction. A life insurance company declared itself a leading pain reliever. My name was called.

A nurse led me into a small, windowless room, weighed me, and took my blood pressure. I handed her the clipboard and repeated my symptoms to her; then she left.

A diagram of the internal workings of the human body—the organs, muscles, veins—hung from the white wall. I studied it as I waited.

Finally Dr. Beyer entered, chart in hand—a slim woman with

short, wavy brown hair. She looked up, introduced herself, and gave a perfunctory greeting before sitting down on a rolling stool. "What seems to be the problem?" she said.

I told her I'd moved to Portland in January and had been diagnosed with mono in July. "The doctor at the clinic told me I should feel better in two to three weeks, but it's been seven weeks and it's not getting better. I'm exhausted all the time even though I'm not *doing* anything. I'm on leave from my job and just lie around in bed all day. It's really depressing. And I have all these other problems . . ."

She wrote something in the chart in her lap. "What other symptoms are you having?"

"Well, I never used to get headaches, and now I get them all the time, even in the morning when I wake up. And I've got this pain in my eyes. Sometimes I get dizzy or nauseous for no reason, and my gut's all messed up." I told her about my night sweats, the aches in my legs, the swollen glands in my neck, the recurring canker sores. "It seems like my body is falling apart, and nothing I do seems to help me get better."

Dr. Beyer scribbled something else in my chart.

When she looked up, I asked: "Do you think it could be chronic fatigue syndrome?"

"We'll run some tests."

And then she was standing up to go.

I knew CFS wasn't diagnosed with a blood test. But maybe she'd find something else, something easy to treat. Maybe there was a pill for it. Maybe there was a cure. Maybe I'd be all right.

———

When I tried to push against the illness, the illness pushed back, and harder. Even a brief game of catch would wipe me out the next day, and I'd have to cancel any plans and stay home in bed.

September 14, 1989

> No to Texas with Tom. No to Toronto with Kieran. No to camping, no to golf, no to bowling, bingo, sleeping out by the ocean, no to volunteering at the retirement home, no to singing and choirs, no to dancing at the Tree Café.

September 15, 1989

> I'm tired from talking on the phone with Gail. My left arm is very tired. I'm shaky. I hope I revive soon. Was it too much? How can that be too much?

September 16, 1989

> Very tired today. Called Drew and asked him to take me grocery shopping, then called him later to cancel. He asked me out to breakfast with him tomorrow; I had to decline. A reading tonight . . . the book he published on his letterpress, he was even going to wear a tie—and I had to decline. . . . A trip to Bangor? No, no. I can't.
>
> Tomorrow is the chronic fatigue syndrome support group. I don't want to go, use up my energy. Have to do my clothes soon.

I moved to Maine for the big YES. But all I got was no. And always that nagging fear: What if it doesn't get better?

I wrote to my friend Gail back in Canada that I had devised a scale to rank my fatigue: "It's a scale of one to ten. Zero is dead." Most of the time, I told her, I charted myself at a one.

But now I was fluctuating between a two and a three . . . perhaps even a four for some brief moments.

Ten was normal: full recovery. It seemed wholly out of reach.

————

The tests Dr. Beyer ran were a complete blood count (CBC) to check for anemia, infection, and leukemia, and a lymphocyte function assay to check my immune function. When I returned for my follow-up appointment, she told me the tests had come back normal and that I should begin a program of light exercise and take vitamin B.

This, I knew, was not the answer. Exercise made things worse. But desperate for anything that would help, I did pick up some vitamin B at the health food store even though I knew that what was happening to me was more than a little vitamin B could fix.

―――

The first written indication of concerns about Alice's health came in the form of a letter to Ralph Waldo Emerson, written by her father, Henry Senior. Alice, thirteen years old and fairly "palpitating" with excitement, had received an invitation to visit with Emerson's daughters, Edith and Ellen. At first Henry Sr. gave her "carte blanche to go at any expense of health," as he described the scene to Emerson. But when her mother saw Alice's "expectations so exalted," she determined that the toll might be too great and forbade the trip. Alice was crushed.

A year later, William, then twenty and studying at Harvard, wrote to her in his inimitable tongue-in-cheek style, "I hope your neuralgia or whatever you made believe the thing was has gone and you are going to school instead of languishing and lolling about the house." Humor aside, his words must have stung. William's joke articulated what Alice couldn't yet know she would be contending with for the rest of her life: although her symptoms were real and debilitating, because their origins weren't understood, their legitimacy was suspect.

―――

By the time I fell ill, Dr. Phillip Peterson, a physician who headed the infectious disease department at the largest public hospital in Minneapolis, had seen enough of the devastation caused by CFS to organize a study to assess its morbidity. Surveying patients in the clinic, he and his colleagues tallied startling results. While healthy people scored an average of 75 out of 100 (with 100 being perfect health) and people with rheumatoid arthritis scored in the high 40s, CFS patients scored an average of just 16. No other illness had ever scored so low.

In a separate study, even people undergoing chemotherapy scored higher. That study found that all its CFS-stricken participants "related profound and multiple losses, including the loss of jobs, relationships, financial security, future plans, daily routines, hobbies, stamina and spontaneity, and even their sense of self because of CFS. Activity was reduced to basic survival needs for some subjects."

Using a different morbidity assessment tool, Dr. Mark Loveless, an infectious disease specialist who treated both HIV and CFS patients in his Portland, Oregon, office, found that even in their last week of life, many of his AIDS patients scored higher on the scale than CFS patients. Twenty years later, Dr. Nancy Klimas, an immunologist who also treated both AIDS and CFS patients, had this to say about the impacts of the two illnesses:

> My HIV patients for the most part are hale and hearty thanks to three decades of intense and excellent research and billions of dollars invested. Many of my CFS patients, on the other hand, are terribly ill and unable to work or participate in the care of their families. I split my clinical time between the two illnesses, and I can tell you, if I had to choose between the two illnesses in 2009, I would rather have HIV.

One CFS specialist said the illness should be called "chronic devastation syndrome."

———

The welfare office was stark: orange plastic chairs in the waiting room, the light hazed a fluorescent, dingy yellow. In a small, windowless office a woman sat behind a desk and began reading off questions from the form in front of her. I wanted to apologize for taking her time, for being the cause of forms to be filled out. I wanted to offer to fill out the forms myself. Show her that I was capable of doing something even if I couldn't pay my bills.

She asked me why I wasn't working and what I paid for rent and said I would need to bring evidence of all my bills before they could help me. "And you'll need to work for your benefits," she said, sliding a form across the desk at me. "Unless you can get this filled out by your doctor."

———

When I didn't recover, my father agreed to continue lending me a small monthly sum, which helped me pay for my medical expenses. I was more fortunate than many, because he and my stepmother could afford to provide this extra support. But the fact that his assistance came in the form of a loan signaled to me that he was afraid my illness was all in my head and that his monthly checks might otherwise encourage malingering. Given the state of things, I didn't know when or how I would ever be able to pay him back.

———

I did some research before my next doctor appointment and arrived armed with a list, along with the form my caseworker had given me. As Dr. Beyer signed the form excusing me from Workfare, I pulled out my list and handed it to her. "I found an article that named illnesses with symptoms similar to chronic fatigue syndrome. Do you think it could be anything on this list?"

She gave it a cursory glance and shook her head, handing the sheet back to me.

"Are you sure? For instance, I was in Belize before I moved here . . . Could it maybe be parasites?"

She shook her head briskly. I looked at the list.

"Multiple sclerosis?"

No.

"Lupus?"

No.

"Lyme disease?"

Nope. No to everything.

"But how do you *know*?" I said.

"Not the right symptoms."

And that was that. She ushered me out of her exam room and back to the plexiglass window to write her a check.

———

I never got over the strange sensation that overcame me as I signed a check to pay for my doctor appointments. That was not something anyone was expected to do in Canada. It just felt so *wrong*.

When I was preparing for my move to the United States, my father suggested I purchase travel insurance in case I got sick. I'd pondered this briefly, but ultimately rejected the idea. I was twenty-one years old and healthy, moving to Maine on a shoestring. I decided to take a chance. For the first time in my life, I would be uninsured.

I moved to the U.S. and promptly got sick—sicker than I had ever been in my life.

In Canada, everyone had health coverage, paid for by the federal and provincial governments through both personal and corporate taxes. The only time Canadians pulled out their wallet in a doctor's office was at their very first appointment, when they presented their government health card. There were no deductibles, no copays, no hidden fees. In Canada, healthcare was viewed as a human right. In fact, both the World Health Organization and the United Nations declared health a fundamental human right in the 1940s.

I was living on welfare, too sick to work, could barely afford hair conditioner or tampons, but in order to get medical care I had to shell out a substantial percentage of my monthly loan. The entire transaction felt a little dirty, a little, well—sick.

———

One afternoon, sitting at the wheel waiting for a light to change from red to green, I spotted a woman I'd worked with at the group home before my leave of absence and tooted my horn. A redheaded woman in her late fifties, she was in the early stages of multiple sclerosis.

"You look pale," she said.

I confessed my despair.

"Are you heading anywhere?" she said. "Why don't we meet at the Victory Deli?"

We ordered tea. She listened for a long time. Then she said, "Sounds like you could use some extra support right now. Do you know about the Feminist Spiritual Community?"

I didn't, and she told me it was a group of women who had been gathering for several years, using goddess spirituality and ritual to celebrate and support one another. They happened to be meeting that very night.

"Will you be going?" I asked.

"No, but I used to go, and I think you'll like it."

When I arrived at the old Quaker meetinghouse where the group gathered, two greeters welcomed me into the sanctuary. Within were twenty women sitting in a circle. The room, lit with candles, felt quiet and sacred. Serendipitously, that night they'd planned a special healing ritual, and invited anyone in need to lie down on the floor, each with a woman sitting behind her head and others by her sides. The women sang songs about the goddesses Demeter and Isis, and I lay in the midst of it all, eyes closed, focusing on allowing the support and healing to enter my body. The sanctuary filled with the harmony of their voices, and the women at my sides laid their hands gently on my arms. This felt like mother love. Or what I imagined mother love must feel like. Tears slid down from the corners of my eyes.

———

After that, I sought out every support group I could find. I tried A.R.T.S. Anonymous; Co-Dependents Anonymous; and a support group for people with depression and bipolar disorder. Eventually I found an attitudinal healing group for people facing life-changing illnesses. There were several regulars. A woman who had lost much of the use of her left arm due to cancer treatment, a young mother facing breast cancer, and a smart, acerbic man whose skin was still a deep indigo after being born blue due to a congenital heart defect.

"While there is not always a cure," said Ken, the facilitator, a kindly man who had retired from his career as a surgeon to form the nonprofit that ran these groups, "there can always be healing." So we learned how to reframe our thinking, how to consider the messages our illnesses might be offering, how to envision a great ball of healing light flowing through our bodies.

I started a journal to try to get at the emotional source of whatever had gone wrong. I read Joan Borysenko's *Minding the Body, Mending the Mind* and Charles L. Whitfield's *Healing the Child Within* and Shakti Gawain's *Creative Visualization* and Louise Hay's *You Can Heal Your Life*. I worked on letting go of resentments. I learned about my inner child. I envisioned a vibrant future. I read Arlene Blum's *Annapurna: A Woman's Place*, because the women facing that treacherous Himalayan mountain reminded me of me, the me in that bed trying to make her way to the top of the mountain, and then back down again.

I found a therapist through a community counseling agency. Her name was Marsha. Since I had no insurance, I paid the agency on a sliding scale, $10 a visit. Marsha had a way of reflecting back every-thing I told her with no expression of her own. It was like talking into a mirror.

I kept going back. She was all I had.

———

In December, Dr. Beyer told me that the latest lab tests had revealed no further evidence of the Epstein-Barr virus in my system. The mono had run its course.

So why was I still sick?

She didn't have any answers for me. I was exhausted, and she was exhausted of me. She disappeared me with her impatience. Every time I went to see her, I felt her irritation.

I endeavored to return to work, failed, and, submitting my letter of resignation, consigned myself to my life in bed.

———

My doctor couldn't help me; but maybe somebody else could. I be-gan seeking out alternative healthcare providers. A woman who studied flower essences told me that these essences worked on a deep vibrational level; she gave me a tincture that she thought would help. I wrote down the tincture's accompanying affirmation: "I transcend apparent limitation and frustration." Four times a day, I diligently added a few drops of the magical elixir to a glass of water and drank it.

———

My bed faced the door to my apartment, which meant that all day I was faced with the means of my escape—which then reminded me that there was no escape: the fatigue followed me wherever I went, and rest was my only means of treatment.

I recorded in my journal one morning that a mysterious acrid odor had seeped into my apartment. I opened my front door to investigate. Whatever it was, it seemed to have permeated the entire building. The odor lingered for the rest of the day, and by bedtime I had a piercing headache that Advil couldn't alleviate.

When I awoke the next morning, the inexplicable smell was gone and my headache had receded.

———

In April 1990, my case manager said she needed an updated form from my doctor verifying my inability to work. I phoned Dr. Beyer. When she returned my call, I explained what I needed.

"No, I can't do that. I can't help you with that," she said.

"But I'm *so* fatigued. I just—" She cut me off.

"You're just depressed. It would be good for you to go back to work. And I recommend psychotherapy."

I hung up the phone, gut-punched. She thought I was just depressed. *Just.* As though what I really needed from her was a firm shove back into the real world.

I wonder now if in med school Dr. Beyer had studied Talcott Parsons's 1951 theory of the "sick role." Parsons, a sociologist, theorized that as unproductive members of society, the ill entered a role of "sanctioned deviance" that disturbed the social function of society. A doctor's job was to police this deviance, to make sure the ill did not benefit so much from their exemption from normal social roles that they refused their duty to get well.

Since she couldn't *see* my suffering, couldn't quantify it, then surely I must be reaping tremendous secondary gains in this great ploy of mine to live on welfare benefits instead of working like a productive

citizen. After all, how many ninety-hour weeks had she pulled to get
through med school?

———

Many years later, when I asked a CFS group on Facebook what kinds
of comments they had gotten from doctors over the years, I was inundated with responses. "You're just depressed" got a callout. Also: "You
need to see a psychiatrist." And: "You don't want to get well because
then you'd have to go back to work."

And these:

"So what is it this time?"

"As long as you can lick a stamp, you can still work."

"You need to join a health club."

"Do cognitive behavioral therapy."

"You don't look sick."

"Force yourself to get out of bed."

"You're not dying."

"I'm not sure how real your symptoms are."

"Oh no, dear . . . it's not curable. What do you want me
    to do?"

"Another neurotic young female."

"You're a mom, that's all. You are just tired."

"Get more exercise. You're depressed."

"You would feel better if you lost some weight and exercised.
    Listen to nice music. Get married!"

"Nothing's wrong. It's all in your head."

When asked about support groups, one doctor sighed and said, "I suppose I can refer you, for all the good it will do."

———

I arrived empty-handed to my next welfare appointment. My case manager mercifully assigned me a low-stress position volunteering for a refugee resettlement program. On my first day, the supervisor took me down to the agency's dim basement, gestured to the metal shelves piled with donated tchotchkes, dishes, and table lamps, and asked me to cull out the useless things and organize what remained. Then she went back to her office.

I pulled out the mugs and glasses one by one, the bowls and the plates, the metal pots and baking pans, my body awash with fatigue. I worked for the allotted two hours, and then went home to bed, exhausted.

The next day I went back to the refugee agency and worked some more. Then I drove home and collapsed. And then I called up Ken, the doctor who facilitated my attitudinal healing group, and asked if maybe *he* could sign the welfare form.

And he did.

———

Another letter of regret penned by Alice's father, this time when she was eighteen, indicated that quashed plans were not unusual for her. The fatigued Alice had to break a date to accompany her friend Annie on an outing to the Museum of Fine Arts. "She is not able even to write to you to say how 'awfully' sorry she is to be forced to disappoint your hospitable intentions once more," wrote her father. "'What a mysterious world it is,' she cries, 'where one's force is never equal to their good-will, or their good-will . . . never equal to their force!'"

Sitting in my car one day after a trip to the grocery store, head tipped back against the headrest, eyes closed as I summoned the energy to lug my bags to the elevator, suddenly I pictured myself an empty corn husk, browning, crackling at the edges. If any more life seeped out of me, I would crumble into dust.

How had my life come to this?

Earlier that day, I'd paged through my photo albums and found pictures from the camping trip I took with my college friends the summer before moving to Maine. We'd had such good laughs, the crew of us—Betty-Anne, the actress; Monica, the social work student; Debbie, who was studying sociology; Karen, the environmental studies major; and me, the writer. One weekend, Karen's blue-eyed mountain climber boyfriend, Jeff, took some of us rappelling, something none of us had ever done.

From my place in my bed, I studied the photo of me leaning off the edge of a cliff wearing a red-striped harness strapped over my track pants. In my gloved hands—right hand in front of me, left hand behind—I gripped a rope. I smiled gamely for the shot, but I made no bones about the fact that I was scared shitless.

"You've got this!" Jeff had shouted from below. And I did.

Now, here, I was alone, exhausted, all crumpled up inside.

I got out of the car, lifted my bags out of the hatchback, and made my way across the street, up the two granite steps in my building's brick courtyard, and through the heavy glass door, a second door, and finally to the black iron gate of the old elevator. I pushed the gate open, set down the bags, pressed the button for the sixth floor, and leaned against the elevator's back wall, waiting for it to take me home.

Cassie was asleep on my quilt. She looked up at me in greeting, and I collapsed into bed and buried my face in her orange fur.

I wanted to die.

I didn't want to die.

I wanted to die.

I didn't want to die.

I picked up the phone and called my therapist.

But Marsha was busy with some other client's crisis. The receptionist told me to go to the emergency room if I needed assistance.

———

I can't remember how I got to the hospital. I do remember the long walk down the ill-lit corridors—everything in shades of gray. I was walking as though asleep on my feet, one foot after the other, looking for the emergency room, thinking it must be just around the next gray corner.

And then I was behind a curtain, waiting for a doctor. Feet scurried in every direction. Finally the curtain opened, and there before me stood a tall doctor who bore a striking resemblance to Richard Chamberlain. He told me his name and shook my hand. In the tunnel of my vision, his hand looked very large and oddly comforting.

I told Dr. Kildare about the illness and all it had taken from me. "My life is slipping through my fingers, and it feels like this fatigue will never go away," I said, and I started to cry. "I'm not going to commit suicide. It's not in me to do that. But I want to die."

Dr. Kildare stood there and listened, in that small moment in that bustling hospital, a look of compassion in his eyes, and I knew then that I could go on.

"We're going to help you," he said. "I don't think you need to go up to the psych ward tonight. But here," he said, handing me a slip of paper, "this is Dr. McCarthy. He's a psychiatrist. I'll schedule an appointment for you to see him tomorrow. I suggest you also go to our walk-in clinic for some more tests to check on the situation with the fatigue."

I was filled with gratitude and hope. I was not alone. Someone said they would help me.

On the way home I stopped at the art store for some fingerpaints. They came in bold colors: red, blue, green, and yellow. I bought a roll of white paper, thirty inches wide. In my room, I unrolled a wide swath of it and dipped my hand into the cool red paint. I smeared the letters, one after the other, onto the paper. I dipped my hand into the blue and slid it over the red paint. Then yellow. And then green. I made another banner, and then another. One for each wall that I could see from my bed. LIVE, I had spelled out. LIVE. LIVE.

CHAPTER 2

Still Waters

A network of entwined lives, theories, and treatment advances runs from Alice and William in the late nineteenth century to my arrival at Dr. McCarthy's office at the hospital in the late twentieth. The room, with its drawn shades, was a quiet sanctum. He invited me to sit down and tell my story. I told him about the fatigue that had shattered my life—how I'd come to Maine to launch my adulthood and how the illness shackled me. How I'd had to quit my job and go on welfare. How I'd barely had time to make any friends before I got sick, and how these new friends were out in the world doing things while I was chained to my bed. How I'd been depressed twice before, in high school, and how this crippling fatigue was another thing entirely. I told him about my mother's depression and about the day she drove away. I told him how this weakness was anathema to me. Unsure of what was relevant, what not, I told him everything I could think of.

When I was done, he said, "I am struck by your fortitude, even in the midst of this hardship."

This was an angle I hadn't considered. I'd been so immersed in my weakness, I couldn't recognize my strength.

"This continued fatigue you've been experiencing could be the lingering effects of mononucleosis, it may be emotional, or it may be both interrelated. In any case, it's clear your symptoms are debilitating. I can see how much you want to get better, and whether it's physical or emotional, you're on the right track," said Dr. McCarthy. "What I *can* do is give you a prescription for an antidepressant that might help you."

I told him I wasn't sure I wanted to take an antidepressant. He shrugged and said, "It's up to you." Then he slid the script across his desk. "Just in case," he said. And I took it.

Driving home, I felt lighter, more hopeful.

I didn't fill the prescription.

———

When Alice regretted that her "force" wouldn't permit her to join her friend Annie at the museum, she was referring to the nineteenth-century notion of nerve-force, what we today would simply call "energy."

Doctors at that time believed that each person was constitution-ally predisposed to a certain amount of nerve-force, and—correlating human biology with capitalism—that overspending one's energy could precipitate nervous collapse. Surging industrialism, the rapid onslaught of modernity, and the ruthlessness of American capitalism were all believed to be responsible for the sudden rise of neurasthenia. Famed neurologist S. Weir Mitchell, in his 1872 book *Wear and Tear: Or, Hints for the Overworked*, wrote that American nervous systems were "sorely overtaxed." He blamed:

> . . . the cruel competition for the dollar, the new and exacting habits of business, the racing speed which the telegraph and railway have introduced into commercial life, the new value which great fortunes have come to possess as means toward social advancement, and the overeducation and overstraining of our young people

for bringing about "some great and growing evils"—namely, neurasthenia—"now beginning to be distinctly felt."

Renowned neurasthenia specialist George M. Beard agreed. Comparing nerve-force to capital, he suggested that some people were "millionaires of nerve-force . . . who never know what it is to be tired out, or feel that their energies are expended, who can write, preach, or work with their hands many hours, without ever becoming fatigued, who do not know by personal experience what the term exhaustion means."

Correspondingly, he found that there were increasing numbers of people who, although they appeared healthy, "are yet very poor in nerve-force . . . and if from overtoil, or sorrow, or injury, they overdraw their little surplus, they may find that it will require months or perhaps years to make up the deficiency, if, indeed, they ever accomplish the task." He called this latter state "nervous bankruptcy."

Alice was nerve-force poor. Bankrupt.

And so was I.

———

At eighteen, Alice surrendered herself for six months to the care of Dr. Charles Fayette Taylor, who, like many of his time, believed that an excess of mental activity and particularly "emotional prodigality," or immoderation, could provoke nervous disorders in women. "I would especially include the *emotions* as the most exhausting of all mental attributes," he said, noting that "women are emotional as a class of human beings," and prone to "excitable temperaments."

So Alice learned to quell her emotional life. "Owing to muscular circumstances my youth was not of the most ardent," she later wrote, "but I had to peg away pretty hard between 12 and 24, 'killing myself,' as some one calls it—absorbing into the bone that the better part is to clothe oneself in neutral tints, walk by still waters, and possess one's soul in silence." She was taught that such restraint would restore her to good health—or at least prevent her further decline. And she wanted to get better.

For a woman who later described herself as a "geyser of emotions," walking by still waters could not have been easy.

In fact, it was not. In a letter to Henry, their mother wrote, "Alice is busy trying to idle, and it is always very hard depressing work, this to her; but I think it will tell in the end."

I'd spent my whole life trying to quell my emotions. One day, while I lay on an acupuncturist's table, splayed in my tan cotton robe like a subdued butterfly, she posed a question. "If you were a body of water, what would you be?"

"A tsunami," I replied. I had always felt myself to be a force of nature. Too much. Something that needed to be restrained.

"But don't you see?" said the acupuncturist. "You can't restrain a tsunami. How exhausting it must be, to aspire to something so fruitless."

Hope can be a tenuous, unstable thing. The copious letters of the James family record a period, roughly from 1868 to 1872, when Alice "improved." Alive at a time when therapies were only beginning to be conceived of by her brother and his fellow psychologists, Alice had sewing bees to join rather than support groups, and books and needlework in lieu of talk therapy. And she rallied, albeit cautiously. William shared his optimism in a letter to Henry celebrating "the slow steadiness of her improvement" and enthusing that "she never thinks now of lying down." One can almost hear a familial huzzah in William's follow-up comment: "If it keeps on at the same rate this summer she'll be as good for social purposes next winter as any one."

———

My own bout of hope carried me to an intake appointment at the hospital's outpatient counseling clinic set up by Dr. McCarthy and requiring a two-month wait. When the date arrived, I sat down in a small conference room across from the intake worker and repeated my story. But when I told her about Marsha, the worker said they wouldn't be able to provide me with a therapist because I already had one.

"But, like I already told you, I don't connect with her. I don't really get anything out of it. It's not helping. I need a different therapist."

She looked at me squarely. "Sometimes people just aren't ready to change. Stick with it. See what happens."

———

If Alice James wrote at all during that time when she first fell ill, there is no trace of it. But twenty-two years later, Alice did write of that period, describing the terrible battle she waged with her own body. She believed that an inherent defect in her nervous system was responsible for her problem.

> I saw so distinctly that it was a fight simply between my body and my will, a battle in which the former was to be triumphant to the end. Owing to some physical weakness, excess of nervous susceptibility, the moral power pauses, as it were for a moment, and refuses to maintain muscular sanity, worn out with the strain of its constabulary functions.

And that was my experience, especially at the beginning. There was my body and then there was me. I wanted to work; my body demanded that I rest. When I disobeyed what my body demanded, it punished me. It pinned me to my bed. I wanted to hear live bands at the Tree Café, to play Frisbee and Wiffle Ball with my friends. My body would allow none of it.

In her journal, at forty-one, when Alice looked back at her early teens, she saw her youthful self standing "crushed and bewildered before the perpetual postponement of its hopes."

I, at twenty-one, didn't know if I would *ever* get better.

——

I stopped seeing Marsha not long after the intake worker at the hospital clinic implied that the sessions weren't helping because of me.

I went without professional support for many months, and then I found a therapist who offered the opposite of Marsha's blank slate. A refreshingly acerbic, sharp-minded feminist and writer, Camilla had a witchy look to her, with her wrinkled angular face and her wild black hair piled on top of her head in a huge tangled mound. She was a fierce woman with a weakness for animals. Sometimes I brought Cassie to our sessions, and Camilla cooed over her when we arrived. Then Cassie settled on my lap and Camilla and I got to work.

——

I applied for Social Security Disability Insurance (SSDI) but was turned down. The denial letter told me that my problem was not disabling.

Chronic fatigue syndrome was not officially recognized by the Social Security Administration until 1999. To this day, it remains difficult to win a claim if chronic fatigue syndrome is the sole complaint.

I was too tired and discouraged to appeal.

——

Denied SSDI and thus Medicare as well, I paid Camilla out of pocket, a sliding scale fee of just $30 a session. I was getting housing assistance and some food stamps, and my father and stepmother continued to send me a little bit each month to help me scrape by. I knew that mental health therapy, no matter how helpful to me psychologically, was not going to cure the CFS, and my former doctor had made it clear that conventional medicine had nothing to offer me, so I tried whatever alternative treatments I could afford: acupuncture, then homeopathy, then polarity therapy.

My progress was so glacial it was hard to see that I was improving at all or to track what helped. Over time I was able to get out of bed more. I adopted a confident little Welsh corgi and took her for short walks. I started swimming laps at the pool. As a teen, I'd regularly swum twenty-five laps; now I swam just six. But my energy waxed and waned inexplicably, and some days all I could do was lie in bed curled up in a ball.

I babysat for a little extra money. On my good days, I played games with the boy in his house or pushed him on the swing in his yard or pulled him in his wagon to the park. On my bad days, I read him stories, then lay on his bed while he jumped on it.

I lived close to the bone, shopping for my clothes at Goodwill and watching my credit card debt mount higher every time my car needed a repair.

———

Almost a year after I tore up that prescription, Camilla convinced me to give antidepressants a try. I knew my problem wasn't "just depression," but I *was* depressed.

Three days after I swallowed my first dose, it seemed like the world had changed. To this day I don't know if it was something about my genetic makeup, the fact that people with CFS tend to be more sensitive to medications, or the placebo effect that prompted such a speedy reprieve. But for the first time in months, I felt happy. It seemed as though the very air around me sparkled. This lasted for four days. And then an uncomfortable agitation crept in, and insomnia. The sparkles dimmed. My doctor and I meddled with the dosage, and I waited and waited and waited for the Prozac to work. I wanted to be happy; I wanted to have the energy to be happy. But the exhaustion remained.

———

"There's something the matter with her," Camilla said.

I had driven Cassie across the city, carried her in my arms up the stairs to Camilla's office, and curled her up in my lap, but Camilla spoke even as I gathered my thoughts.

"What?" I looked down at my ginger cat. "You think there's something wrong?"

"She looks sick. Look at her face. She looks . . . it looks like she's suffering. Is that a new flea collar?"

When my dog brought fleas into the house, I tackled the infestation with pesticide. I believed the government was overprotective, so when the directions on the pesticide canister said to cover all food processing surfaces and utensils and to remove pets from the house before spraying, I thought it was sort of like when the carton of milk was labeled with an expiration date but you could always get away with drinking it a few days later. So I didn't cover the silverware. And I didn't remove the pets; because where would I put them? And I was so determined exterminate the fleas, I also sprayed Cassie with flea spray, and just to be sure, I put a flea collar around her neck, too.

"You need to take her to the vet."

"Really? You think it's that bad?"

"And let's take that flea collar off her."

The veterinarian kept her overnight. When I picked Cassie up the next morning, the vet told me she had made a full recovery, but it was too much—the premise spray, the flea spray, the flea collar. I was more careful after that. But a lifetime of pets meant a lifetime of pesticide exposures. For them *and* for me. Not to mention the annual spraying of my childhood lawn to rid it of dandelions. And the pesticides on all the foods I ate growing up in the sixties and seventies and eighties. I didn't think of it at the time, but I think of it now.

————

Scholars tend to write about neurasthenia as an expression of the cultural dissatisfaction of women—to pigeonhole it as an emotional disorder, just like some doctors to this day do with CFS. Jean Strouse and other critics suggest, for instance, that Alice's illness was the mute dissent of a woman whose voice would not be heard.

True, Alice's father had written that a woman's "aim in life" was "simply to love and bless man." In an 1853 *Putnam's Monthly* article entitled "Woman and the 'Woman's Movement,' " Henry Sr. wrote:

> The very virtue of woman, her practical sense, which leaves her indifferent to past and future alike, and keeps her the busy blessing of the present hour, disqualifies her for all didactic dignity. Learning and wisdom do not become her.

So although he strove to provide his children with a "sensuous education," exposing them to art, theater, and books, Alice got no formal education. While she, too, had access to her father's library, and delighted, in her later years, in spending hours with him in his study, is it any wonder that an eighteen-year-old Alice, with her bright, incisive mind, was sometimes nearly overwhelmed by the secret impulse to "knock off the head of the benignant pater"?

America's feminist movement was birthed the same year as Alice—1848, the year of the first Women's Rights Convention. But neither of her parents was in favor of women's suffrage; indeed, in

Alice's family, for all its eccentricities, gender roles were markedly conventional. Alice's mother, the stout, no-nonsense Mary James, who carried out her role as wife and mother to the hilt of the Victorian ideal—expressing no ideas of her own, no political opinions distinct from her husband's—could not be a model to the uniquely brilliant Alice. In the midst of this suffragist sea change, the first wave of feminism, Mary James was an antifeminist.

So the clever, single, politically astute social critic Alice James never joined the feminist movement, although her later letters and journal entries convey an increasing feminist sensibility and gender pride.

Neither William nor Henry knew of Alice's diary until after her death. Both were deeply impressed by it. In a letter to Henry, William wrote: "The diary produces a unique and tragic impression of personal power venting itself on no opportunity." Henry replied that their sister's "tragic health was in a manner the only solution for her of the practical problem of life."

In the spring of 1993, four years after my collapse, I moved twenty miles inland to become the caretaker of the historic house museum and its formal garden. My job, at least in the summers, was to tend the flower beds and give tours to occasional visitors. I had not yet encountered Strouse's biography, but every time I entered the preserved part of the house with its faded red velvet couch and ornate wallpapers, I was steeped in the material history of Alice's era.

The previous caretakers left me their three sheep, a rabbit, and several chickens. I brought along Cassie, my little Welsh corgi Sadie, and a handsome chestnut-brown guinea pig named Moses. I used malathion on the aphids in the garden and rotenone on the lice I found on the chickens. When I discovered little red mites in my guinea pig's cage and bare patches on his belly, the vet recommended

I powder him with rotenone, too. A few days later, I found him in convulsions, near death. I washed it all off him before he could succumb completely, and miraculously, he lived.

———

The tulips bloomed and faded, the grass greened, the sheep grazed in the pasture, their bells ringing bucolically. I tried craniosacral therapy, nutritional supplements, a different homeopath, a new acupuncturist. My psychiatrist adjusted my meds.

One summer day, I made a trip into the city and stopped to browse a used bookstore. The silver-haired woman who owned the place stood behind an old wooden counter reading the newspaper. Dust motes shimmered in the air. It seemed that the whole shop was bathed in sepia. I scanned the biographies—and stopped.

Alice James. My nineteenth-century doppelgänger.

The owner rang me up, and I tucked my find under my arm and took it home.

———

My bedroom in the ell behind historic house–museum was white with trim the color of cornflowers. From the window I could see the enormous perennial garden and the chickens pecking in the grass. My body, always heavy, pulled me down, down, into the bed. I burrowed in and opened the book.

"When I am gone," Alice James wrote to her brother William a few months before her death, "pray don't think of me simply as a creature who might have been something else, had neurotic science been born."

With these words, Alice's own, Jean Strouse introduced her readers to Alice James.

It seemed like Alice was reaching across time to speak to me. To speak *for* me. The room stilled. After years of feeling pummeled and broken, suddenly I felt something inside me lift and open. Alice, too, rankled at the thought that her lived experience might be distilled into something diminishing. The psychologist's sister did not want her selfhood reduced to a bundle of neuroses. She knew herself to be more than this.

And then, in the next paragraph, Strouse wrote:

[H]er existence had long been dominated by mysterious illnesses for which no organic cause could be discovered and no cure found.

And so it began.

I was no longer alone. And perhaps what I was suffering was not quite so new, so uncharted.

———

In his 1890 essay "The Hidden Self," William referenced French psychologist Pierre Janet's pioneering work with hysteric women to describe what was then a new idea: that in certain cases the human mind may slip into "separate consciousnesses." William wrote that a woman suffering hysteria "abandons part of her consciousness because she is too weak nervously to hold it all together. The abandoned part, meanwhile, may solidify into a secondary or sub-conscious self." When the forty-two-year-old Alice read the essay, she was reminded of her own youthful bout with hysteria, which was at first indistinguishably intertwined with her symptoms of neurasthenia. The phrase *abandons part of her consciousness* provoked a torrent of thoughts and memories, which Alice recorded in her journal. Granting that William's description was an "excellent expression," she added a caveat: "altho' I have never unfortunately been able to abandon my consciousness and get five minutes rest." In a deluge of words and images, she went on to write,

[I]t used to seem to me that the only difference between me and the insane was that I had not only all the horrors and suffering of insanity but the duties of doctor, nurse, and strait-jacket imposed upon me, too. Conceive of never being without the sense that if you let yourself go for a moment your mechanism will fall into pie and that at some given moment you must abandon it all, let the dykes break and the flood sweep in, acknowledging yourself abjectly impotent before the immutable laws. When all one's moral and natural stock in trade is a temperament forbidden the abandonment of an inch or the relaxation of a muscle, 'tis a never-ending fight.

It was exhausting, this constant policing of herself, and Alice believed that her conscious self wasn't ultimately powerful enough to secure a definitive win.

———

Neurasthenia is often confused with hysteria, and this was the case even in Alice's time, but despite some overlap in symptoms the two were distinct illnesses. Hysteria was almost solely a women's disorder, and symptoms could include emotional volatility, hallucinations, dissociative states, tics, and convulsions. Neurasthenia, on the other hand, could strike both men and women, and although patients suffered from a variety of symptoms, fatigue was their primary complaint.

Doctors often blamed "over-education" and emotional expressiveness for causing these illnesses in their female patients, believing that engaging the mind and emotions caused women to divert energy away from where it was needed most: their reproductive organs. They cautioned these patients to put down the books and learn to exercise complete control over their emotions, to focus instead on marriage and motherhood.

Despite dramatic changes in healthcare since Alice was sick, some doctors still default to blaming emotions for certain of their female patients' symptoms and illnesses.

———

During my sessions with Camilla, I had a place to explore possible psychological sources for my depression, beyond the obviously depressing limitations of my illness. I told her about my parents' divorce: how my mother was the one to leave, how she'd suffered from depression. "Even before she was gone," I said, "she wasn't really there."

"Do you remember the first time you felt abandoned by your mother?" said Camilla, her voice strong and direct.

I thought for a moment, and then I told her about the time my mom drove away when I was six. "I was dawdling, and she threatened to leave without me. And then she did. In my memory I stood on our walkway and watched the car crest the hill and disappear from view, then I started to cry—just silent tears at first, but then when she didn't come back, I panicked. But she says that's not what happened at all. She says she just drove up the street for a quart of milk and came right back and she found me sitting on the steps, quiet and still. She thought I was fine. But that night, and for many nights afterward, I woke crying from nightmares, and she would lie with me until I fell back asleep, sorry and ashamed for what she'd done."

Camilla looked at me, her brown eyes soft with compassion. "You were overwhelmed by emotion. You found a way to separate your mind from your body so that you could be okay. You moved right up into your head. You *appeared* fine, but you weren't. You weren't at all fine."

———

What might Jean Strouse, or any biographer for that matter, have to say about this vignette, and what it might reveal about the origins of my illness?

Perhaps:

As early as age six, Jennifer abandoned a part of her consciousness—the vulnerable, feeling part—in favor of an exterior of invulnerability and self-sufficiency. Over time, it became her modus operandi to sublimate her emotions. Like Alice, Jennifer absorbed "into the bone that the better part is to clothe oneself in neutral tints, walk by still waters, and possess one's soul in silence." In time, this style of coping would be her undoing. Her silence, internalized, attacked her own body. Through her body, the silence spoke.

Having written it, I find this psychoanalytical summing up quite satisfying. I want to brush off my hands, as though I've just chopped a cord of wood: Job Well Done.

But the book isn't finished yet. It's only just begun.

CHAPTER 3

Elephant

C ould it be that chronic fatigue was for me—as Henry had said neurasthenia was for Alice—"the only solution for . . . the practical problem of life"?

In 1989, just two months before the first adumbrations of fatigue came creeping into my life, researcher Stephen Straus, of the NIH, published "Psychiatric Diagnoses in Patients Who Have Chronic Fatigue Syndrome" in the *Journal of Clinical Psychiatry*. Straus, who opened all of his med school lectures about CFS with the same slide—a woodcut of a Victorian woman reclining on a fainting couch, hand to her forehead—measured depression and other mental health problems in twenty-eight hospitalized CFS patients and found that twenty-one of those studied "had been or were currently affected by a psychiatric illness." A press release sent by the NIH to five hundred U.S. reporters and news outlets declared, "This rate of psychiatric illness greatly exceeds that reported for the general public." Headlines like "Chronic Fatigue Linked to Psychiatric Troubles" ripped across newspapers around the country.

A year later, *The Mayo Clinic Family Health Book* informed its readers that "emotional and psychological factors may play a role" in CFS. "In most cases," it added, "there is no serious underlying disease causing it." The book was a bestseller.

———

It seems true that what my mind could no longer hold together in silence, my body spoke. My mother had abandoned me long before she drove away that early morning in August when I was eleven. And I bore up. Not just on the outside, but on the inside, too. If I was grief-stricken or angry, I did not know it.

Alice, too, had reason to be carrying around a host of buried emotions. Her gender marked her as a second-class citizen at home just as she was in the outside world. And she wasn't entitled to speak the truth. She wasn't even entitled to *know* the truth. She, like many Victorian women, became powerless in the most literal of ways—through her body's collapse.

Both Alice and I, in order to get through life, had to disconnect our minds from our bodies and repress our emotional truths. Is it any wonder that we collapsed? Our histories, separated by more than a century, suggest that both neurasthenia and chronic fatigue syndrome are psychosomatic ailments of the divided self. In order to survive, we learned to live in our heads.

That, it turns out, is not a good idea. Because what's held captive in your head must eventually express itself through your body.

I understood Alice. And although she was long gone, I felt understood by her. And it was more than our illnesses that twinned us. Both of us specialized in what psychologists call isolation of affect. I hadn't realized how early or how thoroughly I had disconnected from my emotions. Maybe that *was* what made me sick.

———

But it's not that simple. After years of study I've come to see that CFS research is like the parable of the blind men and the elephant. In the story, each man touches a different part of an elephant's body and, based on what he learns of that individual part, erroneously declares the animal's essence. None of them understand the animal to be an elephant. They can't perceive the whole.

Of course, blind people are savvier than the depiction in this story, but it's a telling analogy for the challenges faced by those studying multisystem diseases. In the case of CFS, teams of researchers, each studying the illness through the parameters of their own specialty, have found markers of disturbance in an astonishing array of bodily systems. Why, then, is the physiological basis of CFS still even a question? Why are so many people with CFS still being told by their doctors that their symptoms are all in their heads?

I found some answers in journalist Hillary Johnson's doggedly reported *Osler's Web: Inside the Labyrinth of the Chronic Fatigue Syndrome Epidemic*. With this book, Johnson gets to the very foundation of the problem.

I have a photo of myself from a few years back, reading *Osler's Web* in a zero-gravity chair on a cabin deck two hours up the coast from my apartment in the city. Years had passed since my body had first broken down. I'd appealed the second denial of my Social Security application and won, so I no longer had to sit in those hard orange plastic chairs at the welfare office. I'd moved out of the historic house. Left the weedy beds behind and returned to the city. I'd spent years managing my body's every need—resting frequently, adhering to a strict diet, downing handfuls of supplements, and consulting with a multitude of healthcare providers. My energy was slowly returning, but I had to be careful not to overextend myself.

It was summer but it was cold, and I'd bundled up, with my hoodie tied under my chin. I had a pillow behind my head and a pencil in my hand. *Osler's Web* is a 720-page tome, and I hadn't expected to spend my vacation so fully engrossed in it. My pile of lighter fare lay untouched because I couldn't believe what I was reading or stop turning the pages. By the time I finished the book, it was clear to me that we don't understand the physiology and treatment of chronic fatigue syndrome because unthinkable levels of bias and malfeasance at the nation's top public health agencies have gotten in the way of good science.

One of the worst offenders was Stephen Straus.

According to Johnson, problems with Straus's study were numerous. The size of the study, just twenty-eight subjects, was tiny. But in addition, Straus included common phobias such as fear of heights in his catchall of "psychiatric illnesses." And he failed to compare CFS patients with people who suffered from other disabling illnesses, completely ignoring the likelihood that having a disabling illness might negatively impact a person's mental health.

Several doctors wrote to the *Journal of Clinical Psychiatry* to complain. One of them, Cecil Bradley, noted that depression pre-occurs or co-occurs in a number of diseases—among them diabetes, Hashimoto's thyroiditis, and carcinoma of the stomach. (Multiple sclerosis is another.) However, in these cases, doctors viewed depression as an inherent component of the illness.

On the very same day that Straus's study was released, the *Annals of Internal Medicine* published a letter by two doctors dealing with outbreaks in their communities: Paul Cheney, who practiced in Incline Village, and David Bell, in Lyndonville, New York. They reported inordinately high levels of interleukin-2—an immune system protein that makes infection-fighting cells multiply and mature—in 104 CFS patients. The doctors theorized that the molecules, also known as T-cell growth factor, might be elevated in response to an as-yet-unidentified pathogen. Other disorders, they knew, including multiple sclerosis, were marked by similar results. The levels of interleukin-2 in CFS patients, however, were much higher than those in even the most severe cases of MS.

But there were no headlines about this promising direction for research into a physiologic basis for the illness.

———

In 1990, a year after Straus's damning study, another group of researchers showed that before contracting CFS, people were no more depressed or anxious than the general population. "Patients with CFS were not excessively hypochondriacal," they wrote. "We conclude that psychological disturbance is likely to be a consequence of rather than an antecedent risk factor to the syndrome."

That same year, the CDC sent out a bulletin stating that most CFS patients do not have any immunologic abnormalities, an assertion that was patently false. Reams of studies had found immune system dysfunction. Since that time, a number of papers have shown that natural killer cells are in short supply in people with CFS, and the ones that remain have consistently low killing power in their response to infection.

———

CDC psychologist Dr. Walter Gunn didn't need to see these kinds of laboratory results to know that something unmistakably physiological was happening to the CFS patients who consulted him. As he told Johnson when she was researching *Osler's Web*, "Maybe it takes a psychologist to realize these patients don't have a psychiatric disease." (Straus was not trained in psychology or neurology.) It was clear to Gunn that they were truly ill.

Eighty percent of people with depression have co-occurring fatigue, but unlike people with CFS, the fatigue is not their primary complaint. People with depression feel *depressed* and lack interest in doing things they once loved. In contrast, people with CFS still have the interest; what they lack is the energy they need to do those things. As psychology professor and CFS researcher Leonard Jason, PhD, points out, "If you want to do a quick diagnostic test, you could say, 'If you were well tomorrow, what would you do?' And the person with CFS would give you a list of things that they want to get back to in their life, and the person with classic depression would probably say, 'I don't know.'"

On a biological level, research has found that one of the markers of depression is an enlarged adrenal gland and an increase in cortisol production, says CFS doctor and researcher Nancy Klimas, but "in CFS, the adrenal gland is smaller than normal and makes less cortisol."

———

I'd been depressed before, but not until I came down with mononucleosis had I ever experienced such a debilitating exhaustion. Even when lab results indicated that the mono was gone, the fatigue seemed to have made my body its permanent residence.

Much later, as I researched the physiology of CFS, I learned that about 10 percent of patients who contract mononucleosis still experience disabling fatigue six months later. Why did I stay sick while others get better? Turns out genetics may have something to do with it. Research to identify genes that may predispose people to ME/CFS is still in its early stages. But in a small 2006 study a team of Australian researchers led by Andrew Lloyd found that in response to a variety of infectious illnesses, people with certain gene variants, or polymorphisms, were significantly more likely to experience severe symptoms and to develop CFS. And a 2009 study linked polymorphisms in several genes related to the autonomic nervous system to CFS, indicating that a genetic predisposition to heightened stress reactions may play a part in the disease.

Could it be that my genes predisposed me to CFS?

The more I read, the clearer it became that all the bodily systems are interconnected. Erica Verrillo succinctly summed up these complexities in *Chronic Fatigue Syndrome: A Treatment Guide*:

> When clinicians describe [CFS] as a multisystem illness, the primary systems they are referring to are the nervous system, the immune system, and the endocrine system. . . . To a great extent, the division between these three systems is artificial. The cell receptors of each of these systems are shared, which means that it is impossible to have a dysfunction in one system that does not alter the other two. The central nervous system releases neurochemicals that regulate the immune and endocrine systems; the immune system releases cytokines that regulate the nervous system; the endocrine system releases hormones that affect the nervous and immune systems, and so forth, in an endless web of interactions.

Accumulating research indicates, for instance, that something may be awry in the autonomic nervous system (ANS) of people with CFS. The ANS is the part of the brain, spinal cord, and peripheral nerves that controls vital functions, such as heart rate, blood pressure, body temperature, sweating, and breathing rate. Studies suggest that the sympathetic nervous system—the fight-or-flight branch of the autonomic nervous system—may be overactivated, and the parasympathetic nervous system—the rest-and-digest branch—may be underactivated. For people with CFS, this can mean that even when they're at rest, their fight-or-flight system is switched on. Their bodies are never able to achieve true rest. This is certainly what it felt like in the earliest, most devastating months of my illness. Even when I was lying down, I could feel the fatigue coursing through my body. It's like the fatigue itself was toiling.

The hypothalamic-pituitary-adrenal axis, or HPA axis, controls reactions to stress and regulates the immune system, energy storage and expenditure, mood and emotions, digestion, and more. In the early 1990s, a team from the National Institutes of Health discovered a disturbance in the HPA axis in people with CFS. Most studies since then have seen similar results and have found relatively low levels of cortisol, which normally rises during times of stress. This is consistent with the theory that the systems of people with CFS go into overdrive, depleting their cortisol. A 2008 lab test showed that my daytime cortisol levels were severely depleted, basically flatlined.

————

So there are solid studies indicating immunologic, ANS, and HPA problems in people with CFS, others that clearly distinguish CFS from depression, and still more that indicate a genetic involvement. Further research could lead to effective treatments. But CFS research has been difficult to corroborate because a number of different case definitions of varying degrees of rigor have been published over the years.

The first, published in 1988 with CDC researcher Gary Holmes as the lead author, was a research definition designed to include a very narrow group of patients to ensure that all those who qualified for the diagnosis really did share the same disease. The criteria specified that the illness was characterized by a "new onset of persistent or relapsing, debilitating fatigue or easy fatigability in a person who has no previous history of similar symptoms, that does not resolve with bedrest, and that is severe enough to reduce or impair average daily activity below 50% of the patient's premorbid activity level for a period of at least 6 months." Back in 1989, in the early days of my illness, I certainly met the requirements for this part of the diagnosis.

To qualify for the Holmes definition, patients had to have amassed a number of additional symptoms. These included fever, sore throat, painful lymph nodes, generalized muscle weakness, muscle discomfort, exercise intolerance, headaches, sleep disturbance, difficulty concentrating, and other neuropsychologic complaints—all of which I suffered.

But my depression excluded me from the Holmes definition.

By Holmes's criteria, the presence of any of a wide range of conditions ruled out a diagnosis of CFS. That list included psychiatric illnesses such as depression and anxiety, as well as autoimmune diseases, HIV infection, chronic bacterial diseases like Lyme, chronic inflammatory diseases, endocrine illnesses such as hypothyroidism, substance use disorder, and effects from toxicants such as pesticides or heavy metals. Critics of the criteria argued that CFS was a multi-system illness, that many of these problems could be co-occurring symptoms of CFS, and that excluding patients with these problems may have been throwing the baby out with the bathwater.

There are now at least eight different case definitions for CFS, some of which are better for clinical diagnosis and some, the more rigorous ones, better for research. But researchers may choose to use any of the eight definitions to determine their catchment group. So some teams use one definition, some use another, and that makes it entirely possible that they aren't always studying the same disease.

———

In addition to determining the case definition, it fell to Holmes, the government's principal investigator in charge of researching the perplexing disorder, to give the illness a name. He opted against myalgic encephalomyelitis, the term used by the British (who nicknamed it ME). It was, he determined, "overly complicated and too confusing for many nonmedical persons." As Johnson commented, "It's difficult to imagine other situations in which scientists' criteria for a disease's name included a stricture that it not be 'overly complicated' or 'too confusing' to the lay public." But there is another reason the medical community has declined to call the illness myalgic encephalomyelitis. According to Julie Rehmeyer, who lives with the disease and is the author of *Through the Shadowlands: A Science Writer's Odyssey into an Illness Science Doesn't Understand*, "There's only a small amount of evidence that neuroinflammation even exists in ME/CFS patients— that is, that their brains and spinal cords are inflamed—though it sure as hell feels like that."

Holmes settled on *chronic fatigue syndrome*. But that name, according to Johnson, cast the illness's victims in the role of "shirkers who chose to defy the nation's Protestant work ethic." It is, she argues, a name that sets up CFS sufferers for aspersions and disregard. "If diseases were named after symptoms," she notes, "leukemia too might well be called 'chronic fatigue syndrome' and diabetes 'chronic thirst syndrome.'"

For some people, like Julie Rehmeyer, the neurocognitive symptoms can be even more disabling than the fatigue. In her book, she describes sometimes being incapable of forming words, sometimes being unable to walk but only to stagger or crawl, and sometimes experiencing moments of near paralysis.

For those most severely affected, the disease can be life threatening. A British woman, Sophia Mirza, developed CFS after two bouts of malaria and then a 1999 case of flu at the age of twenty-six. Her condition deteriorated rapidly and soon she was bedbound, unable to tolerate light, sound, or human touch. In 2003, a state-appointed doctor visited her at home, where her mother was caring for her, and without performing any kind of physical exam, reported that he "detected major psychological causality precipitating Ms. Mirza's illness. . . . Her illness could best be understood in terms of severe regression and conversion/dissociative disorder." She was involuntarily committed to a psychiatric facility for two weeks, where she was not adequately protected from stimulation, and her condition deteriorated irrevocably. She developed sensitivities to all foods and then even to water, which caused her glands to balloon and a feeling, she said, that the circulation in her legs was being cut off. In 2005, Mirza became the first person on record in the UK to die from CFS. A postmortem found inflammation of the dorsal root ganglion in 75 percent of her spinal cord and stated that the cause of death was acute renal failure resulting from CFS.

For every CFS victim, no matter where they fell on the spectrum of severity, Holmes's chosen name negated the magnitude of the problem.

In the early 1990s, when immune abnormalities had been proven, epidemiologist Seymour Grufferman proposed renaming the illness "chronic fatigue and immune dysfunction syndrome" (CFIDS). The name was used by many in the CFS community who felt that *chronic fatigue syndrome* was not adequate to the illness, but ultimately sufferers chose to refer to the illness as myalgic encephalomyelitis/chronic fatigue syndrome, or ME/CFS.

In her book *Hystories*, Elaine Showalter takes pains to point out that "myalgic encephalomyelitis," while it "*sounds* impressively medical. . . . The acronym ME also ironically emphasizes the patient's self-absorption."

———

What's in a name? A study of over a hundred med students and residents found that the name of the illness affected their perception of it. When it was called myalgic encephalopathy in case studies, 39 percent of the trainees attributed the symptoms to medical causes; when it was called chronic fatigue syndrome, just 22 percent did so. Even the wholly fictitious "Florence Nightingale Disease" fared better, with 30 percent determining that the illness was biologically based.

Neurologist Marshall Handleman, who was skeptical of the illness until he found abnormal brain scans in forty-nine of fifty subjects in a small study, told Johnson, "I want them to change the name—stop with this 'chronic fatigue' crap. It does a *great* disservice to these people. Doctors associate this term with malingering, and doctors work hard; they don't like malingerers."

Just as neurasthenia is often now derided as a "fashionable" illness of the nineteenth century, some viewed ME/CFS in a similar light. In their introduction to a 1992 conference on the illness, Arthur Kleinman and Stephen Straus reflected: "In our times, the metaphor of being exhausted by the multiple, competing demands of work, family and play is a badge of success and achievement, a lifestyle that demonstrates that one has prestige, position, and power." In other words, ME/CFS was the new fashionable malaise.

———

But did the "yuppie flu" really strike mostly yuppies? Epidemiologist Sandra Daugherty was the first to do a community-based prevalence study to find out. Performed in Incline Village and nearby Crystal Bay in 1993, it found that people with less money were actually at increased risk of the disease. Daugherty suggested that ME/CFS sufferers in the lower economic brackets might have been largely uncounted simply because they had no access to healthcare. After all, previous government surveys had relied on doctor reports. As Johnson notes, "Certainly many clinicians had suspected for some time that the appellation 'yuppie disease' had arisen because it was only the upper middle classes whose education gave them the financial ability and self-confidence to negotiate the nation's health care system to the point of accurate diagnosis."

When poor people say they are tired, they're more likely to be seen as shirkers than as patients worthy of a diagnosis. But in fact, according to Daugherty, "Practically every illness you can name hits the lower classes harder."

———

In Alice James's time, doctors believed neurasthenia was primarily a malaise of the yuppies of the Victorian era—the urban professional and upper classes. As the gears of industrial capitalism ground on, one doctor opined, "those influences which demand an exhaustive expenditure of nervous energy . . . are all the time rapidly increasing in professional, business and social life. The march of scientific progress is so rapid that the professional man has to maintain a high state of mental tension in order to keep pace with it." Some just didn't possess the nervous capital necessary to sustain their health under these conditions.

This presumption of class-related neurasthenia perpetuated until the 1980s, when historian Francis G. Gosling performed a comprehensive study, analyzing virtually all the medical literature published on neurasthenia during its peak years—a total of 332 articles. In *Before Freud: Neurasthenia and the American Medical Community, 1870–1910*, Gosling shared his discovery that in fact Americans across the economic spectrum were diagnosed with neurasthenia—bankers and lawyers and their wives, sure, but also schoolteachers, seamstresses, housekeepers, and servants.

The notion that neurasthenia struck primarily the upper and upper-middle classes emerged because the physicians most prominently writing about neurasthenia made their livings by treating that population—the ones who could afford to see them. Gosling notes that "physicians sympathized most with those patients with whom they identified—the middle-class business and professional men most like themselves." He adds that doctors, "like most middle-class Americans, believed the upper classes to be hardworking and ambitious while the lower classes were of grosser, more animal-like sensibilities, and their diagnoses reflected their opinions." So among the professional classes, doctors most often identified the source of their neurasthenia to be overwork; but among laborers, "sexual excess" was most often blamed.

So when researchers early in the ME/CFS epidemic dubbed the illness the "yuppie flu," they were falling prey to the medical establishment's long-standing history of class bias.

———

ME/CFS does strike more women than men—as many as two to four times more—which might explain why the illness has been trivialized. It's well documented that women's concerns are more often dismissed in the doctor's office. To cite just one example, a 2006 study showed that when doctors were asked to evaluate two hypothetical cases, one man and one woman, each with symptoms of coronary heart disease, they gave an accurate diagnosis to both genders—unless stress was also added as a factor. Suddenly, even though both individuals were suffering from identical symptoms, doctors identified heart disease in 41 percent fewer women than men. In other words, if women admit to being stressed, doctors become more dismissive of their symptoms, while men's symptoms are perceived as organic whether stressors are present or not.

If it's that hard for women with symptoms of heart disease to be taken seriously, it's not much of a leap to see why women with ME/CFS are so often sent by their doctors to psychiatrists.

———

For many years after my first dose of Prozac, I saw a psychiatrist who adjusted or replaced my antidepressants every time they stopped working. After a decade of this, I wondered how much cumulative good the drugs were doing to improve my mental health. Each day I began marking down on a calendar whether I was depressed or not depressed. Likely it would have been even worse without them, but ultimately the math didn't work out in my favor. Extrapolating from a few months' calculations combined with my memories of the many years of grinding fatigue and depression, I realized that in the decade that I'd been ill, I'd been depressed far more days than not. Which was pretty depressing.

———

Like me in the first year of my illness, between 35 and 60 percent of people with ME/CFS are unable to work at all. Seventy-seven percent report significant economic hardship due to the illness. And because these ME/CFS sufferers are unable to engage in social activities, they describe "marked feelings of isolation." A 2005 study found that only 5 percent of those stricken fully recover.

The illness is financially devastating for individual sufferers, but it's also astronomically expensive for the country, costing more than $9.1 billion annually in medical expenditures and lost productivity. For two decades after I was finally able to return to work, I could work only part time. I relied on food stamps, a housing subsidy, Medicaid, Medicare, and Social Security Disability Insurance (SSDI) to help me get by. I barely made ends meet. When I went to grad school, I requested the maximum in student loans and used that to pay my extensive out-of-pocket medical expenses. Unable to keep ahead of the interest rates, I am thus saddled with a growing $178,000 student loan debt, and at the time of this writing, at fifty-four, I've accumulated a grand total of $1,800 in retirement savings. I will forever be behind.

———

Considering the profound impact of the stigma of ME/CFS and lack of support from doctors, combined with the continuous grief from the ongoing losses that accompany this illness, therapist and researcher

Patricia Fennell says that she has found that many with ME/CFS suffer from "a post-traumatic stress disorder (PTSD)-like syndrome because of the social context in which they are sick." I know this is true for me. I can feel the trauma in my body. I clench up protectively when I think of the doctor who told me I was just depressed; of the Social Security Administration, which twice told me I was not sick enough to receive help; of the well-meaning healthy people who used to tell me they got tired, too. The illness is the biggest trauma I've ever faced. Bigger than my parents' divorce, than my mom's leaving. The economic devastation, the feeling of being utterly alone, of being shunned by my doctor, the omnipresent message that my illness wasn't real, that it was all in my mind, that I was a malingerer, that I *wanted* to be sick in some subconscious way (probably because I didn't really want to be working, or because of some emotional need the "sick role" was fulfilling): it often seemed the whole world was telling me about me . . . and I myself even joined the chorus.

When I was first diagnosed with mono, I wrote a friend: "Phew. . . . I was beginning to worry that it was Yuppie Disease." I didn't even put "yuppie disease" in quotes. It was just a thing. A thing I called it. A thing I feared I might have. I wasn't even aware that in doing so I was oppressing *myself.*

To this day, when I get excessively tired, I flash back to that fatigue, to that time in my life when all was lost. Later, when I became a therapist, I worked with trauma survivors. What I told them was that people who've endured trauma know the truth: that bad things can happen. They know it in their bodies. *We* know it in *our* bodies. Everyone else walks around in the happy (and desirable) delusion that they are safe, that nothing bad can happen to *them.*

———

In the decades since I first fell ill, ME/CFS has wreaked havoc on the lives of millions of Americans, and we still don't have a biomarker to legitimate the illness and help with diagnosis and directions for treatment. One reason for that is that neither the CDC nor the NIH has invested in finding one. It's a vicious cycle: officials at these agencies believed the illness was psychological, so they didn't invest in studying it, and as a result, they created the impression that the illness was psychological because there was no biomarker, and so on.

At the CDC, even when ME/CFS did get some funding specifically earmarked for research, the money was diverted for other uses. In 1988, the year before I fell ill, fierce patient lobbying induced Congress to appropriate $407,000 to fund ME/CFS research. Gary Holmes was put in charge of the project. But from day one, he found the funding mysteriously evaporating. As he told Hillary Johnson, "The $407,000 was immediately chopped up, *sizeably*, as soon as it hit the door. From all the way at the top on down, people are chopping out little sections for their own use. . . . I'm sitting here, and I'm just watching it disappear!"

Two years later, in 1990, Walter Gunn requested $730,000 in funding for a case-control study to look for organic markers of ME/CFS. He had made many such requests for other illnesses and was astonished when his request was denied. Congress had earmarked $1.4 million for ME/CFS research that year, but Gunn was told there was no money to fund his request. "I asked them where the money was," he told Johnson. "They said it just wasn't there. This was the first time I was alerted that there might be a problem."

In 1991, Congress allocated $2.1 million dollars for ME/CFS research, but Gunn learned the CFS division would be granted just $683,000. As he told Johnson, agency employees were in agreement "that people with chronic fatigue syndrome are mentally ill and that Congress was forcing them to perform research on a non-disease. As a result, CFS became the division's golden goose."

Hillary Johnson's assiduous reporting in the 1996 edition of *Osler's Web* led to an independent audit by the Inspector General of the Department of Health and Human Services, which concluded that even between the years of 1995 and 1998, $8.8 million that had been earmarked by Congress for ME/CFS was instead spent on other diseases, such as measles and polio, and that an additional $4.1 million could not be fully accounted for due to dubious bookkeeping.

———

Even as recently as 2011, the biased research and damning headlines continued. In the PACE trial, a team of researchers, some of them psychologists with ties to the disability insurance industry, did some statistical acrobatics to produce results showing that a program of cognitive behavioral therapy combined with exercise was an effective treatment for ME/CFS. At a press conference, one of the researchers declared that compared to the controls, "twice as many people on graded exercise therapy and cognitive behavior therapy got back to normal." In a follow-up paper, the researchers claimed that 22 percent of participants recovered by the end of the yearlong trial.

But in a sweeping critique of the study (which had been funded by British government agencies and published in *The Lancet*), David Tuller, who has a doctorate in public health, exposed its multitude of flaws. Most significant, the investigators made a number of critical mid-trial changes. Perhaps the most problematic was their altering of the baseline scores for the two primary measures—physical function and fatigue. "While a physical function score of 65 was considered evidence of sufficient disability to be a study participant," writes Tuller, "the researchers had now declared that a score of 60 and above was 'within the normal range.' Someone could therefore enter the trial with a physical function score of 65, become more disabled, leave with a score of 60, and still be considered within the PACE trial's 'normal range.'"

At the beginning of the trial, investigators collected data on a number of objective measures of fatigue and disability—a walking test, a step test, and data on employment and financial status. At the trial's end, a year later, when these objective measures failed to offer much in the way of evidence of recovery, the team dismissed all but one of those outcomes and otherwise relied solely on subjective measures—which was especially problematic since the study was not double blinded to prevent biased results.

The only objective measure that made it into the final paper was the six-minute walking test, which did indicate a slight improvement for participants who exercised. On average, they were able to walk 67 meters farther than they'd been able to at the start of the trial the year before—from 312 meters at baseline to 379 at the end of the trial. In other words, study participants could walk only about a fifth of a mile at the beginning of the study, but after treatment they were able to walk almost a quarter of a mile. However, as Tuller points out, this modest gain pales in comparison to the mean performances of relatively healthy women between the ages of seventy to seventy-nine years (490 meters), patients with Class II heart failure (558 meters), and people with cystic fibrosis (626 meters).

The CDC adopted the PACE treatment recommendations, as did Kaiser, the Mayo Clinic, and others. Headlines like "Pushing Limits Can Help Chronic Fatigue Patients," "Got ME? Just Get Out and Exercise, Say Scientists," "Talk and Exercise Helps Sufferers Beat Chronic Fatigue Symptoms," and "ME/CFS: Pacing Yourself Isn't the Answer" set the recovery movement back by decades.

Not only did the PACE trial fail to provide evidence for its claims, but it may have done the opposite. As science writer Julie Rehmeyer points out, "the PACE trial is the most convincing evidence we have that ME/CFS isn't fundamentally psychological. They used the best psychological techniques they could find, and they failed. NONE of the techniques we have for treating psychological illnesses, either talk therapy or medication, have done much of anything for patients with this illness." The CDC has since removed graded exercise and cognitive behavioral therapy from its treatment recommendations.

———

ME/CFS has devastated the lives of as many as 2.5 million Americans, and yet in 2014, the National Institutes of Health set aside just $5 million for studies of the disease, a million dollars less than its budget for hay fever. By 2019, funding had increased to $15 million, which seems like a lot—comparatively at least—until you find out that headaches got $40 million that year; Crohn's disease, which impacts the lives of 780,000 Americans, got $76 million ($97 per person); chronic pain got $856 million; HIV/AIDS, which infects about 1.1 million Americans, was allotted $3 billion (about $3,000 per person); and cancer received $6.5 billion in funding ($3,700 per person diagnosed that year). The allocation for people with ME/CFS adds up to somewhere between $6 and $15 per person.

What might have happened if ME/CFS had actually received its fair share of the funding? How many answers might have been discovered? What biomarkers? How many treatments?

———

Studies by the CDC and Dr. Leonard Jason of DePaul University indicate that 80 to 90 percent of patients with this disease are undiagnosed. These astronomical numbers may be explained by a 2010 CDC study in which 57 percent of doctors admitted their belief that "a diagnosis of CFS can inhibit a patient's motivation to get better." Perhaps these doctors were bolstered by psychiatrist Simon Wessely's remarks about CFS in a 2006 paper: "Diagnosis elicits the belief the patient has a serious disease," and becomes "a self-fulfilling prophecy. . . . Diagnosis leads to transgression into the sick role, the act of becoming a patient even if complaints do not call for it, the development of an illness identity and the experience of victimization."

Contrary to Dr. Wessely's beliefs, what's clear from the research is that ME/CFS is a complex multisystem disease that has a devastating impact on the people it strikes. As far back as 1996, this was evident to some researchers, such as Paul Cheney, who told Hillary Johnson in an interview for *Osler's Web*:

> All great avalanches start with something very small. It is not unlike the theory of chaos in which a butterfly flaps its wings in Japan and starts a hurricane in Florida. It becomes like a snowball going downhill. One doesn't necessarily care what the little pea was that caused all this. . . . You can find the pea, but what do you think that is going to do? *Nothing*. . . . [T]his disease is a *multiple* injury—there are *many* injuries. If I disregulate your immune system, and that disregulates your brain and injures it, and the injured brain now makes hormones that become toxic to you, which further injure you so that your natural killer cells drop and allow the reactivation of viruses you caught in childhood, which further injure you. . . . Systems break down, problems beget more problems. . . . This disease is made up of complex networks of interacting systems.

In 2015, a quarter of a century after I first fell ill, and two decades after Cheney said as much in an interview with Johnson, a panel of experts appointed by the Institute of Medicine (now known as the National Academy of Medicine) announced that after a close examination of over nine thousand studies, it had come to the conclusion that chronic fatigue syndrome is a "serious, chronic, complex and systemic disease."

CHAPTER 4

Territories

When we speak of Mother Nature, we evoke the ancient perception of our planet as a living—and female—organism. In 1605 the cosmologist Johannes Kepler turned that perception on its head. The world, he said, should instead be recognized as a celestial machine, more accurately compared to clockwork. René Descartes was nine when Kepler wrote these words. He was a sickly child. His doctors didn't hide the expectation that he would die young, and his father despised him for his weakness. Later, as an adult, Descartes—whose mother perished when he was just one, and whose only child, a beloved five-year-old daughter, died from scarlet fever—was determined to solve the puzzle of the human body, and with it, the problem of disease.

I imagine that Descartes did not have the best relationship with his body, the betrayer. How else could he have come up with the ultimate repudiation of the body, *Cogito ergo sum*, "I think, therefore I am"? In his 1641 *Meditations*, Descartes wrote,

> From this I knew I was a substance whose whole essence or nature is simply to think, and which does not require any place . . . in order to exist. Accordingly, this "I"—that is, the soul by which I am

what I am—is entirely distinct from the body, and indeed is easier
to know than the body, and would not fail to be whatever it is, even
if the body did not exist.

And thus dualism, the idea that the mind and the body are two
separate entities, was born.

Descartes had long been fascinated by machines, in his youth even
building some that simulated animal activity, such as a dog chasing
a pheasant. He was an avid student and would have studied Kepler.
But Descartes, a brilliant mathematician, took Kepler's idea to the
nth degree. Not only was the entire universe a mathematical system,
but so were all the animals in it. In other words, bodies, too, were
simply complex clockworks that could be dismantled, analyzed, and
understood. With study—with the proper *kind* of study—all answers
could eventually be found.

———

When Descartes put quill to paper in the mid-1600s and declared
that people were essentially machines, he forged the path to modern medicine. In the centuries since, the scientific method, with its
emphasis on objective observation, has enabled researchers to learn
a lot about how our parts work, all the way down to the cellular and
molecular level.

This view of the world as a giant mechanism that can be taken
apart piece by piece and then put back together again paved the way
for innovations like X-rays, CT scans, and robotic surgery equipment.
It enables us to diagnose and treat illnesses like pneumonia, cancer,
and heart disease. We've become masters at breaking things down to
their smallest components so we can study them, but our fragmented,
mechanistic way of viewing the world comes at a cost.

Descartes's legacy glorifies the mind and repudiates the body. It
advocates the extraction of emotion from the acquisition of knowledge,

privileging thinking over feeling, the objective over the subjective. I like how biographer Richard Watson puts it:

> [Descartes] has cursed us with the belief that what is important is not the subjective sensations and emotions we have within us but rather the objective things in the outer world that cause them. Descartes is the father of machismo, of the ideal of the big tough hard stoical rational man. Grin and bear it. Emotions are subjective, trivial, useless, meaningless, and misleading. There are no emotions in the material world, so they should not be allowed to interfere with man's serious, objective work of controlling nature.

In medicine, this manifests as a kind of medical colonialism, the patient's body a territory to be claimed by the medical authorities. Talcott Parsons, the sociologist who brought us the concept of the sick role, observed that the core expectation of the ill is that they surrender themselves to the care of a doctor. Think about the use of the word *compliance* when physicians assess patient engagement. They prefer patients who will do what they're told. Like S. Weir Mitchell, who believed that wise women trusted their doctors and the "wisest ask the fewest questions," they tend to be less enamored of the patient who doesn't comply, asks too many questions, or doesn't get better. In this model, the doctor is the authority, the engineer of bodily repair.

But in a medical culture that privileges the doctor's voice over the patient's, something gets lost. In *Illness and Culture in the Postmodern Age*, David B. Morris remarks on the difference between disease and illness. Disease is objectively substantiated by diagnostic tests; illness is the subjective experience of the sick person.

> Medicine gives greatest value to knowledge that can be verified as objective. Thus disease as objective and illness as subjective are categories that convey a powerfully divided sense of worth. What the patient reports is subjective (and untrustworthy), what the lab

reports is objective (and true). Numbers are objective (and serious), stories are subjective (and trivial). Doctors are the authorities on disease, while patients remain the more or less unreliable narrators of their own unruly illnesses. The distribution of power within the traditional doctor/patient couple is tellingly one-sided. One knows, the other feels; one prescribes, the other complies; one is paid, the other pays.

As social critic Ivan Illich puts it, "The patient is reduced to an object being repaired" rather than "a subject being helped to heal." In this paradigm, treatment no longer involves the entire individual, and the experience is thus fragmented, isolating, and disconnected.

What gets lost in the healing relationship when the patient's story, and its attendant emotions, are subordinated?

———

When Alice was advised to keep her emotions in check, that was a Cartesian intervention. We now know that health is compromised when emotions are suppressed.

When I think of how Alice described herself as "bottled lightning" and "an emotional volcano," I wonder at who she might have been— how she might have experienced her body—if she'd been encouraged, instead, to *feel* and even to *express* what she was feeling.

———

It's an awfully phallic image, this scene plucked from our national psyche: the golden spike proudly hammered into a pre-drilled hole in the last railroad tie under the last rail that would finally join America's urban-industrial East to its fertile and untamed West. A crowd of about six hundred people, mostly men, had gathered at Promontory Summit, Utah, to witness the official act that would signal the people's triumph over America's formidable landscape. It was 1869, the year George Beard introduced the term *neurasthenia,* and America's love affair with industrial capitalism was thrusting full steam ahead.

Americans believed it was their manifest destiny to colonize the country, civilizing the rugged land, imbuing the entire nation with a distinctly American triumvirate of ideals: independence, democracy, and a mentality of unflagging forward progress. The transcontinental railroad would unite the nation's economy, transporting machines, tools, building materials, coal, and other goods from sea to shining sea.

Train after train steamed through this wild nation. As settlers fanned out across the country—hacking their way through the brush, felling trees, planting fields, driving out the Indigenous people who already lived here—women's bodies also fell under the rubric of wild and inexplicable territories men sought to colonize.

Take, for instance, Dr. J. Marion Sims, inventor of the duck-billed speculum, who performed his gynecological experiments—including surgery without anesthesia—on enslaved women, many of whom he bought and kept in the back of his private hospital. Of the new worlds opened up by his creation, Sims wrote that he could see "everything as no man had ever seen before. . . . I felt like an explorer in medicine who first views a new and important territory." Another gynecologist, Dr. Robert Battey, saw himself as a Daniel Boone of the female body, "carving out for myself a new pathway through consecrated ground, upon which the foot of man has not dared willingly to tread."

Women and their bodies were generally correlated with nature in all its mysterious power, and men sought to master women's bodies as they were striving to master America's "virgin" landscape.

―――

And what an awesome power women possessed. As one nineteenth-century physician marveled, it seemed "as if the Almighty, in creating

the female sex, *had taken the uterus and built a woman around it.*"
Another doctor, with what seems a combination of admiration and
dismay, declared, "From the foundation of the world man has been
born of woman, and notwithstanding that his inventive genius has
discovered steam . . . and harnessed him to his chariot, and sent
lightning to do his bidding over the almost boundless extent of the
world; yet we cannot hope that any change may be effected in this
particular." Men would be forever beholden to women for their very
existence.

Perhaps it's to be expected, then, that men began to diminish
women by correlating the uterus with emotional instability. The word
hysteria derives, after all, from the Greek word for womb. Men saw
the uterus as the seat of a woman's power, and the source of her (or
perhaps *their*) undoing.

The most common of all surgical interventions for nineteenth-
century women was removal of the ovaries—officially known as
ovariotomy, but also called "desexing" or "spaying." Popularized by
Dr. Robert Battey, who recommended it for treating a wide range of
health and mental health problems, including insanity, "nymphoma-
nia," epilepsy, and what we now colloquially call premenstrual syndrome (PMS), the operation had a mortality rate somewhere between
18 and 33 percent. While a number of physicians registered concerns
about the overuse of the procedure, some doctors proudly claimed to
have removed between 1,500 to 2,000 ovaries, passing them around
at medical society meetings "on plates like trophies," according to the
scholar Ben Barker-Benfield.

Another doctor in support of the procedure rationalized thus:
"Why do we alter our colts and calves? Not that we expect to abate
strength or endurance, nor yet to render them less intelligent; but that
we may make them tractable and trustworthy, that we may convert
them into faithful, well disposed servants."

Sigmund Freud's specialty was hysteria, but most of his earliest patients, including those whose cases he described in *Studies on Hysteria*, came to him with what would now be considered organic complaints. According to Richard Webster, author of *Why Freud Was Wrong*, both Lucy R, who sought help for olfactory hallucinations, and Katharina, who described attacks of throat constriction with an accompanying buzzing in her head, probably suffered from temporal lobe epilepsy. Emmy von N's facial tics and involuntary vocal exclamations were likely the result of Tourette's syndrome. And Elisabeth von R's disabling chronic leg pain was, as Freud himself said, "rheumatic in origin."

Freud, however, believed that these women's symptoms were caused by suppressed trauma expressing itself symbolically through their bodies. The process of talking about their experiences, he claimed, would cause a cathartic release and heal them. When his patients denied experiencing any trauma, well, that was called "denial," and there was, he wrote, "no harm" in making suggestions: "It is of use if we can guess the ways in which things are connected up and tell the patient before we have uncovered it"—something that present-day therapists are firmly advised *not* to do because of the risk of planting false memories.

Webster offers a long list of illnesses that might have been misdiagnosed as hysteria in the nineteenth century and beyond: epilepsy, head injury, brain cancer, multiple sclerosis, Parkinson's disease, Tourette's syndrome, autism, syphilis, viral hepatitis, and more. Maya Dusenbery, author of *Doing Harm: The Truth About How Bad Medicine and Lazy Science Leave Women Dismissed, Misdiagnosed, and Sick*, adds endometriosis and autoimmune disorders to this list.

Freud later admitted to a colleague that he had exaggerated the success of his treatments. Not one of the women he wrote about in *Studies on Hysteria* was in fact cured. But his pseudoscience still lives, predisposing an entire medical system to distrust women's reports of their own bodily experiences.

———

Even before Freud sailed to the United States to deliver his 1909 lectures on his theory of psychoanalysis, doctors in the late 1800s were already beginning to experiment with psychotherapeutic techniques of their own. By the 1920s, however, psychiatry had become a distinct specialty, and, as researcher F. G. Gosling notes, Freudian psychoanalysis, "because it emphasized mental processes exclusively and required substantial investment of time and money in specialized training, was especially instrumental in ending the more holistic approach to health care that had been traditional in American medicine." Some scholars theorize that neurasthenia "disappeared" in the early twentieth century because it was relegated to the psychological sphere.

———

In the time between neurasthenia and chronic fatigue syndrome, there were a number of outbreaks of illnesses with similar profiles. The first to be put on record struck 198 healthcare workers in a Los Angeles hospital in 1934. Because it followed on the heels of a poliomyelitis epidemic, the illness's victims were initially diagnosed with polio. But when it did not cause paralysis or death, the illness was dubbed "atypical polio."

All told, between the 1934 epidemic in Los Angeles and the 1984 epidemic in Incline Village, fifty-three outbreaks were documented from all over the world. Dr. Anthony Komaroff, now an ME/CFS researcher, first noticed patients with the flu-like symptoms of what came to be called ME/CFS in the late 1970s. The numbers increased in the early eighties. By then, other doctors—in Atlanta, Denver, New York, and Beverly Hills—were also seeing an upswing of patients with these confounding symptoms.

Alice never sought the care of S. Weir Mitchell, but the visionary social worker Jane Addams did, along with a host of other prominent women, including Charlotte Perkins Gilman, the author of "The Yellow Wall-Paper."

Mitchell believed that a successful cure depended on the neurasthenic's acquiescence to male authority. Certain patients in particular needed a commanding male doctor "who can insure belief in his opinions and obedience to his decrees." He believed the symptoms were real, but that some women *were* shirkers. As he put it in *Fat and Blood*, his book describing the Rest Cure:

> To lie abed half the day, and sew a little and read a little, and be interesting and excite sympathy, is all very well, but when they are bidden to stay in bed a month, and neither to read, write, nor sew, and to have one nurse,—who is not a relative,—then rest becomes for some women a rather bitter medicine, and they are glad enough to accept the order to rise and go about when the doctor issues a mandate which has become pleasantly welcome and eagerly looked for.

Part of what he called his "moral medication" included directing the thoughts of his patients "to the lapse from duties to others, and to the selfishness" of "a life of invalidism." Dr. S. Weir Mitchell repudiated the sick role long before Talcott Parsons ever gave it a name.

Like me, and most of us with ME/CFS, Alice found that her symptoms fluctuated. When her health was good, she loved to ride and drive horses, kept a greenhouse, and even organized a women's luncheon club for intellectual discussion. In the fall of 1876 she wrote to her friend Sara Sedgwick (who later married Charles Darwin's eldest son), that she was doing so well "that to be any better would be quite superfluous." A year and a half later, however, at the age of twenty-nine, she relapsed. Her mother described it to Alice's brother Robertson as "a nervous breakdown of a very serious character—an aggravated recurrence of her old troubles." In addition to her other symptoms, Alice was depressed to the point of suicidality.

Seven months later, when she was finally well enough to at least write letters, she wrote to her friend Fanny Morse of the emotional toll of her confinement: "When one can only take a passive part in life, the base, crude, blankness of nature here with nothing to call one out of one's self, plays upon the soul, and makes the process of getting well a task and not a pleasure." She believed she could have tolerated her bodily ailments had she not been depressed. Reflecting on the circular nature of the illness, she said, "My physical sufferings would have given me no concern, but my patience, courage & self-control all seemed to leave me like a flash & I was left high and dry." The depression took her under, and she no longer had the emotional resilience to shore herself up each day and get on with it as best she could. And so the fatigue kept her bedridden, taking "a passive part in life," and that was nothing if not depressing. As she quipped to Sara Sedgwick in August 1879, "ill-health though not an exceptional or tragic fate inevitably brings a certain monotony into the lives of its victims which makes them rather sceptical of the much talked of and apparently much believed-in joy of mere existence."

Jean Strouse tied the collapse to her brother William's engagement to another Alice—Alice Gibbens, a rival for his affections. The siblings had always had a close relationship, and Strouse implied a manipulative aspect to the breakdown, writing that it "constituted . . . a dramatic objection" and that Alice took "spectacularly" to her bed, thus preventing her mother from visiting William's fiancée. Elsewhere, Strouse described Alice's "tyrannical helplessness."

I can remember myself at my sickest. It was the illness itself that felt tyrannical. It ruled my life. It stole my body from me. It contradicted my will.

———

Women have a long legacy as healers; starting in the late fourteenth century, they were burned as witches for it. Feminist scholar Silvia Federici argues that the witch-hunts were an integral part of Europe's transition to capitalism.

In feudal Europe, says Federici in her book *Caliban and the Witch*, women had more financial power than they would see again for hundreds of years. I learned of her work from Eula Biss, who writes in *Having and Being Had*:

> Peasant women were often partners in holding land, and they could inherit property. The work they did in their homes and gardens was considered real work with real value. They produced cloth and soap and medicine. Later, as cities grew, women worked in hundreds of professions, as smiths, butchers, bakers, ale brewers, and retailers.

But during the fraught and jagged push toward capitalism—at the same time that communal land formerly used for harvesting herbs and berries, gathering wood, and grazing livestock was expropriated from the peasants—women lost important economic rights. For instance, the wages of married women who worked were paid to their husbands, and even single women lost the right to make business contracts. Women's primary role now, according to Federici, was as "a machine to produce more workers." Those punished as witches were often childless women or those past reproductive age, midwives who provided birth control, and other herbalists, and, as Biss points out, "notably, poor."

Biss writes of learning from *Caliban and the Witch* that "the witch hunts in Europe reached their peak as slave ships sailed to the

Americas and feudal relations gave way to capitalism. The burning of women, the enslavement of Africans, and the theft of indigenous land were all . . . part of the same process."

A few hundred years later, with help from their household cookbooks, pioneer women in the New World used folk remedies to care for their families and other community members. But these healers were relegated to the domestic realm; by the nineteenth century, men protected their status and their economic interests by forming medical societies and keeping women out, making the unlicensed practicing of medicine punishable by fine or imprisonment. These men, known as "regular" doctors, commodified medicine, and they distinguished their treatments from the gentle herbs dispensed by those who were disparagingly called the empirics by turning instead to "heroic" measures like bloodletting, blisters, and laxative purges, which, as Barbara Ehrenreich and Deirdre English noted in *For Her Own Good: 150 Years of the Experts' Advice to Women*, offered "something activist, masculine, and imminently more salable than the herbal teas and sympathy served up by rural female healers."

———

One of the very few female doctors of the nineteenth century, Mary Putnam Jacobi, took S. Weir Mitchell to task for his overgeneralizations about women, whom he adamantly believed were not fit for education or careers. In an 1891 letter to him, she suggested that he was constructing his theories on an unrepresentative sample population: the neurasthenic women he treated. Perhaps she based this observation on something she likely read in his 1888 book *Doctor and Patient*, in which he wrote, "the man who does not know sick women does not know women."

Mitchell conceived his treatments in accordance with his gender biases. For women, predominantly, he devised the Rest Cure. His female patients more often convalesced at his sanitarium, where they were restricted to complete bed rest and spoon-fed a diet consisting primarily of milk and beef broth, returning to a state of "childlike acquiescence," as Mitchell put it. But as my friend Jennifer Tuttle, the Dorothy M. Healy Professor of Literature and Health at the University of New England, noted in her paper "Rewriting the West Cure: Charlotte Perkins Gilman, Owen Wister, and the Sexual Politics of Neurasthenia," while Mitchell saw women as constitutionally delicate, he viewed the neurasthenic men who came to see him as having temporarily overtaxed their brains as a result of their professional careers. Instead of being sent to their beds, these "feminized" men were frequently sent into the outdoors, sometimes out West, to reclaim their manly vigor.

Many years later, Mitchell expressed regret that he had only recommended what he called the "Camp Cure" to men, saying that he had not understood that this treatment was "also in a measure attainable by many women."

―――――――

In December 1875, Alice found a productive way to engage her prodigious intelligence despite the limitations imposed on her by her illness: she began teaching for today's equivalent of an online university—a correspondence course for women. The Society to Encourage Studies at Home, brainchild of Anna Eliot Ticknor, embraced a philosophical foundation in direct contradiction of the medical claim that intellectual stimulation was harmful to women's health. On the contrary, Ticknor maintained, education was critical to women's overall physical and mental health. In an 1878 tract sent to all students, Ticknor referenced the machinelike "motor power seated in the brain and the nerves," but added her view of the body-mind as an interconnected system: "If the mind needs a healthy body for its service, the body also needs an active, healthy mind to act upon it," and "The best preventative of mental disease, even in those predisposed to it, is education, or wisely directed mental activity."

The society's teachers organized themselves into several departments, including history, art, literature, and natural science, and pulled books from their own shelves to establish an extensive lending library. Instructors worked collaboratively to co-create a curriculum with each of their students. Alice was recruited to teach history. Her department head was Katharine Peabody Loring, whom four years later Alice described to her friend Sara Darwin as having "all the mere brute superiority which distinguishes man from woman combined with all the distinctively feminine virtues."

In her second year of teaching, Alice wrote to her friend Annie Ashburner that she had students from California, Kansas, Missouri, Michigan, Kentucky, Florida, Iowa, and Illinois. "We who have had all our lives more books than we know what to do with can't conceive of the feelings that people have for them always. They look upon them as something sacred. . . . Now this is the sort of being that we want to help and that we do help." She told Annie she wrote thirty to forty letters per month, "but I have nought else of importance to do" and "it is what I most care about just now."

While her friends were getting married all around her, with no prospects in sight for Alice, in 1876 she confessed to Annie, "I am becoming ardently matrimonial, and if I could get any sort of man to be impassioned about me I should not let him escape." That never happened.

But just three years later, in that 1879 letter to Sara Darwin, the clearly besotted Alice wrote of Katharine Loring: "She is the most wonderful being. . . . There is nothing she cannot do from hewing wood and drawing water to driving run-away horses and educating all the women in North America."

Until legislation was passed in the early 1990s, women were rarely included in medical studies. So almost all scientific knowledge up until that point was gained by studying men, whose bodies were considered normal and representative. The research community justified this decision by arguing that women's hormonal fluctuations complicated research results, and that women could get pregnant and potentially put a fetus at risk. As Maya Dusenbery points out in *Doing Harm*, it seems that nobody stopped to consider that women's different biochemistries might also cause them to react differently to medical treatments, to suffer different disease symptoms, and even to contract different diseases.

A 2006 review published in the *Journal of Women's Health* found that although things have improved significantly since the 1990s, women are still underrepresented. Of studies that included both genders, women made up only 37 percent of the sample. (A 2011 update found that there had been no change.) This number fell to 24 percent in drug trials, which might explain why women are 50 to 70 percent more likely than men to suffer an adverse drug reaction. Eighty-seven percent of studies did not break results down by sex. Early studies of the COVID vaccine also failed to categorize results by sex, and perhaps this is the reason that women tend to suffer worse side effects.

———

When twenty-nine-year-old Emma Eckstein sought Freud's help for agonizing menstrual pain, gastrointestinal distress, and disabling leg pain, he diagnosed her, predictably, with hysteria. This time, however, Freud put his patient, a feminist socialist from a prominent family, in the hands of his good friend Wilhelm Fliess, a proponent of the peculiar theory that female troubles could be caused by nasal anomalies. Fliess diagnosed her with "nasal reflex neurosis." He believed the problem was best treated with topical applications of cocaine to the mucous membrane in the nose, and if that didn't work and cauterization of the nasal tissue didn't, either, sometimes a surgical intervention was in order.

According to Frederick Crews, author of *Freud: The Making of an Illusion*, it was an admittedly experimental surgery, with Eckstein as Fliess's second guinea pig—the first being the cocaine-addicted Freud himself. Fliess removed an area that he later said was often inflamed in women who masturbated, something Eckstein had guiltily confessed in her sessions with Freud. Of course, another possibility is that the *cocaine* had something to do with the inflammation.

Fliess performed his surgery in Vienna in February 1895, and then immediately returned to his home in Berlin, leaving Eckstein at the sanatorium where she had already been convalescing. Freud visited her regularly to continue her psychoanalysis.

Just a little over a week after the procedure, Freud wrote to Fliess that Eckstein was suffering from painful bleeding and other confounding complications. He eventually called in a surgeon, who, as Freud wrote in a grisly follow-up,

> cleaned the area surrounding the opening, removed some sticky blood clots, and suddenly pulled at something like a thread, kept on pulling. Before either of us had time to think, at least a half a meter of gauze had been removed from the cavity. The next moment came a flood of blood. The patient turned white, her eyes bulged. . . . Immediately thereafter, however, he again packed the cavity with fresh iodoform gauze and the hemorrhage stopped. It lasted about half a minute, but this was enough to make the poor creature, whom by then we had lying flat, unrecognizable. . . . At the moment the foreign body came out and everything became clear to me—and I immediately afterward was confronted by the sight of the patient—I felt sick. After she had been packed, I fled to the next room, drank a bottle of water, and felt miserable. . . .

[Eckstein] had not lost consciousness during the massive hemorrhage; when I returned to the room somewhat shaky, she greeted
me with the condescending remark, "So this is the strong sex."

Two months later, Freud confided to Fliess that Eckstein continued to suffer from intermittent bleeding and he worried she was
"rapidly moving toward a bad ending." With the help of several
doctors, however, Eckstein survived her ordeal. All the while, she
continued psychoanalytical treatment with Freud, and he continued
to pursue an unconscious motivation for her bleeds. On April 16,
1896, he crowed in a letter to Fliess that he had determined that
"her episodes of bleeding were hysterical, and occasioned by *longing*." Two weeks later he elaborated, writing that he had extracted
from her a story of getting a nosebleed "when she had the wish to
be treated by a certain young doctor who was present." Here is his
interpretation, then, of her most recent bleed:

> When she saw how affected I was by her first hemorrhage. . . . she
> experienced this as the realization of an old wish to be loved in her
> illness, and in spite of the danger during the succeeding hours she
> felt happy as never before. Then, in the sanatorium, she became
> restless during the night because of an unconscious intent of long-
> ing to entice me to go there; since I did not come during the night,
> she renewed the bleedings, as an unfailing means of rearousing my
> affection.

In a searing summary, Crews points out that Freud "was accusing
a mutilated patient, led into danger by himself and nearly killed by
his bosom friend, of having emitted quantities of blood in the service
of typical female wiles."

Eckstein, whose nose was permanently disfigured, nonetheless
continued therapy with Freud until at least the next year, and then
returned to him for about six months in 1909–1910. Around that

time, she sought help for excruciating abdominal pains from a surgeon who found and removed several abscesses from her uterus. Although the pain persisted, Eckstein, long suspicious of Freud's diagnosis of hysteria, was relieved to have an organic explanation for the troubles she had experienced since adolescence.

Freud disagreed and sent her for a second opinion to a Viennese surgeon he believed would support his diagnosis. But the surgeon, Dr. Dora Teleky, later told a journalist:

> I saw that the abscesses still persisted, or that a fresh abscess had formed on the site of the incision. I made a new incision and at one stroke freed the patient of her pains. When I later told this to the master at his home, he blew up. With biting scorn he asked me whether I actually believe that hysterical pain could be cured by the knife. Quaking, I objected that an obvious abscess must be treated. Despite the fact that the patient was cured of all complaints, Dr. Freud became so unfriendly to me that I was obliged to break off the discussion and leave him.

It seems likely that Eckstein suffered from what we now know as endometriosis, a painful disorder caused by uterine tissue growing outside of the uterus. Eckstein improved for a short time and even regained her mobility, but—as commonly happens in cases of endometriosis when new growths form—the disabling problem returned. As Freud later put it, she "remained abnormal to the end of her life."

———

In a 2001 article for *Psychiatric Services*, licensed clinical social worker Nancy Hedrick—referencing an earlier paper by Mary Lou Ballweg called "Blaming the Victim: The Psychologizing of Endometriosis"—makes a strong argument that Alice suffered from endometriosis.

Ballweg, the president of the Endometriosis Association, points out that a patient with endometriosis could easily be diagnosed with somatization disorder—basically, a psychiatric euphemism for hysteria—per the *Diagnostic and Statistical Manual of Mental Disorders* (DSM), which is *the* professional reference book of psychiatric diagnosis. Endometriosis symptoms that overlap with symptoms of somatization disorder, and with those that Alice suffered, include irregular periods and excessive menstrual bleeding, pain in the abdomen even when not menstruating, abdominal bloating, diarrhea, and back pain.

The most recent version of the DSM has changed the name to *somatic symptom disorder* and, wisely, has drastically changed the list of symptoms, removing menstrual symptoms altogether. However, it would still be easy for a doctor to prematurely and erroneously decide that a patient fulfills another criterion: "disproportionate and persistent thoughts about the seriousness of one's symptoms."

A 1993 study advising doctors on how to manage somatization and hypochondria took pains to point out that about 25 percent of patients diagnosed with a somatization disorder are eventually found to have an organic basis for their symptoms. I suspect this number is actually much higher, particularly now that so many more autoimmune disorders are being identified. For instance, one very small 2018 study found that of twenty people diagnosed with psychogenic illnesses and sent to the psychosomatic department of a clinic, fourteen were later found to have organic illnesses.

Hedrick notes that the episodic nature of Alice's symptoms does indicate a possible menstruation-related disorder. Indeed, when she was forty, Alice wrote in a letter to William that many doctors had suggested she would feel much better after menopause, which, she said, "seems highly probable as I have had sixteen periods the last year." Hedrick also remarks that women who suffer from endometriosis are at a higher risk for female cancers, and thus Alice's eventual death from breast cancer could be another clue.

Hedrick's analysis makes no mention of the fatigue that was Alice's predominant symptom throughout the decades of her illness. It's possible that Alice suffered from endometriosis and ME/CFS as co-occurring illnesses. One survey of endometriosis patients found that one in five had been diagnosed with a second disease; for one in three of those women, the second illness was either ME/CFS or fibromyalgia.

Echoing what Jean Strouse and other researchers have written about neurasthenia, in 1994 a psychologist at the Fourth World Congress on Endometriosis commented, according to Ballweg, "that endometriosis is the result of modern women's conflict over her role in society." This is also what several doctors said to me when I interviewed them in 2002 for a research class paper about doctors' perceptions of ME/CFS.

———

As Maya Dusenbery suggests in *Doing Harm*, "Many general physicians seem to have more extreme ideas about the limitless range of physical symptoms that they can pass off as psychogenic—even in the absence of any psychological symptoms—than those held by trained mental health professionals." She quotes Stanley Finger, vice chairperson of the board of the American Autoimmune Related Diseases Association, who says that "even as late as 2000, mental health professionals were often the first to make a correct diagnosis" of autoimmune disease.

All told, more than 75 percent of people with ME/CFS were misdiagnosed as "psychological cases" by one or more of their doctors, according to one 1999 study.

Ballweg, in her piece on the psychologizing of endometriosis, describes the thrust of a paper published in *American Family Physician* in 1989, one that might have been read by Dr. Beyers the very year that I went to her desperate for a diagnosis and a cure:

The article . . . suggests that somatization allows patients to avoid blaming themselves for their problems, "as in the patient who is convinced that her pain is due to some disease and that the physician is at fault for not diagnosing the disease."

But *then* Ballweg turns that idea on its head:

The converse is surely worth considering: Perhaps the physician who wishes to avoid being blamed for not recognizing symptoms or keeping up with medical advances is choosing to exonerate himself or herself by labeling the patient with a psychiatric diagnosis.

To that end, I consulted with an expert in ancient Greek for help with a *new* diagnosis—for the doctor. Rather than offering up dustbin diagnoses like somatic symptom disorder (née hysteria), doctors who don't know what is causing their patients' symptoms should have to give a diagnosis that says just that. I have one to suggest: iatraporiueretia (pronounced ee-AT-ra-POR-you-REE-sha). It means "doctor being at a loss for discovering the cause." Say it a few times and it will almost roll off your tongue. Iatraporiueretia. Iatraporiueretia.

Imagine how different things would be if instead of blaming the patient, doctors had to point to the real source of the problem. Medicine doesn't have all the answers; research is an ongoing process. But when a doctor tells a patient her mysterious symptoms are the result of mental illness, that doctor is presuming an exhaustive knowledge of all disease.

A little humility would actually improve medical outcomes. It would decrease the risk of physician error (because a diagnosis of somatoform disorder or somatization disorder or somatic symptom disorder—or whatever nom du jour doctors give it—is often an error, but a diagnosis of iatraporiueretia would actually be an honest representation of the problem), reduce the anti-therapeutic experience of gaslighting, and let patients know that although the source of their troubles is currently unidentified, there might yet be an answer out there.

———

Strouse gave us a brilliant biography that brought Alice out of the shadows and revealed the sister of William and Henry James to be a woman with a voice of her own. But there are places where I think Strouse gets it wrong. Her analysis of Alice's 1878 breakdown is one of them.

In a 1981 *New York Times* article, Strouse revealed that even before starting the book, she had determined that Alice was not someone she could ever admire. "There was a period when Alice was in her late 20's. And she was making decisions which were limiting her life, ruling out meaningful work or serious relationships with men. The whole thing horrified me and I just really didn't like her. I had to stop." She took a month away from the project and found herself having little conversations with Alice in her head. Finally she realized something: "Alice spent her whole life getting from others what she felt she lacked. She made passive demands. And I felt she was doing the same to me; that here I was, after 100 years, taking care of Alice. I felt I was being manipulated from beyond the grave."

That word: *manipulated.*

I wonder: How did Strouse's personal response to the effects of Alice's illness influence the writing of her biography?

Let me review the "decisions" that Strouse told the interviewer were limiting Alice's life. First, that she ruled out meaningful work. But for a time, Alice did work: she began teaching for one of the country's earliest correspondence courses, something she could do without exerting herself unduly. Alice loved the work. As she wrote to a friend shortly after joining the society, "I am enjoying the feeling that I dare to be busy, for the first time in many years, during which I have been an invalid." Although Strouse does not say when or why Alice stopped teaching, and I couldn't find a record of it in Alice's letters or diary, presumably this happened when she found she was just too ill to sustain it.

And given that no men expressed any romantic interest in Alice, I think it's unfair to say she "ruled out" serious relationships with them. And toward the end of her brief life, she did indeed invest her heart in a serious relationship—with her former department head, Katharine Loring.

Strouse referred to Alice's illness in several places as her "career." Here, too, I read her judgment. A career is something you *choose*. An illness is foisted upon you.

Strouse could just as easily denigrate my years of illness as my "career"—all the time spent in bed convalescing, all the time I spent seeing healthcare providers in a desperate bid for recovery.

When I improved enough to work part time, I had to fit all my healthcare appointments into my schedule. Often there were two or three a week—a therapist, a doctor, and an alternative healthcare provider. People with healthy bodies have no idea how much *time* it takes to be sick.

Strouse wrote:

The intelligence and energy Alice might have used in some productive way went into the intricate work of being sick. . . . Her miserable health *was* her career. It grew out of her particular, troubled existence, just as Henry's novels and William's psychology grew out of their moral concerns and personal conflicts. All three careers expressed private experience, but two addressed themselves to the world and were crowned with public success, whereas Alice's "work" affected only herself—and by anybody's standards, a life of incapacitating illness denoted failure and waste.

I have a different experience of Alice. I *do* admire her. What fortitude she had, what grit! Alice was smart, edgy. Her indomitable wit delights me. She cracked it like a whip.

She kept on.

Of course, defining the life of a person with an incapacitating illness as "failure and waste," as Strouse did, is an ableist comment steeped in the ideology of capitalism. Alice was more than her disability. Like each of us, she had an ineffable spirit. Could that be enough? For her, and for me, too?

Strouse fell victim to the same impulse as many doctors. *I don't know what this is—so it must be psychological.* It's satisfying to do so. We hate a vacuum. And without answers, we are asked to stand in the unknown.

PART II

Body Burden

Every Truth passes through three stages before it is recognized. In the first, it is ridiculed. In the second, it is opposed. In the third, it is regarded as self-evident.

—attributed to philosopher
Arthur Schopenhauer

CHAPTER 5

Minefield

And then something new: headaches.

They came when the waitress sprayed detergent on the table next to mine, when I entered a public bathroom that reeked of air freshener, when I rode in a car with a hole in the exhaust. They came when someone wearing perfume sat down next to me at the movie theater. Or a reading. Or a concert. When I breathed in the cloying chemical sweetness of lit scented candles at the podiatrist's office and the potpourri on display at the department store. They came at the tire store and on airplanes, when I passed through the pesticide aisle at the hardware store and the laundry aisle at the supermarket. They came when I stayed at hotels that had just installed new carpet or laid down a fresh coat of paint. They came when I was exposed to the fumes from the toner in my printer and the chemicals off-gassing from my new TV or even a new pair of shoes. They came from the fabric softener I couldn't scrub out of the jeans I bought from the consignment store and the perfume I couldn't get out of the shirts.

The world became a minefield.

———

Before I fell ill, headaches were a rarity and easily relieved with a couple of aspirin. But these new headaches were something different. They started behind my eyes—a pressure, subtle at first. Soon, though, it felt as though my entire brain was pressing against my skull. A fog rolled in. My capacity to juggle a number of thoughts at once—an ability I had taken for granted—dwindled. Everything closed in. The pain was dull, grinding, relentless. Tylenol didn't touch it. Advil didn't touch it. Hydrocodone didn't touch it. I was helpless to repulse this pain. The lymph nodes in my neck swelled up. My throat got raw and sore. The only thing that stopped the onslaught was separating myself from the offending agent, or it from me, and that required first that I identify the source, which wasn't always easy. For instance, who knew a new desk would off-gas chemicals? I didn't smell anything, but it turns out most desks are now made with particleboard, and particleboard contains formaldehyde.

It was a clingy pain. And even when the offender was gone, the pain lasted. Sometimes for hours, sometimes till the next morning, sometimes longer.

———

I can't remember the first occurrence. Not unless it was the time in that first year of illness when my building filled up with a rank chemical odor that gave me a dull, stubborn headache.

The time I remember came when I was visiting a friend and had just washed my hands with apricot-scented liquid soap. The manufacturer probably called it "Sun-Kissed Apricot" or "Honey Apricot," something to evoke images of nature, but really it was scented with chemicals designed in a lab to remind consumers, however faintly, of apricots. I thought nothing of it at the time; just lathered and rinsed. But then came the pressure behind my eyes and the full-on headache, and I wondered *what* it could be. I took a whiff of my hands. It was such an artificial, chemical smell.

But how could it be that I was getting a headache from something as innocuous as liquid soap? I went back to the cramped little bathroom to try to wash the off the odor. But there was no scrubbing it away.

Eventually I discovered that my new problem had a name: multiple chemical sensitivity (MCS)—and that 80 percent of those who suffer from it also meet the major criteria for ME/CFS. Fatigue is in fact one of the most prominent complaints of people with MCS.

The first time I used the premise spray or the rotenone or the malathion, I didn't react noticeably, but maybe they primed me. Because my immune system was already compromised by the virus that caused the mononucleosis, it probably wasn't a good idea to be exposing myself to these pesticides. But I was innocent: I believed the government was keeping us safe. I washed my fruit like I'd been taught, but other than that I didn't give chemicals much thought.

Synthetic pesticides are products of World War II chemical weapons experimentation. They work by disrupting insects' neurotransmitters and thus destroying their nervous systems. Humans share many of the same neurotransmitters, which means pesticides can also damage our nervous systems.

The authors of a study published in the *Archives of Internal Medicine* concluded: "Despite their different diagnostic labels, existing data, though limited, suggest that these illnesses [MCS and ME/CFS] may be similar, if not identical, conditions. . . . In fact, the diagnosis assigned to patients with one of these illnesses may depend more on their chief complaint and the type of physician making the diagnosis than on the actual illness process."

If I had known that as many as 67 percent of people living with ME/CFS report adverse reactions to everyday chemicals, I would have done things differently. That is the siren call of hindsight.

Now, no matter where I went or what I did, this new iteration of my illness came with me. After several years of country living, I moved back to Portland, dated, learned to play the bass guitar and joined a punk rock band, turned thirty, and finally, after seven years of part-time attendance, finished the second half of my English degree, graduating in the spring of 1998. To have done all this while avoiding chemicals in commercial goods would have been impossible.

———

In the United States, an astonishing 35 percent of people experience health issues when exposed to fragranced products like perfumes and lotions, air fresheners, cleaning supplies, and laundry products. Chemical sensitivity afflicts 57 percent of Americans with asthma and asthma-like conditions, and 80 percent of people on the autism spectrum.

And hazardous chemicals are everywhere. When researchers in a 2010 study analyzed twenty-five fragranced products—including laundry detergent, dryer sheets, fabric softeners, cleaning supplies, air fresheners, baby shampoo, and personal care products—they found a total of 133 volatile organic compounds (VOCs), with each product containing an average of 17 VOCs, including at least one known to be toxic or hazardous. VOCs permeate the brain and bloodstream directly through the nasal passages.

———

The doctor who ultimately diagnosed me with chronic fatigue syndrome was kind and sympathetic but didn't have any answers for me. Eventually I learned of a physician, Dr. Joseph Py, who practiced environmental medicine. This subspecialty came into being in the 1950s when Dr. Theron Randolph, a groundbreaking allergist now known as the father of clinical ecology, discovered that petrochemical products were making some of his patients sick. Winning my Social Security case entitled me to Medicare, but because its reimbursement rates were so much lower than private insurances, it was hard to find good doctors who took my insurance. Dr. Py's receptionist told me that he required full payment up front, but she would then bill Medicare, which would in two or so months send a partial reimbursement to me.

Dr. Py's intake paperwork was like nothing I'd ever seen before. In addition to the standard questions, it asked which industries were prominent in the area where I grew up and whether I'd had any known exposures to toxicants. The form triggered a series of newly connected memories. My city in Canada was home to a General Electric plant; when I lived in Belize, DDT (an organochlorine that Monsanto continued to sell to that and other developing countries after the United States banned its use) was used for pest control in the house where I slept and the school where I taught; and when I returned to Canada, I worked for three months around Freon in a refrigerator tubing factory.

A compact man with falcon-like features, Dr. Py greeted me with a warm smile, ushered me into his office, sat down behind his large wooden desk, and looked over my intake paperwork with interest. I told him I'd been sick for nine years. I said that I did my best to avoid sugar, and that it seemed like my body was reacting to other foods, like wheat and maybe dairy. And then I broke down in tears. "I try so hard to do everything my body wants. But it's never enough." He handed me some tissues and I held them over my eyes and sobbed. Dr. Py sat quietly, fully present, witness to my pain.

When I was able to go on, I looked up and said, "I allow myself one sugar treat a week. But maybe I shouldn't even do that. Do you think if I could just do it *perfectly*, I could get better?"

Dr. Py smiled gently. "It's not your fault you're not better, Jennifer. This is a really complex illness and we don't have enough answers yet. I'm going to do my best to help you." I put my head in my hands and wept some more.

———

On the bulletin board in Dr. Py's waiting room I discovered a flyer for a monthly support group for people with multiple chemical sensitivity. They met in a multipurpose room at a community center. When I arrived, several women were already seated around a large conference table, smiling and chatting. They welcomed me in, and one by one we introduced ourselves and shared our illness stories. A former teacher said that she got sick after she and her husband renovated their kitchen. "The new cabinets smelled something awful, but we just figured it would fade over time," she said.

"But when I woke up the next morning the room was spinning and I could barely walk to the bathroom. At first I thought I was just sick. But this was something different. It didn't go away. It took weeks to figure out it was those cabinets. We tried opening the windows to air it out, we bought an ozone machine to clean the air, we tried painting them with a special paint to seal in the formaldehyde. . . . Nothing worked. Eventually, we replaced them. But by then the damage had been done. That was three years ago. And here I am. I'm a stay-at-home mom now. My energy's better than it was for a long time, so I can come to this group now, and I'll be able to go pick up some groceries after this, but then I'll be toast."

There were general nods all around, and then someone else spoke up. Her hair was trimmed in a tidy bob and she wore a pink button-down shirt with a floral scarf neatly tied around her neck. "You know, sometimes I wonder if we have it all mixed up. We think we're the sick ones, but maybe our bodies are smart. Maybe our bodies are warning us about a real danger. I mean, the formaldehyde in those cupboards is a neurotoxin. Should anyone really be inhaling it?"

"That's right," said another woman. "We're all canaries in a coal mine. These chemicals aren't good for *anybody.*"

This was a perspective I hadn't considered. Suddenly the feminist dictum "the personal is political" made sense to me.

———

Fragranced products can restrict people's access to social settings. Consider the simple universal need of a safe, usable restroom. Forty percent of people with chemical sensitivities find air fresheners a barrier to accessing public restrooms, and even 14 percent of the general population say they have been reluctant to enter a public bathroom due to its air fresheners. Air "fresheners" emit over a hundred different chemicals, including volatile organic compounds like formaldehyde and benzene, both known carcinogens.

A survey by Anne Steinemann, an internationally known expert on the health effects of indoor pollutants, found that 67 percent of Americans are unaware that fragranced products typically emit hazardous chemicals, and that 60 percent would not continue to use a fragranced product if they knew it contained toxicants. Comparing synthetic fragrances to cigarettes, she used the term *secondhand scents*. In the United States, manufacturers are not required to disclose the ingredients in "fragrance."

Thanks to synthetic fragrances, people with chemical sensitivities are often shut out of schools, churches, hotels, gyms, Laundromats, stores, libraries, taxicabs, and public transportation, and the list goes on and on.

———

My years of therapy made me want to help people the way my therapist had helped me, so I enrolled in a master's in social work program.

When I walked into the classroom that first day, the fragrances from people's shampoos, fabric softeners, body washes, and perfumes hung conspicuously in the air. Soon I noticed the pressure building behind my eyes. And then the headache. And the brain fog.

I wanted to flee the room.

But if I intended to become a social worker, I had to stay. Realizing I was going to have to say something, I gathered my thoughts for a minute. Then I raised my hand and spoke up: "This is kind of hard to do on the first day of class, but I need to ask for your help. I have multiple chemical sensitivity, which means that scented products give me terrible headaches that aren't relieved by any painkiller. The chemicals in these products also make it hard for me to think clearly. I know it's a lot to ask, but if you could avoid wearing scented products as much as possible on the days you have class with me, that would be a big help."

I was fortunate to be in a room full of aspiring social workers. If there's one thing this set wants to do, it's help. I saw expressions of compassion on the faces around me, and when I was finished our professor, a tall, bearded man who told us we could call him Steve, launched into his lecture.

Far too often we pathologize the individual without considering contexts. But human behavior doesn't happen in a vacuum. In this class, we will be looking at problems on a societal level that contribute to problems on an individual level. We'll explore how capitalism, which reduces people to commodities with a specific economic value, causes disconnection, alienation, and fragmentation, and how this is the source of so many of the problems people face in society today. We'll also discuss the concept of "normality" as a form of social control.

Social workers are generalists, so it's important that we look at the whole picture when we consider our clients—that means the biological, the social, and the psychological. In other words, people are biopsychosocial beings. You'll be hearing that term a lot in your career as a social work student.

I could see I had a lot to learn.

I detested it, starting each new course with that speech. I hated drawing attention to myself, to my weakness. But invariably, my announcement elicited a wave of sympathy from my fellow students. And often it generated questions. I found suddenly that my illness afforded me, for those brief, condensed moments, a soapbox. Instead of being pulled under by the illness, I could use it as a sounding board for discussion about the hazards of our society's dependence on synthetic chemicals.

"More and more people react adversely to common chemicals," I told my classmates. "And every time I give one of these speeches, at least one person comes up to me later and thanks me, because they, too, get headaches from scented products. Or some other problem, like constricted airways. Or they have a friend who does."

It was during this time, when I was delivering those speeches and learning about the interconnections between people and systems, that I first began to understand that my illness was not just about me, my weakness, my infirmity. My illness was about *us*, about what we're doing wrong, about what we are being called to rectify.

———

The day before the start of the second semester, I returned to the community center to sit with my fellow canaries.

"I'm really nervous about class tomorrow," I said. "The first day of classes is always the worst."

"You should get a mask," said Marge, in those days long before COVID-19 made masks ubiquitous.

Everybody nodded.

"No, no, no," I said, shaking my head from side to side. "I don't want to wear a mask. That's where I draw the line."

"Oh no," said Marge. "Get a carbon filter mask. It makes a world of difference. If you carry it with you in your purse, you can go anywhere and you don't have to worry about getting sick."

"Ugh. I don't want to look like a weirdo."

"I know," said Marge. "But it's worth it. Trust me."

Nods all around the room.

———

The first thing most people are inclined to do, often unconsciously, when faced with someone who has a disability or a chronic or life-threatening illness is differentiate themselves. *I'm not like her. It could never happen to* me.

There's also a moral dimension. That person must have done something wrong. Probably she wasn't going to the gym, or she was eating Hostess Twinkies all the time, or she had too many negative thoughts. *I'm not like that, so it won't happen to me.*

Once I went out to lunch with a woman I met at the library. I thought we might become friends. When she expressed curiosity about the illness, I told her more. She listened intently, exuding warmth and presence. She was a vibrant, creative woman, her short gray hair framing an intelligent face. When I was finished, she said, "I've always believed that if I take good care of myself and think positively that it would protect me. And so far that's worked for me."

So what did that say about me?

For a moment, we sat with that unspoken question hanging in the air between us. Then I said, "You're lucky. That doesn't always work for everybody."

———

The disadvantage of a disabling invisible illness is that people think that since you don't *look* sick, you must not *be* sick. When you say,

I have an illness, they hear, *I have an "illness."* The advantage is that you can avoid stigma by passing as non-disabled. You can keep your health issues private.

In considering a mask, I was considering making my invisible disability visible in an all-too-conspicuous way.

"Here," said Lenore, with a friendly smile, "I have an extra one in my purse you can buy from me." She pulled out a fabric carbon filter mask in battleship gray, and the women passed it down the table to me. The package read, *I Can Breathe!*™ I pulled out the mask and turned it over in my hands, trying to imagine myself wearing it in class. Frankly, the thought horrified me.

"That's your freedom, right there," said Marge. "That's your health you're holding in your hands."

I pulled the elastics over my ears and adjusted the mask over my mouth and nose. Everyone smiled and nodded approvingly.

"How do I look?"

"You look great!" said Lenore. And we all laughed.

———

The next day, I raised my hand at the beginning of class and asked the professor if I could say something before we began. Trembling, I pulled out the mask and held it up for everybody to see. I explained my condition, offering my standard speech with a new twist.

"This is a carbon filter mask. If you see me pull it out today or anytime this semester, it's not because I have some communicable disease; it's because I'm starting to feel a headache coming on and the mask will help protect me from the chemicals in the room. I know that sometimes people forget and dab on a little perfume or whatever. I know you'll do your best."

This time, when I felt the first pressure behind my eyes, I pulled out the mask and put it on. I felt conspicuous and strange, but I also felt like it was important, what I was doing. I often wished people could somehow *see* the headaches I was getting because it would help them remember to leave their scents at home. The mask was a physical representation of my invisible illness. I knew that by being open about my MCS I was helping others who would come after me.

But also . . . what a relief. I could *breathe*. I was *safe*. With this little mask, I could keep my brain clear and stave off the headache.

———

The women in my support group were right. The mask was a godsend. It saved me on airplanes and buses and at concerts and movie theaters. But I hated that without an explanation from me, people didn't know what the mask was for. What I *really* wanted was a mask appliquéd with a symbol that stood for "your toxic products are making me sick."

My energy was on a gradual upswing, but even with my trusty mask ready at hand to protect me, and despite my ongoing efforts to recover my health, the chemical and food sensitivities were only getting worse and worse.

I tried holotropic breathwork. I consulted a medical intuitive. I worked with a spiritual teacher. I tried a different acupuncturist and a new chiropractor. I tried colonics—a treatment of last resort that involved allowing a stranger in a tidy trailer home to insert a tube into my rectum and inject water all the way up into my colon until I felt I was going to burst, while another tube carried out the waste, purportedly flushing out toxins.

Once I went to a church to be blessed by a faith healer, but I was toward the end of a very long line, and perhaps by then she'd been emptied out.

Meanwhile, Dr. Py and I tried a variety of interventions: a very restrictive elimination diet to help cut down symptoms related to food sensitivities, vitamin B injections, vitamin C IVs, even a system of daily coffee enemas combined with liquid vitamin supplementation that I inserted rectally.

By this point my energy was charting around four or five on my scale of ten, and I was interning at an after-school program for a group of sweet and vivacious girls, refugees from Somalia and the Sudan. I loved the work. I gave the girls disposable cameras and they photographed their lives. Then they cowrote and performed a play. But in February 2000 I sank into an inexplicable depression, and now I couldn't bear the thought of facing them. I felt dead inside.

Depression is a thief of meaning and connection—and loss of meaning and connection can also be a trigger for depression. On those depressed days, every morning I woke up with the thought: *What is the purpose of any of this?*

Then one morning I awoke with a different, even darker thought: *I don't want to be alive.*

This thought frightened me.

Or maybe that's not it: I don't feel alive. Maybe I just want to be unconscious.

It was too painful to be disconnected from the world. From everything. From those delightful, smiling girls at my internship. From the maple tree outside my window. From the strangers I passed in the street. From my own self.

I'd been off antidepressants for well over a year, but I called Dr. Py and asked for a prescription, then took a week's leave from my internship and lay in bed watching nature documentaries. The depression lifted enough for me to return to work. A few months later, when my mood had stabilized, I found I no longer needed the meds.

———

In 1878, Alice's plunge into depression was so deep and unbearable that on many days she found herself contemplating suicide. Sitting with her father in his study, she asked if he considered suicide a sin. He replied, as he later wrote in a letter to her brother Robertson, that it was absurd to think it sinful when one was driven to it in order to escape bitter suffering. . . . I told her so far as I was concerned she had my full permission to end her life whenever she pleased; only I hoped that if ever she felt like doing that sort of justice to her circumstances, she would do it in a perfectly gentle way in order not to distress her friends.

Alice expressed great relief at his approbation. She told her father that by granting her this freedom to end her life should it become unendurable, he had alleviated her of the drive to do so. But mustn't she have felt a little empty inside when her father expressed greater worry about the potential distress to her friends than he did for what might also have been a great loss for him?

———

In September the depression returned. By November, I was contemplating suicide.

I called my mother.

There was a deadness in my voice when she picked up the phone. My mother knew this deadness. Most of our relationship had taken place over the phone, and she could recognize my mood just by listening.

I started to talk. "Things are really bad, Mom. I'm just so tired of trying. Nothing is working. I've been sick forever. I have tried everything I can think of to get better, but I'm getting headaches all the time from the chemicals. And the food sensitivities are just getting worse and worse. I feel like I'm getting painted into a corner. Soon there'll be nothing left to eat."

She listened.

"And, Mom, I've been thinking about suicide again. And the other day I had this sudden flash that it seemed like a very rational solution. This isn't going away. I've tried everything in my power to get better, and it just isn't. What if it's never going to get better? I've been sick for *eleven years*. It just seems so right, just to end it. It scares me, how rational it seems, but I can't live like this for the rest of my life. I just can't take it much longer. I'm tired. I'm so tired. I'm tired of fighting. I want to raise the white flag."

My mother was quiet for a long moment. And then she said, "I understand."

My body relaxed in a sudden flood of relief. She said, "You have been fighting a long time, and you're not getting better. I understand that you want to die. And I want you to know that I will accept whatever decision you make."

I let out a great sigh. I was relieved to hear her say it. She would accept whatever I chose. If there was an emptiness, I did not notice it.

––––––

I went back on the antidepressant, and by mid-December the suicidal thoughts had dissipated, and I was left with the low-grade depression that had dogged me since I'd first fallen ill.

That same month, Dr. Py suggested we test my blood for heavy metals, and the lab results revealed that my mercury levels were off the chart. This was the first test to show something was out of whack since the discovery of the Epstein-Barr virus that caused my mononucleosis. Could it be the source of all my problems? High levels of mercury can cause fatigue, depression, and other symptoms. Dr. Py prescribed a chelating agent that would bind with the mercury so that I could pee it out. I followed his protocol rigorously, and when we retested six months later the mercury, although still elevated, was reduced. I continued chelation, but when we tested seven months later, it was again off the chart. Seven months after that, despite following the protocol, my mercury levels had not come down at all. It seemed that no matter what I did, I couldn't eliminate the mercury.

I watched what I ate, giving up tuna completely, and consumed trout just once a week. But I had a mouthful of dental amalgams, and by then I had done enough reading to suspect that perhaps the mercury in my teeth was leaching into my body. I decided to do something drastic: I asked my dentist to replace all my amalgams with composite resin fillings. We followed a careful protocol, removing just two or three at a time over a period of many months. I used my student loans to pay for it.

And finally, my mercury levels came down.

I was not cured. The lethargy, the sensitivity to chemicals, remained. But gradually the depression lifted. Completely. The darkness had been with me through the many years of my illness, casting a pall over everything, or, in the better times, crouching in the shadows. Now it was gone.

———

In January 2002 I placed a personal ad in the local alternative weekly.

> Creative, smart, strong woman seeks fun,
> companionship, warmth and support from grounded,
> irreverent, unconventional man. Surface appearance
> of calm . . . powerful emotional life roils underneath.
> Do you love words, new adventures, passionate
> exploration of the sacred and the profane?

One day, there was a message from a man who said his name was Frank and that he was a visual artist and musician. I was pretty sure this was the Frank who used to work at Amadeus, a legendary music store in town. When I had first moved to Portland, he cashed me out a couple times. He had a thick head of auburn hair and horn-rimmed 1950s glasses, and his skin looked as smooth as a baby's. I used to see him zipping around town on his bike, even in winter, when he wore a brown tweed bomber hat that I found fetching. More recently, my friend Jill, also an artist, had said, "You and Frank Turek should go on a date. He's totally your kind of guy."

He played sax in a surf band called Shutdown 66; once I'd had an almost mystical experience listening to them play live at the Free Street Taverna. He made intricate, delicate boxed assemblages. I'd seen them at a group show at the Local 188, an artist-run restaurant with brick walls and high ceilings that sometimes hosted poetry readings and live bands.

These shadow boxes were complex, mysterious, and playful, and I stood studying each of them for a very long while. One piece, made out of an old wooden drawer, contained an etching of a heart, to which he had pinned five words gleaned from some old found text: *converge, osculate, pretend, circle, freeze.* On a small green shelf atop the etching was a tiny lightbulb, and below that the word *electricity.* In a box constructed within the box, a gray plastic knight holding an olive fork sat—or floated—against a backdrop of a fancy 1960s living room. Surrounding the knight's box were four gray plastic spacemen clutching various tools, and when I bent my knees, I found myself looking into a mirror. The drawer was lined with text from a story about a girl named Alice, and behind that the artist had glued a clipping of a photographic print of a monarch butterfly on a sunflower.

The label gave the title: *Elusive Dying Embers.*

I thought, *Who's* this *guy?*

When I called him back, I gave him the name my friends called me, Lunden, and said, struggling with the awkward grammar, "I think we might know who each other is . . ."

"I think so," he said, and I quickly replied, "Is that a *bad* thing or a *good* thing?"

"It's a good thing," he said.

And so it was.

———

In May 2002, my father and stepmother drove across the country to celebrate my graduation. Frank and I had been together for four months, and he joined us after the ceremony. We decided on an early dinner at a colorful Mexican restaurant, but when we arrived the place reeked of cleaning chemicals. I stopped in my tracks. *Oh no.* I really didn't want to trouble everybody. But I knew I would regret it if we stayed. I turned to my folks, wincing. "I'm really sorry. I don't think I can stay. Can we go someplace else?"

"No problem," said my dad, and we all turned around and piled back into the car.

———

A year before graduating I'd asked the university's research librarian if she could help me locate some articles. I wanted to know if anyone else had made the correlation between neurasthenia and chronic fatigue syndrome. I learned that a handful had. And then I wanted to know about nineteenth-century gender constrictions and the effects of early industrialization. I was consumed with the thrill of the hunt, and in an ever-widening web of research, I used the interlibrary loan service to order one paper after another and then drove to pick up my piles of booty. I brought it home, climbed back into bed, and began to read. Endnotes led me to more articles and to entire books, and off I went, farther and farther down the rabbit hole.

Now that I'd graduated, I had more time for this research. It had been eight years since I'd first read about Alice James, but now I was ready to look for some answers.

CHAPTER 6

Our Domestic Poisons

I took a job as a therapist at a small agency a mile from my apartment. I worked part time and didn't earn much, and thus my SSDI continued. As a per diem employee, I could set my own schedule and work the few hours my body would allow. To start, I saw six clients a week, a very small caseload. Most therapists, I learned, saw closer to twenty-five.

The agency was housed in an old brick building with several offices on each of its three floors. I walked to work or rode my bike, since my car had died and I couldn't afford a new one. I was well enough now to do this, and I liked seeing the skate kids attempting flip tricks on the median and the punks sprawled out smoking cigarettes in the park, and the guy with the cart selling hot dogs rain or shine.

My boss, who wore ties with designs drawn by children, decorated each floor with hearts. He'd just bought the building and was in the process of renovations. I told him about my chemical sensitivity and asked him to paint with no-VOC paint, explaining that volatile organic compounds were bad not just for me but for all of us. I gave him a brand name and told him where I had found it in the past, and he assured me he would take care of it.

But one morning I opened the front door and was slammed by

the acrid odor of fresh paint. Workers had painted the hallways and stairwells on every floor. The reek was everywhere; there was no escape. My first client was on her way, and I couldn't exactly move the session to a coffee shop, so I sat down in my office and waited. The sharp odor in my nostrils quickly became pain behind my eyes and the sensation that my brain was pressing against my cranium.

When she arrived, a middle-aged woman with a face wizened by years of cigarettes and drink, I smiled warmly through my headache and welcomed her in. She told me about her week and the things she was trying to understand, and I felt the fog roll in and wrap itself around my head. Still, I kept smiling and listening, nodding and listening, trying to hold the threads in my mind, jotting things down so I would remember, so I could bring her back to the important points, so I could ask the right questions, so I could help her find a way to a better life. And after her, the next one. And after him, the next. By the end of the day, my throat was seared and it felt like someone had pumped up a beach ball inside my head.

I fled as soon as I could, swung my leg over my bike and rode away, gulping the fresh air, pumping the pedals, thinking, *Escape, escape, escape.* In the distance, I saw a white metro bus, and soon I was riding in its wake, inhaling the exhaust, trying not to breathe, then running out of oxygen and sucking in more fumes. The air was heavy with heat and all the chemicals roiling around the city streets. *Get home. Get home. Get home.*

A few days later when I saw my boss, I asked him what had happened. "Oh, I'm sorry," he said. "I was away at a retreat and my business partner took it upon herself to hire a crew and get the place painted. I guess we got our signals crossed." He clasped his hands in front of him and bowed his head in a gesture of remorse.

The paint fumes lingered for weeks. And so did the headache. And then somebody from the MCS support group lent me an ozone machine, and room by room, night after night, the machine cleaned out the last of the VOCs, and finally I could safely breathe again.

———

When we smell something, molecules drift through the air and into our noses, where they attach to cell receptors. The cells then send signals via the nervous system into a region of the brain called the olfactory bulb, which hangs just behind our eyes and helps us identify odors. There is no blood-brain barrier in the olfactory system, so this is an access point for chemicals. Could this be why my headaches always started behind my eyes?

From my research, I learned that I got off easy compared to some. Almost 13 percent of Americans have been diagnosed with MCS. Some have seizures when exposed to chemicals. Their airways close. They suffer joint and muscle pain. They experience disabling fatigue, nausea, insomnia, heart palpitations, and loss of coordination. Unable to work, some become homeless, living in their cars and tents. Some, struggling to find safe places to breathe, move to the deserts of Arizona.

On the other side of the spectrum was the vast gamut of people who reacted to certain chemicals but didn't identify as chemically sensitive. My own father, for instance. When I was a kid, I learned he couldn't use Irish Spring soap because it made him itchy. In more recent years, he developed a host of sinus issues that he finally traced to a new allergy to newsprint. Sometimes when I told people about my chemical sensitivities, they mentioned that although they'd never identified as having multiple chemical sensitivities, they, too, reacted to certain cleaning products or perfumes or other chemicals.

And these percentages are growing. In a 2018 study, Anne Steinemann found that over the previous decade, the number of people who reported having chemical sensitivities rose by over 200 percent, and those who had been diagnosed with MCS by a provider shot up by 300 percent.

―――――

I continued to fight for full recovery. I tried a tapping treatment called the emotional freedom technique. I consulted with a medical intuitive who told me that I had a fungal infection in my intestines and that my blood-brain barrier was damaged as a result of getting the wind knocked out of me as a child. She gave me a handout and recommended that several times a day I do an exercise that involved twisting my wrists clockwise and counterclockwise, which I did for two days because I was willing to try anything, and then gave up because it was so patently ridiculous.

―――――

And I kept thinking about Alice.

In 2005, at a downtown vegan café, I told my friend Jennifer Tuttle, the English professor whose work introduced me to the "West Cure," about the books and research articles that were like a trail of bread crumbs leading me to answers. "But I'm searching for the missing link," I said, holding my fork above a plate of lentil casserole and sautéed kale. "Do my illness and neurasthenia have more than fatigue in common? Might there have been a chemical component in the nineteenth century as well? And if so, what was it? I mean, weren't things cleaner and simpler a hundred and fifty years ago?"

"Well," said Jennifer, who specializes in nineteenth-century literature and health, "I wouldn't exactly associate that period with cleanliness. . . . That's when the modern industrial economy really started taking shape, driven by fossil fuels and corporate greed."

"But there were no plug-in air fresheners then," I said, "no—you know—stinky dryer sheets and scented *toilet paper* and *vacuum bags*, for god's sake. I mean, I know all the researchers say that neurasthenia was a 'fashionable' illness, a form of depression or a somatoform disorder or an unconscious resistance to patriarchy, but I think something physical was undermining people's ability in that time to be well. But if so, *what*?"

A few months later, Jennifer and I met at a coffee shop. It was a sunny day in July, and while we stood in line waiting to make our orders, Jennifer handed me a clipping from *The Boston Globe*: "Death by Wallpaper."

Here was something.

––––––

The clipping Jennifer gave me has yellowed with age. On it, I later scrawled the date of publication—June 22, 2003—and the author's name, Joshua Glenn. The entire clipping, barely larger than a postcard, has frayed at the edges. I've stapled it to a sheet of paper so that it doesn't get lost amid all the other articles that have come since.

Underneath the photo of the earnest, bearded, wild-haired Arts and Crafts designer William Morris and the abutting sample of one of his wallpaper designs is this caption: "William Morris: toxic utopian?"

> While studying arsenic mine spoils on the Scottish border, Andy Meharg, a researcher in the University of Aberdeen's school of biological sciences, learned that Morris owned shares in Britain's most profitable copper and arsenic mine. The mine probably owed its success to the mid-19th-century popularity of a brilliant green arsenic-and-copper compound used by the British in everything from tinted glass to medicine.

Meharg, a professor of biogeochemistry, wondered if it was possible that the renowned environmentalist had used the chemical element in his own products. So he got hold of some samples of Morris's wallpapers and ran some tests. The results confirmed his suspicions. Nine of the first eleven papers Morris designed contained arsenic.

———

I read every single thing I could find about Alice—her published journal and letters, scholarly papers, other James family biographies—and while I never found direct evidence linking Alice's sufferings to arsenical wallpapers, I did unearth a number of other accounts of illness and even death from toxic wallpapers.

In an 1872 Massachusetts state health report ominously entitled *On the Evil Effects of the Use of Arsenic in Certain Green Colors*, I read the story of a woman who fell ill when she and her family moved house—how, after two months in her new home, everything had mysteriously changed, how she'd been fine but suddenly was not, how she was so fatigued she could barely leave her bed, succumbed to brain-numbing headaches, suffered from fainting spells, had terrible indigestion, and couldn't bring herself to eat much of anything. By the time she called a doctor in, she was emaciated. Her doctor couldn't fathom what was making her sick.

In the spring, she and her family moved to the country for a few months and her health returned to her. But when she went home, all her symptoms came back. And then more: diarrhea, severe cramps, frequent paralysis, a loss of sensation in her extremities.

She left; she got better. She returned; she got worse.

When she moved out the third time, this time just for three weeks, she and her husband hired workers to remove the lead pipes and replace the copper tank in their house—just in case. Immediately upon her return, however, she fell ill again.

One day, her stymied doctor noticed the wallpaper, a large floral pattern with a profusion of green leaves, and a suspicion arose: Could it be arsenic? He urged his patient to leave the house again and to hire someone to remove the paper that covered the walls of both her bedroom and parlor. I can imagine her feeling hopeless, but desperate enough to try even this—removing the green wallpaper that graced those two rooms, stripping the walls clean, just to see what would happen, whether this desperate measure might be the answer.

Miraculously, it was. When she returned to the house, her head cleared and her body grew stronger.

When she returned, this time it was for good. She would never fully recover her health, it turns out, but finally she was safe in her own home.

Her story, so long lost to time, sounded so familiar, so contemporary.

———

The entrepreneurial William Morris, a masterful designer of textiles, wallpapers, and stained glass, built an empire out of his aesthetic, leaving his mark on the decor of his era and those that followed, even to this day. Morris was also an acclaimed poet, and the author of several fantasy romance novels that influenced the likes of J. R. R. Tolkien, C. S. Lewis, and even James Joyce.

In 1861, he and six friends set up shop in London, determined to revive the art of craftsmanship, which they saw being ground down by the unrelenting machine of the Industrial Revolution. They called themselves Morris, Marshall, Faulkner & Co., but eventually the firm came to be known simply as Morris & Co., and Morris came to be called the founding father of the Arts and Crafts movement.

The young visionaries rebelled against mass production. They believed that a return to pride in craftsmanship would restore the dignity of workers. Men and women worked side by side. They built furniture; wove fabrics, tapestries, and carpets; and printed textiles and wallpapers. They made architectural carvings, stained glass, metalwork, ceramics, and light fittings. Henry James met Morris in 1869 and wrote to Alice of Morris's "exquisite" taste: "Everything he has and does is superb and beautiful."

Ten years later, the successful craftsman began to take an active

interest in politics, and in 1883, embodying the long-held ideals of
Morris & Co., joined Britain's fledgling Socialist party. A tireless
orator and coauthor of the Social Democratic Federation manifesto,
he soon emerged as a leader in the movement, and before long he was
speaking out against the environmental destruction wrought by the
forces of capitalism.

> Is money to be gathered? cut [*sic*] down the pleasant trees among
> the houses, pull down the ancient and venerable buildings for the
> money that a few square yards of London dirt will fetch: blacken
> rivers, hide the sun and poison the air with smoke and worse, and
> it is nobody's business to see it or mend it: that is all that modern
> commerce, the counting-house forgetful of the workshop, will do
> for us herein.

But William Morris had a dirty little secret. His design business—
which prided itself on its anti-industrial form of craftsmanship—was
bankrolled by one of the largest mining operations in the world.

———

Alice was forty-three years old and two months from dying of breast
cancer when her neurasthenic contemporary, Charlotte Perkins
Gilman, published her gothic masterpiece, "The Yellow Wall-Paper."
Gilman's friend, William Dean Howells, the former editor of *The
Atlantic*, had tried to help her get it published there, but his successor
declined it and it went to *The New England Magazine* instead. The
story, which fell into obscurity until it was revived in the 1970s, is now
a feminist classic, studied by college English majors like the younger
me. In it, a nameless woman and her husband, a physician, leave the
city and move into a country mansion for the summer. The woman
writes in her forbidden journal that she's ill but her husband doesn't
believe her. He tells friends and family there is nothing the matter

save a "temporary nervous depression—a slight hysterical tendency," and confines her to her room—a former nursery—for the summer.

But the wallpaper—"one of those sprawling, flamboyant patterns committing every artistic sin"—drives her to distraction. Before long, she sees a figure in the paper, a woman who appears unable to get out. Haunted by that figure, she writes: "There are things in that wallpaper that nobody knows but me." I wondered if Gilman might have embedded allusions to arsenical wallpapers in her cautionary tale.

The next time Jennifer and I got together, we sat down to dinner at a quiet Japanese restaurant. As we sipped our miso soup, I told her all about my arsenic obsession, which she had launched when she handed me that little clipping from *The Boston Globe*. As we talked, she remembered a scholarly paper by Heather Kirk Thomas that suggested that "The Yellow Wall-Paper" was more than the story of a woman's decline into a madness induced by postpartum depression and the constraints of patriarchy. Thomas argued convincingly that the wallpaper described by Gilman's heroine was a William Morris design. She makes brief mention of arsenical wallpapers, but quickly dismisses the possibility that Gilman's story was alluding to them, quipping that it was more likely that the yellow wallpaper's "distasteful design and color affronted [the protagonist's] postpartum despondency." But in the words of Gilman's nursery-bound heroine, "It strikes me occasionally, just as a scientific hypothesis, that perhaps it is the paper!" Arsenic, it turns out, tainted a variety of colors, including yellow.

———

I kept digging. I discovered a long-out-of-print 1862 story published anonymously in the popular English weekly *Chambers's Journal of Popular Literature, Science, and Arts* that illustrated my burgeoning thoughts about arsenical wallpapers. Set against a backdrop of dingy industrialism, in "Our Best Bedroom"—possibly the only story in history of attempted murder by wallpaper—the wealthy young nephew of a man who will benefit by his demise falls mysteriously ill after being assigned a bedroom papered in emerald-green velvet flock. Fatigued and pale, he takes to his bed, delirious with fever. Soon his hired caregiver, sitting bedside, also develops headaches and fatigue. She and her husband send for an eminent London physician, who, observing the decor, suspects that the *wallpaper* is in fact to blame. He tests the paper, and his suspicions are confirmed. It bears what he describes as "poison enough to be the death of generation after generation."

"Our Best Bedroom" reflected the heated debate playing out in British medical journals of the time (those interested can read the story in full on my website, https://jenniferlunden.com). The controversy was first sparked by an 1857 letter by Dr. William Hinds, which was published in *The Medical Times and Gazette*. After redecorating his study, Hinds found himself plagued by a host of mysterious symptoms—including severe depression, nausea, abdominal pain, and faintness—beginning the very first time he occupied the room. Finally, Hinds speculated that his new wallpaper was making him sick. He subjected it to laboratory analysis and found the paper tainted with arsenic. He removed the paper, and sure enough, his symptoms disappeared.

————

The mine that subsidized Morris's Arts and Crafts enterprise belonged to his father, a successful discount broker who speculated in copper and hit pay dirt—literally—when a party of miners he and his fellow investors bankrolled struck what was then the greatest copper lode in the world. Devonshire Great Consolidated Copper Mining Company—Devon Great Consols for short—was registered as a joint stock company, and by the end of just one year of trading, stock values had shot up by 800 percent. Morris's father and uncle were appointed directors, and when the board was formed, they soon joined.

Just three years later, when Morris was a mere thirteen years old, his father died suddenly. Thanks to stock dividends, Morris nonetheless grew up in financial ease. He had his father's mining enterprise to thank for a life of privilege that allowed him to pursue his many creative interests.

When Morris and his siblings reached adulthood, their mother, Emma, parceled a portion of the shares out to each of them. Morris sold two of his thirteen shares back to her in 1861–62, and used the dividends to launch Morris, Marshall, Faulkner & Co.

His first wallpapers came out in 1864—the same ones that researcher Andrew Meharg found tainted with arsenic. One of the designs, Trellis, would one day be used to paper the nursery in the adult Morris's own home.

———

Arsenic, originally a waste product of the copper mining industry, was once so worthless that it was left in piles that pocked the countryside. But when copper values plummeted, the Devon Great Consols board of directors sought a new source of profits, and in 1867 began to capitalize on what had previously been seen as nothing more than a nuisance. Suddenly, many new uses for arsenic were discovered in the domestic and agricultural realms. Devon Great Consols had plenty to go around; its arsenic works quickly grew to be the largest in the world.

A few years later, in 1871, William Morris was named a director of Devon Great Consols. The man who would in twelve years declare himself a Marxist celebrated his appointment, says Meharg, by investing in a top hat to wear to meetings.

Morris and his board, dressed in their fine apparel, sat in their well-appointed offices and made decisions about how their operation would run. Decisions that affected the laborers at the mines. Some of the board's less savory choices had hit the newspapers a few years earlier, when Morris's uncle Thomas was the resident director. A study performed by the Royal Commission learned that at Devon Great Consols, girls as young as eight worked ten-hour shifts hand-sorting the arsenic minerals from the copper ore. Boys who started down in the mines at age ten were destroyed by thirty or forty, their lungs wracked with silicosis, their bodies wrecked by dust and toil. Miners worked without benefit of any protections from the toxins they touched and breathed. They lived in poverty. A monthly fee was deducted from their pay to cover healthcare, but if a miner became too sick to work, his medical coverage was lost. At Devon Great Consols, the board's first concern was profit.

In 1871, industry was largely unregulated. Noxious fumes snuffed out the greenery and caused livestock to lose their hooves and crawl their pastures on their knees. When it came to health, safety, and fair wages, workers at Devon Great Consols were on their own.

Morris resigned his directorship in 1875, marking the occasion by sitting on his top hat. Perhaps there had been family pressure to accept that role in the first place, and, says Patrick O'Sullivan, editor of *The Journal of William Morris Studies*, perhaps his experience there influenced both his socialism and his environmentalism.

———

At Morris & Co., the partners dedicated their careers to an egalitarian, anti-industrial approach. In 1883, Emma Lazarus, the American poet who wrote the famous lines that now grace the pedestal of the Statue of Liberty—"Give me your tired, your poor, / Your huddled masses yearning to breathe free"—sailed to England and made an appointment to meet Morris at his Surrey workshop. She was impressed with what she found there, an atmosphere quite different from the strain and clatter of other factories.

> The exquisite fabrics to be found in his workshop, which have so largely influenced English taste in household decoration, are

intended to perform another service less conspicuous but still more important than the first. That the workman shall take pleasure in his work, that decent conditions of light and breathing-space and cleanliness shall surround him, that he shall be made to feel himself not the brainless "hand," but the intelligent cooperator, the *friend* of the man who directs his labor, that his honest toil shall inevitably win fair and comfortable wages, whatever be the low-water record of the market-price of men, that illness or trouble befalling him during the term of his employment shall not mean dismissal and starvation,—these are some of the problems of which Mr. Morris's factory is a noble and successful solution.

She added: "In accordance with these ideas, one is not surprised to find his factory a scene of cheerful, uncramped industry, where toil looks like pleasure, where flowers are blooming in the windows, and sunshine and fresh air brighten the faces of artist and mechanic."

She learned, too, that Morris scrupulously paid above standard wages and engaged in profit sharing with some of his higher-ranking employees.

During Lazarus's visit, Morris showed her the workshop gardens from which he harvested plants for dyes. "One of the clear, brilliant yellows frequently employed in his fabrics is procured from the bushes of his garden," Lazarus enthused.

That very year at the Boston Trade Fair, Morris & Co. distributed a pamphlet assuring buyers "that the colours used in the printing are entirely free from arsenic." But many manufacturers were still using arsenical dyes in their wallpapers, and they were fighting any attempts at legislation, arguing that the arsenic in their products was completely safe.

By the late nineteenth century, the interests of business had become a powerful social and political force.

———

Never before had the United States seen such growth. Between 1850 and 1900 the population tripled. Productivity skyrocketed. The nation's wealth rose by a factor of thirteen. Innovations in the mass production of steel and the invention of steel cables made elevators possible, as well as skyscrapers and the Brooklyn Bridge. Steel was used to lay down the tracks that joined East to West in the first transcontinental railroad, opening the country up for commercial farming and setting the stage for a mining boom. The invention of the telegraph meant that people could communicate in minutes what in the past might have taken days to deliver by Pony Express. Thomas Edison invented the filament lightbulb and then, two years later, threw the switch on the first ever power plant, lighting up the square mile of real estate that serviced the country's largest newspapers, the New York Stock Exchange, and the offices of his benefactor, J. P. Morgan. The steam turbine was invented. The telephone. The typewriter. In New York Harbor, the Statue of Liberty was erected, her lustrous copper slowly oxidizing to a patina of green.

In this atmosphere of unregulated industry and laissez-faire economics, the first of the great commercial banks were born. Wall Street rose to be America's financial hub. Industrialists were called "captains of industry" by some and, for the unscrupulous ways they obtained their vast wealth, "robber barons" by others. Cigars rolled in hundred-dollar bills were passed out at parties while the nation's poor lived in filthy tenements and died of typhoid, dysentery, and cholera. Social Darwinism gained steam among the wealthy elite, who justified their success—and their spurning of the poor—as "survival of the fittest."

Mark Twain called the decades between the end of the Civil War and the turn of the century the Gilded Age because all the opulence of the period was but a thin layer of gold covering a world of grime and strife. The cityscapes were gray with soot from the smoke pouring out of the chimneys of coal-burning factories and from the smokestacks of trains and steamships bearing goods for the multiplying masses surging to the cities. The smoke was so thick in some cities that streetlights blazed even in the day to light the way through the pall. The rich were very rich; the poor were very poor. And everything seemed to move very, very fast.

———

Tapping into the zeitgeist of the day, in the late nineteenth century a mechanical engineer named Frederick Winslow Taylor innovated a system he called scientific management, which revolutionized the Industrial Revolution. He broke each job down into its component parts and then used stopwatch time studies to measure each motion to a hundredth of a minute. He analyzed his data using flowcharts and set quotas to keep workers producing at top capacity.

Workers who had once been proud craftsmen were reduced to the role of "mere feeders of machines," in the words of one Gilded Age writer. It was as though the people themselves had become interchangeable parts in the monolithic machine of progress—seen first and foremost for their productive value, easily replaced when they failed to keep up. Doctors and researchers intensified their view of the body as machine, set in motion all those centuries ago by René Descartes. Neurologist George M. Beard, for example, in his pioneering treatise, *American Nervousness*, explained neurasthenia by comparing the weakened body to a machine with a poor electrical conductor.

Beard blamed the stresses of modern civilization for triggering the epidemic of neurasthenia. People were feeling a new kind of pressure: the pressure to keep up. He called the illness that was laying waste to a wide swath of Americans "the cry of the system struggling with its environment."

———

In this time of gray cityscapes, perhaps it's not surprising that two brilliant green dyes came into vogue on both sides of the ocean.

Reminiscent of the colors of new-leafed forests and the grassy, dew-bright hills now getting trampled by the footsteps of progress, emerald green and Scheele's green painted the increasingly industrialized nations a bright, stirring hue—and left behind a vast secret swath of destruction.

I bought Meharg's book, *Venomous Earth: How Arsenic Caused the World's Worst Mass Poisoning*, and learned that by 1863, between 500 and 700 tons of Scheele's green and emerald green were being produced in England every year. The dyes were beautiful and cheap: an irresistible mix. These arsenical greens were used to dye clothing and curtains, candles and tablecloths and lampshades, toys and stuffed animals, playing cards, soap, and even candies and puddings. They were painted on the walls of bakeries and candy shops and grocery stores. They colored grocery bags and the linings of cupboards and drawers and boxes of dried fruit. They tinted the paper used to wrap chocolate bonbons and other candies.

When gas lighting replaced candles, homeowners could cover their white walls with colorful wallpapers without fear of darkening their rooms. With the invention of machine printing, papers became affordable to more people, and soon arsenical wallpapers were decorating houses throughout England and then the United States.

In both countries, industrialists conceptualized products, factories turned them out, and then those products were purchased by merchants and sold to people who most likely never stopped to wonder if their soap or their candles or their new wall coverings were safe.

As I read about the profusion of arsenic in nineteenth-century commodities, I thought about all of the chemicals in all of the products that I had once assumed were safe but which now gave me headaches. I'd thrown out my mass-marketed shampoo and laundry detergent and dish soap. I'd given away my perfume. I did my best to avoid toxicants, but it wasn't always possible.

———

As far back as 1857—the year that Dr. Hinds published his provocative story in the *Medical Times and Gazette*—British forensic toxicologist Alfred Swaine Taylor registered his own concerns about arsenical wallpapers in testimony to the Select Committee on the Sale of Poisons. He said he considered them to be "very injurious," but believed that resistance from industry would foil any efforts to prohibit their manufacture or sale. Then, as now, manufacturers had a vested interest in denying people's lived experience of harm. So instead, Taylor recommended a massive public information campaign to warn people away from the toxic papers.

That same year, when administrators at one British government agency learned that the wallpapers in some of the rooms in its newly occupied buildings were tainted with arsenic, they summoned government chemist George Phillips to investigate. In his report, Phillips concluded that since arsenious acid could not be "volatized" (vaporized at room temperature), the only risk was from the dust, and good housekeeping would take care of that. Taylor minced no words in his rebuttal, writing: "If the manufacture of arsenical papers is to be continued, the Prussian poison-symbol of a skull and cross-bones, with the motto *memento mori* ["Remember that you must die"], should be printed as a pattern upon it." A few years later, the scientific rigor of Phillips's tests was called into question.

Meanwhile, anecdotal evidence kept pouring in. Newspapers like *The Times* reported a number of stories of children dying from arsenical wallpapers, and *The Lancet* and the *British Medical Journal* became vocal advocates for reform. *Lancet* founder Thomas Wakley may himself have been poisoned by arsenical wallpapers after the journal's offices were redecorated, and one of his journalists lost two children to tainted wallpapers.

In 1879, a British writer named Henry Carr published a pamphlet entitled *Our Domestic Poisons; or the Poisonous Effects of Certain Dyes and Colours Used in Domestic Fabrics*. In it, he called for legislation to end the "free trade in poisonous dyes." A year later, after he had delivered a paper on the subject to members of the Royal Society of Arts—a group devoted not only to the encouragement of the arts but also to the support of manufacturing and commerce—the society joined forces with the Medical Society of London to propose government regulation.

The project stalled. Carr put things succinctly in the next edition of *Our Domestic Poisons*: "That Society was, in fact, too much associated with trade and manufacture to be altogether a suitable medium for action '*in restraint of trade*'."

In 1885, two years after declaring his own wallpapers arsenic free, William Morris himself joined the chorus of naysayers in a private letter to his dyer, Thomas Wardle. "As to the arsenic scare a greater folly it is hardly possible to imagine: the doctors were bitten as people were bitten by the witch fever. . . . My belief about it all is that the doctors find their patients ailing[,] don't know what's the matter with them, and in despair put it down to the wall papers."

France had banned arsenic as "a pigment in certain manufacture" as far back as 1740. Russia passed legislation in 1876; Germany in 1882; and Sweden in 1883. But in Britain, manufacturers insisted the arsenical dyes used to decorate their papers were inert, and in the end, with no well-organized interest groups, demands for reform were not adequately coordinated or insistent, and legislation wasn't passed.

———

Industrial capitalism was slower to reach American shores, and as a consequence, it took longer for wallpapers to become affordable and popular on our side of the Atlantic. By the time of Alice's illness, however, the controversy over arsenical papers had reached America. The lengthy 1872 Massachusetts Board of Health report *On the Evil Effects of the Use of Arsenic in Certain Green Colors* devotes the bulk of its pages to concerns about arsenical wallpapers, noting that "the columns of the medical and of the general press of the last ten years contain the histories of numerous instances" of illness attributable to the toxic wall coverings.

In 1887, the American Medical Association estimated that 54 to 65 percent of all wallpapers sold in the United States between 1879 and 1883 contained arsenic, and that of those a third harbored dangerous amounts. Another study found arsenic present in the urine of 43 percent of a random sample of forty-eight people. In Massachusetts, doctors, chemists, and other concerned citizens spearheaded a movement to legislate arsenical wallpapers. Four attempts at legislation were made, starting in the year of the Massachusetts report on the evil effects of arsenic. In the report, the Board of Health wrote, "The cases are too numerous and too unequivocal to be thrown aside, and constitute a mass of evidence which cannot well be refuted."

But in the laissez-faire culture of nineteenth-century industrial capitalism, the interests of business ran rampant over the concerns of the people, and legislators were loath to impose regulations. "The rights of individuals and of industrial pursuits are deemed too sacred to allow of excessive restriction," the board opined, and like Britain's Alfred Swaine Taylor, it proposed, instead, enlightening the public, suggesting that "reasonable people, informed concerning the risks, will not be likely to test their own tolerance of arsenic or to subject their children to it."

But even those who duly avoided emerald-green colors were not safe, because arsenic contaminated a wide range of colors. In a campaign to educate the public about the danger lurking on the walls of their homes, Dr. Robert Clark Kedzie, then president of the Michigan Medical Society, cut pieces from seventy-five wallpaper specimens known to be arsenical and collected them in an 1874 book called *Shadows from the Walls of Death*. He included stories of "authenticated cases of poisoning from many of these papers," according to an 1889 article in *Science*, and sent copies of the book to a hundred Michigan libraries. One patron was said to have been poisoned by paging through it.

Two decades after the 1872 report on the ubiquity of arsenical products, with still no legislation passed, Dr. Frederick C. Shattuck, in an article in the *Boston Medical and Surgical Journal*, argued again for regulation:

> Some manufacturers and dealers argue that the diminution in the amount of arsenic contained in papers and fabrics during recent years shows in itself that no law is necessary. But this diminution cannot be attributed to anything except the agitation of the subject, a continuance of which demands considerable public spirit on the part of the agitators whose ranks are not generally largely recruited from the monied class.

In the end, the United States did little better than England. Using tactics familiar to any twenty-first-century advocacy groups fighting to protect us from dangerous chemicals, industrialists were able to convince legislators that arsenic was essential to the production of certain colors (although that was not true), and that trade would be hindered if they were prohibited from using it. When nobody could provide solid evidence as to *how* arsenical wallpapers were poisoning people, it prompted some to question whether arsenical wallpapers actually *were* poisoning people. This made it difficult to persuade lawmakers of the importance of legislation. Massachusetts was the first state in the country to regulate arsenic in manufactured goods, but despite several efforts over a span of decades, that law—which merely lowered the permissible concentrations—didn't pass till 1900.

————

As far back as 1839, a German chemist named Leopold Gmelin noticed that arsenical wallpapers induced illness more often in damp rooms. He described a mouselike odor and proposed the idea that the arsenic in wallpapers was converting into a volatile gas. Other researchers had similar suspicions, but the theory was not generally accepted and fell into obscurity. Even three decades later, the State Board of Health of Massachusetts, in its exhaustive 1872 report, stated: "These hypotheses are not accepted by the majority of chemists at the present day. It is the general belief that the poison escapes from the paper into the atmosphere in the form of dust, mechanically disengaged."

But in 1891, Italian chemist Bartolomeo Gosio made a momentous discovery. His experiments revealed that certain molds converted the arsenic in wallpapers into a gas. He reported that the gas, which came to be known as "Gosio gas," could be distinguished by its garlicky odor, and he suggested that it could be the cause of the mysterious illnesses and deaths that people had been reporting. English chemist Frederick Challenger identified the gas as trimethylarsine in 1932. Damp rooms were the most likely to carry dangerous levels of the gas.

Interestingly, Gilman's nameless protagonist describes a pattern in the yellow wallpaper as "a florid arabesque, reminding one of a fungus." Then she writes,

> But there is something else about that paper—the smell! I noticed it the moment we came into the room, but with so much air and sun it was not bad. Now we have had a week of fog and rain, and whether the windows are open or not, the smell is here. . . . It creeps all over the house. . . . Such a peculiar odor, too! . . . The only thing I can think of that it is like is the color of the paper! A yellow smell.

But what were the symptoms of trimethylarsine poisoning, and did they match the symptoms of neurasthenia?

I reviewed five nineteenth-century American research articles on arsenical wallpapers to glean a representative list. Symptoms presenting with highest frequency included fatigue/weakness, digestive problems, poor appetite/weight loss, nausea/vomiting, headache, poor sleep, and dry mouth and throat. Other symptoms listed more than once included vertigo, pain, faintness, diarrhea, depression, and paleness.

I found a systematic list of neurasthenia symptoms in F. G. Gosling's 1987 text, *Before Freud*, which analyzes results from the author's review of 332 articles by 262 doctors, offering a broad picture of neurasthenia. He reports that "symptoms fell into two not-altogether-separable classifications, 'physical' and 'mental.' Excessive fatigue from slight exertion was the primary sign of neurasthenia and characterized the illness. . . . Other physical symptoms cited were gastric disturbances and headache. . . . The most prominent mental symptoms were insomnia, lack of concentration, depression, fears, and irritability."

The symptoms are strikingly similar.

———

In 1871, Alfred Swaine Taylor wrote that arsenical wallpapers may account for "many of the mysterious diseases of the present day which so continually baffle all medical skill." A year later, the State Board of Health of Massachusetts declared that it seemed likely that "a very great number of instances" of illness and death from arsenical wall-papers had escaped detection due to the "anomalous character" of the symptoms. The lack of "well-defined signs . . . readily traced to their cause," gave rise to "doubt concerning the course to be followed." The report stated that symptoms of chronic arsenical poisoning "follow little regularity of manifestation," and added:

> It is a fact well recognized by physicians that different organisms vary exceedingly in their susceptibility to the action of drugs, and this idiosyncrasy will explain much of the diversity of effects observed in connection with the mode of chronic arsenical poisoning we are studying. An agent which is comparatively inert as regards one organism is to another an active poison.

Dr. Frederick C. Shattuck, in his 1893 paper for the *Boston Medical and Surgical Journal*, suggested: "Some of the cases which have been reported and observed suggest that arsenic may be but one of two or more causes tending to produce ill-health, and that a person already debilitated from some other cause may then be more susceptible to the supposed injurious influence of this poison."

These descriptions sounded familiar to me. Both ME/CFS and MCS are complex, multisystem illnesses that "continually baffle all medical skill," and having ME/CFS could make an individual more susceptible to developing a sensitivity to chemicals, as I did. In addition, chemicals that might be "comparatively inert" to one person might be "to another an active poison."

And if diseases like ME/CFS and MCS presented "well-defined signs . . . readily traced to their cause," they would be easier for people to identify, understand, and accept. But that is not the nature of these illnesses.

———

Two twenty-first-century scientists, William R. Cullen, a chemist, and Ronald Bentley, a biologist, studied what research they could find (which amounted to two papers, one published in 1899, the other in 1914) and came to the conclusion that trimethylarsine has very low toxicity, that the amount of trimethylarsine produced under even optimal conditions is minimal, and that the mold that converts arsenic into trimethylarsine does not grow well in high concentrations of arsenic. They suggest the possibility that it wasn't the arsenic that was making people sick—it was the mold. Mold is a common culprit in contemporary "sick building syndrome," and some people with ME/CFS and MCS find that mold remediation helps reduce their symptoms, sometimes significantly. Cullen and Bentley cite a book put out by the Institute of Medicine of the National Academies, which states, "Exposure to various mold products . . . has been implicated in a variety of biologic health effects."

But Andrew Meharg argues that Cullen and Bentley's paper misses "the key point" that trimethylarsine "could have been a sensitive indicator to the general presence of arsenic in Victorian homes." People were exposed to arsenic from so many sources, it's possible that the trimethylarsine may have tipped some over the threshold from health into illness. Meharg also points out that in addition to trimethylarsine there are several other arsenical gases produced by fungi. Under most conditions, trimethylarsine predominates, but another gas, called simply arsine, "is usually the second most abundant, and arsine is highly toxic." At high enough levels, arsine also has a telltale garlicky odor. Like the chemicals in many of our contemporary pesticides, arsine was studied for use in chemical warfare during World War II.

———

Perhaps there were several toxicants contributing to the ill health of Victorians. Toxicologist Albert Donnay makes an interesting contention that the symptoms of neurasthenia listed in the International Classification of Diseases (ICD) are "remarkably consistent" with carbon monoxide (CO) poisoning. He notes that "illuminating gas," the fuel used for gas lights, contained 4 to 6 percent carbon monoxide, and sometimes much more, depending on the type of gas. Gases contained other toxicants as well. These included xylene, benzene, toluene, and other volatile organic compounds. Leaks in gas lines and fixtures averaged 20 percent nationwide in 1862, according to one nineteenth-century trade publication.

Donnay suggests that although the risks of acute carbon monoxide poisoning were amply recognized and reported in the nineteenth century, the detrimental effects of low-level exposures were not widely understood. In "A True Tale of a Truly Haunted House," he shares excerpts from a gripping story penned by the protagonist herself and originally published in the *American Journal of Ophthalmology* by her eye doctor, William Wilmer, after whom the Johns Hopkins Wilmer

Eye Institute is named. The woman, a Mrs. H, wrote that shortly after moving into their new home—an 1870 fixer-upper—in November 1912, her entire family, as well as its servants, grew fatigued and depressed. Mrs. H developed severe headaches.

The family felt better during a weeklong holiday away from the house, but soon after their return, "the gloom of the house began to cast a shadow over us once more." Mrs. H's headaches came back. The children grew pale and sickly. However, when she sent them outside, their symptoms improved.

And then something truly unsettling happened. Despite carpets so plush that "not a foot-fall could be heard," she began to hear footsteps, even when there was no one to be found. She and the members of her household heard other frighteningly inexplicable sounds, such as the clang of pots and pans crashing together in the middle of the night—and on a number of occasions Mrs. H glimpsed a dark-haired woman dressed in black moving toward her.

When even the servants started to complain of ghosts, Mrs. H and her husband decided to trace the history of the house. "The last occupants we found had exactly the same experiences as ourselves. . . . Going back still further, we learned that almost everyone had felt ill, and had been under the doctor's care, although nothing very definite had been found the matter with them."

When, two months after they had moved in, they described their predicament to Mrs. H's brother-in-law, he remembered reading an article several years earlier about a family that had "the most curious delusions and experiences," and were found to have been poisoned by gas. That very day, Mrs. H and her husband called in an expert. "He found the furnace in a very bad condition, the combustion being imperfect, the fumes, instead of going up the chimney, were pouring gases of carbon monoxide into our rooms." Later that day, their doctor also arrived, and upon examining the children agreed that they were being poisoned and declared that none of the occupants should stay in the house another night.

When the problem was repaired, the family returned. Most of their symptoms cleared up, and the "ghosts" never came back.

Unfortunately, some victims of chronic carbon monoxide poisoning continue to suffer symptoms years after their initial exposure. In 1921, the same year that the *American Journal of Ophthalmology* published the "ghost story," Mayo Clinic researcher Dr. Georgine Luden published a detailed description of the carbon monoxide poisoning she and several others suffered due to a faulty furnace. She divided the symptom clusters into three periods, the third being hypersensitization to even minute amounts of carbon monoxide—a whiff of exhaust from a passing car, for instance, or smoke from a chimney. This symptom is reminiscent of what Dr. William Osler said of neurasthenia in the first edition (1892) of his influential textbook *The Principles and Practice of Medicine*: "The entire organism reacts with unnecessary readiness to slight stimuli," he wrote. Osler's description could easily be mistaken for a definition of multiple chemical sensitivity.

Another 1921 study of carbon monoxide poisoning—this one conducted for the U.S. Department of Labor by Dr. Alice Hamilton, the physician known as the mother of modern occupational medicine—echoes the Massachusetts Board of Health's description of the elusory nature of chronic arsenical poisoning,

> There is a marked variation in the way different individuals are affected by long exposure to small quantities of carbon monoxide. One person will suffer from ill-health, constant headache, neuralgic pains, perhaps albumen in the urine, after a few months' work in a room where others have passed several years with no trouble at all.
>
> There is great difficulty in diagnosing this form of occupational poisoning, because so rarely are the symptoms at all characteristic.

In other words, unidentified chronic low-level exposure to carbon monoxide, like poisoning by arsenical wallpapers, was found to cause a wide swath of potentially confounding symptoms.

It appears that neurasthenia may have had many chemical triggers, just like the illness now bearing the name multiple chemical sensitivity.

———

Once, I thought of the Victorian age as a cleaner, purer, simpler time. But the world was speeding up, and the by-products of industrialization were infiltrating the domestic sphere. Is it any wonder so many people were falling ill? The more I read, the less clean, pure, and simple things seemed. Carbon monoxide and other volatile organic compounds leaked from gas lights, and arsenic was everywhere. But those weren't the only toxicants people were exposed to in the nineteenth century. Home interiors were painted with lead-based paint. Many medicines were made with mercury, arsenic, and other treacherous ingredients. Even cosmetics often contained dangerous toxicants, including arsenic, mercury, and lead.

Today we have carpet laced with benzene and particleboard furniture off-gassing formaldehyde. We have "fresh scent" tampons, "beachside breeze" scented garbage bags, and even lemon-scented duct tape, and consumers don't know what these products contain or whether they're harmful to our health. *Memento mori.*

CHAPTER 7

Our Domestic Poisons, Redux

There was a time before illness. When I was a kid, I used to lock myself in the bathroom so I could experiment with the substances on the counter and in the cupboards under the sink. I pulled a Dixie cup out of the dispenser and squirted some toothpaste into it, then poured in some calamine lotion, and then added a couple of dashes of my dad's Old Spice and a couple of spritzes of my mother's Charlie perfume. I mixed it all together with a Q-tip and peered into the cup, wondering what kind of magic my concoction would effect. Nothing ever happened, but I liked being an alchemist, and when friends came over, I invited them to join in my experiments.

Like most kids, I watched an average of 19,000 television ads a year. We were deluged with commercials, and also with the chemicals in the products advertised.

Strong enough for a man, made for a woman. Get a little closer, don't be shy, with Arrid Extra Dry! Aren't you glad you use Dial? Fresh as an Irish Spring morning! I'm gonna wash that gray right out of my hair. And they told two friends, and they told

*two friends, and so on, and so on, and so on.... Don't hate
me because I'm beautiful. Only her hairdresser knows for sure.
Calgon, take me away.... We wear short shorts! I can bring home
the bacon, fry it up in a pan, but never let you forget you're a
man, 'cause I'm a woman. Softens hands while you do dishes.
Tide's in ... dirt's out. Easy-Off makes oven cleaning easier! This is
a good place for a Stick Up. Mr. Clean! Mr. Clean! Raid kills bugs
dead. Anything less would be uncivilized. Never let them see you
sweat. Because you're worth it.*

At eight, I ran barefoot through our weedless lawn while my father paced the property with his weed and feed broadcast spreader.

At eleven, I began spraying my underarms with powder-scented Secret.

At thirteen, I started spraying Cassie with pesticide.

At sixteen, boy-crazy, I was intoxicated by the scent of Polo cologne. Then, at nineteen, I was convinced by the ads in the women's magazines that I needed to choose my "signature scent," which one day I found when I whiffed a sample of Fendi in an issue of *Vogue*. Spicy and sophisticated, Fendi was for me.

I liked the smell of exhaust.

I cleaned with Windex, lemon-scented Pledge, and Mr. Clean.

Only much later did I come to think of the chemicals in products like these as stealth toxicants.

———

The active ingredient in the premise spray that made my cat Cassie so sick was permethrin, which is a member of the pyrethroid class of pesticides. Permethrin was not put on the market till 1979, and was at first licensed by the Environmental Protection Agency to be sold solely to cotton farmers. But in 1982, the EPA gave the go-ahead to expand its reach to livestock and produce.

Permethrin is considered one of the safer pesticides, and the U.S. Agency for Toxic Substances and Disease Registry (ATSDR) describes it as having a "relatively low mammalian toxicity." In other words, not so very toxic to humans. (Or cats.) But with a bit of digging, I discovered that the Reagan era decision to expand the registration to food sources was marked by controversy. Senior EPA science advisor M. Adrian Gross roundly condemned the decision, which he said would significantly increase cancer incidence in the U.S. "I should think that risks of cancer of this order for a relatively new insecticide are unacceptable to any rational person," he wrote. But they were acceptable to the EPA.

How could this happen? In 1982, the EPA quietly lowered its standards, that's how. Before 1982, an "acceptable" risk of cancer was considered to be one in a million. But the EPA's new standard allowed for one cancer per ten thousand people. And just like that, the road was cleared to approve permethrin for residential use.

Seven years later, in 1989, indelibly imprinted in my mind as the year my body crumbled, the research compelled the EPA to classify permethrin a "possible human carcinogen." In 2006, the agency upgraded it to a "likely" human carcinogen. It's also toxic to bees and fish. But the pesticide is still on the market, still used in home gardens and sprayed on commercial wheat, corn, and other crops, still recommended for killing fleas and repelling ticks and other biting insects.

If permethrin is considered one of the less toxic pesticides, imagine what damage the others might wreak.

————

When it comes to researching chemicals for safety, what's important, of course, is not simply that studies are done, but that the *right* studies are done. Most of those conducted for regulatory purposes examine carcinogenicity but fail to explore effects on the brain or immune system.

In the case of permethrin, however, these studies do exist. Mammalian research shows permethrin to cause "significant neurobehavioral deficits and neuronal degeneration in [the] brain," even when there were no overt signs of neurotoxicity, and "significant effect on learned behavior," as well as hyperactivity and "increased sensitivity to external stimuli."

Other studies indicate a possible impact on immune function. There are also signs that permethrin might increase the risk of breast cancer. One of these studies found that lower doses of permethrin were actually *more* likely than high doses to cause changes leading to risk of breast cancer. Another concluded that permethrin "can modulate the dopaminergic system at low doses, in a persistent manner, which may render neurons more vulnerable to toxicant injury."

Very few studies examine the synergistic effects of multiple chemicals. And of course no study is able to quantify the synergistic effects of *all* the chemicals to which we are exposed on a daily basis. Thousands of synthetic chemicals infiltrate our domestic and natural environments, mingling in our air, our water, our soil, our food, our bodies—an inconceivable chemical soup beyond anything I mixed in my bathroom experiments. And we know literally nothing about the interactive effects of these stealth toxicants.

———

The other active ingredient in the premise spray I used when I was trying to rid my apartment of fleas was piperonyl butoxide, which is not a pesticide but a potent inhibitor of an enzyme that helps mammals to detoxify pesticides. This means that higher concentrations of the permethrin remained in my ginger cat—and perhaps me—far longer than they otherwise would have.

Another of our bodies' enzymes, called plasma butyrylcholinesterase (BuChE), acts like a scavenger, culling out foreign invaders such as permethrin and other unwanted chemicals. Multiple doses of toxicants, however, can overwhelm the BuChE supply. When that happens, the toxicants accumulate in the bloodstream and make their way to the brain (where they can damage the blood-brain barrier) and the nervous system.

———

To trace the modern chemical industry to its beginnings, I realized that I would need to study benzene, which was first isolated from coal tar in 1825. This led me to the remarkable story of William Henry Perkin, a promising young student and lab assistant at London's Royal College of Chemistry. In 1856, the year Alice turned eight, Perkin stumbled upon the benzene-based recipe for a sumptuous mauve dye that would hurtle purple into vogue and launch the synthetic chemical industry.

At the time, the efforts of the British empire to colonize Africa were being thwarted by malaria, and the natural substance used to treat the disease, quinine, was hard to obtain and expensive. Perkin's mentor had asked him to search for a way to synthesize quinine, but, as Perkin explained fifty years later, "I failed, and was about to throw a certain black residue away when I thought it might be interesting. The solution of it resulted in a strangely beautiful color." Who would have thought that such a stunning dye could be produced from coal tar? Perkin, who was also a painter, knew the value of a good color. Perkin mauve—the world's first synthetic dye—broke the dye industry wide open.

Before Perkin's discovery, purple was a rare and costly color made from the glandular mucus of snails. Soon, however, chemists were synthesizing a vast palette of aniline (benzene-based) dyes. Commercial production soared, decimating the market for thousands of acres of indigo, madder, and other plants.

Perkin, who had the foresight to patent his dye, built a factory in Greenford, West London, on what is now known as the Grand Union

Canal, and formulated other synthetic dyes. According to the locals, the water in the nearby canal turned a different color each week, depending on which dye was being produced. The wunderkind went on to synthesize coumarin and cinnamic acid, chemicals that birthed the synthetic perfume industry. He sold his business in 1874 at the age of thirty-six, retiring a very wealthy man.

The first-generation aniline dyes were wildly popular, but people were disappointed to discover that the dazzling new colors in their textiles faded terribly. Soon a new, more lasting synthetic dye came to the fore—this one made from a chemical called anthracene. Like aniline, anthracene was a by-product of coal tar. But unlike aniline, anthracene was not a derivative of benzene.

With aniline dyes being replaced by anthracene dyes, there was a sudden surplus of benzene. What to do with it all? Benzene, now a useless industrial by-product, was in need of a new industrial home.

Then, around the turn of the century, scientists found that the solvent could dissolve rubber, transforming it into an adhesive—rubber cement. The discovery marked the first significant technological change in glue making in more than three thousand years.

Benzene went on to become a critical ingredient in the production of TNT and other munitions when World War I broke out. In the United States, industrialists invested in coal tar distillation factories and cranked out the benzene, reaping their profits from the boon of war. But then the war ended, and again benzene was an undesirable chemical in need of a product.

The wait wasn't long. Soon the chemical would become a ubiquitous ingredient in the manufacture of a wide swath of consumer goods. Vinyl, nylon, Styrofoam, and plastic are all made with a little help from benzene. It's also used in the production of detergents and pharmaceuticals. It's in fertilizers. It's in new carpet and carpet padding. It's in cosmetics, especially nail polish, and one 2021 study discovered the chemical in seventy-eight popular sunscreens. Gasoline fumes, car exhaust, air fresheners, and cigarette smoke all emit benzene.

Its derivatives have also made their way into America's domestic environs. Phenols are found in hair products and cleaning supplies. Toluene is an ingredient in pesticides. Bisphenol A (BPA) is in plastic containers and the linings of almost all food and beverage cans. Other benzene derivatives are found in perfumes and other scented products.

———

When I first started reacting to chemicals, I didn't know anything about them. I had heard of benzene, but I was unaware that it was a known health hazard, that it and its derivatives are in so many consumer goods, and that efforts to ban it from household products—much like attempts to ban arsenical wallpapers over a hundred years earlier—had failed. I had never heard of phenols or bisphenol A or toluene. I didn't know that just a tiny fraction of the 86,000 chemicals in commerce have been tested for their effects on human health. All I knew was that I was getting headaches and that they happened when I was exposed to the products that most people considered harmless.

The more I read, however, the more I believed that my body was a messenger.

———

The first benzene was derived from coal tar, but in the United States, benzene and other synthetic chemicals were made from the by-products of oil and natural gas refining. After World War II, the synthetic chemical industry mushroomed, shooting up from fewer than a billion pounds produced per year in the U.S. to over 54 billion pounds now produced in or brought into the country *per day*. It is a $486-billion-a-year industry.

In the flush of postwar prosperity, in an economy built on shopping, leisure, and convenience, Americans embraced the motto of "better living through chemistry." There was a boom in sales of new homes, new cars, and new televisions, and the commercials on those televisions told America's budding consumers what else they needed to buy.

And buy they did. They bought refrigerators and stoves, washing machines and vacuum cleaners. They bought dishwashers and, later, microwaves and toaster ovens. They bought vinyl flooring and wall-to-wall carpeting and latex paint. They bought Super Glue and Saran wrap. Teflon cookware and Tupperware and Bakelite dishes. Ajax and Lysol and Drano and Tide. They bought aerosol air fresheners, then solid air fresheners, then plug-in air fresheners. Aqua Net hair spray, Aqua Velva aftershave, Prell shampoo, Chanel No. 5. They bought the Pill, and Valium, and, later, Prozac. They bought disposable diapers, Frisbees and hula hoops, Barbie and G.I. Joe, Etch A Sketch and Easy-Bake Ovens. Styrofoam coolers and takeout coffee in Styrofoam cups and bicycle helmets lined with Styrofoam. They bought antifreeze and paint thinner, turpentine and Turtle Wax. They bought DDT and Raid and Roundup. Revlon and Avon and Estée Lauder. Nylons and rayon blouses and polyester pants. Princess phones and then cordless phones and cell phones and smartphones. They bought furniture made out of particleboard. They bought VCRs and DVD players, PCs and Macs and ink-jet printers. Even the credit cards they increasingly used to buy these products were made out of plastic.

Stop for a moment. Look around you. Count the number of products that are made possible because of Perkin's pretty little mauve discovery.

———

In 1947, just over a hundred years after the discovery of benzene, a physician named Theron Randolph was sought out by a woman suffering from a long list of symptoms, including chronic fatigue, depression, chronic rhinitis, coughing, frequent headaches, and reactions to perfume and certain scented cosmetics. For four years, Dr. Randolph, an allergist, was unable to offer much help to Mrs. N.B., a doctor's wife and former cosmetics saleswoman. But by 1951, he had come to an understanding of the ways that chemical exposures can trigger symptoms that she and many of his patients exhibited. He sometimes referred to it as the "petrochemical problem," because the number of people suffering from the illness seemed to be rising in direct proportion to the growth of the petrochemical industry since World War II. He called this new branch of medicine "clinical ecology." It became the foundation for what is now known as environmental medicine, and one of the components of the growing field of functional medicine.

Mrs. N.B. was particularly sensitive to car exhaust. She told Dr. Randolph about an experience that echoes one of my own. While riding in a car with a defective muffler, she began to feel symptoms coming on and suspected an exhaust leak. The other passengers detected no fumes whatsoever, but Mrs. N.B. grew progressively sick, then stuporous.

Reading this account, I was reminded of my old beater and the weeks-long stretch when I developed headaches every time I drove it. I suspected an exhaust leak and took it to my trusted mechanics, but they could find nothing wrong. The headaches persisted. I was certain there must be a leak in the exhaust and brought the car back a second and even a third time. They finally dismantled the entire exhaust system and found a tiny hole in the Y-pipe, fixed it, and my headaches went away. I was vindicated. This is when I began to think of my body as an early warning system, my sensitivity to toxicants an alarm bell for others, if only they would listen.

Another patient reminded me of the Victorian woman who fell ill every time she returned to her house until her doctor advised her to remove her toxic wallpaper. K.S. suffered debilitating chronic fatigue, chronic headaches, repeated bouts of the flu, asthma, and other symptoms. One doctor who examined her wrote: "I would strongly suspect hysteria."

When she moved into an old house, things only got worse. Finally a gas leak was discovered. But by then she had become so sensitized to gas that even when she spent time away at a ranch in Arizona, whenever the weather grew cold enough that the gas wall heater had to be turned on she found herself afflicted with headaches, asthma attacks, and arthritis.

Both women reacted to the fumes from turpentine, shellac, varnish, fresh paint, and rubber cement. They reacted to detergents and air fresheners. They suffered severe respiratory symptoms when they ate food stored in plastic and also when exposed to perfume. They couldn't wear clothes made out of nylon or other synthetic textiles without triggering symptoms. They reacted to sponge rubber in furnishings and mattresses. And to artificially colored foods, to foods grown with pesticides, and to certain pharmaceuticals.

As I read this list, I was struck by how many of these products are made from petrochemical derivatives like benzene.

———

In the summer of 1909, forty years before Dr. Randolph's discovery, a fourteen-year-old girl was admitted to the hospital with bleeding from her nose, gums, and throat. Tests revealed severe anemia. Her white blood count was low as well, and she had very few blood platelets. Doctors tried desperately to save her, going so far as to attempt a blood transfusion—a risky procedure at that time—to no avail. Eight days after her admission, she passed away. The day she died, two more fourteen-year-old girls appeared at the same hospital with similar symptoms. One survived; the other died within the week.

All three girls had worked in the same canning factory, operating machines that sealed cans shut with a mixture of rubber, natural resin—and benzene. This was the first American medical report of benzene-triggered toxic aplastic anemia, which is the diagnosis given when the bone marrow fails to produce enough blood cells to sustain health. Further research confirmed the link between benzene exposure and aplastic anemia. Soon the chemical was also implicated in leukemia.

In 1948, the American Petroleum Institute conceded, "It is generally considered that the only absolutely safe concentration for benzene is zero." Thirty years later, in 1978, the Consumer Product Safety Commission (CPSC) finally proposed a ban on benzene for all household products, but it never went into effect. By 1981—the dawn of the Reagan administration—the government agency announced that it was withdrawing its proposal, instead simply mandating that all glues containing solvents bear warning labels stating *Danger, Vapor Harmful,* and *Poison,* along with the skull and crossbones. The risk of cancer and other benzene-related diseases was left off. In 1987, the International Agency for Research on Cancer (IARC) classified benzene as a known human carcinogen. The chemical was not regulated by the Occupational Safety and Health Administration (OSHA) until 1988, and not by the EPA until 1989.

———

A 2004 study found an average of 91 industrial compounds, pollutants, and other chemicals in the blood and urine of nine volunteers, with a total of 167 chemicals found altogether. Researchers refer to this contamination as a person's *body burden.* The study, released by the Environmental Working Group, concluded: "Of the 167 chemicals found, 76 cause cancer in humans or animals, 94 are toxic to the brain and nervous system, and 79 cause birth defects or abnormal development. The dangers of exposure to these chemicals in combination has [*sic*] never been studied."

Another study showed that eleven toxic compounds, including benzene, were present in significantly higher levels in indoor air than outdoor. "Remarkably," write Nicholas Ashford and Claudia Miller in *Chemical Exposures: Low Levels and High Stakes*, "these sources present in indoor air are the same ones individuals with multiple chemical sensitivities identify as provoking their vague and seemingly inexplicable symptoms."

———

Who's in charge of protecting us from all this stuff? In *Amputated Lives: Coping with Chemical Sensitivity*, Alison Johnson tells the stories of several Environmental Protection Agency employees who developed MCS after being exposed to toxicants in the agency's own building. I dug into the research, and what I learned was even more preposterous than I could have imagined.

CHAPTER 8

Spin

The Environmental Protection Agency officially launched operations December 2, 1970, during the Nixon administration, opening its doors at Washington's Waterside Mall in 1971. The first EPA administrator was a thirty-eight-year-old rising star, Assistant Attorney General William D. Ruckelshaus (R), dubbed "Mr. Clean" for his strong stance on environmental issues. The appointment was even lauded by the Democratic Party's leading environmental advocate, Senator Edmund Muskie (D-Maine).

It was a time of heady idealism, and the new agency's scientists were dedicated to environmental welfare. However, when Ronald Reagan came to power in 1981, he appointed Anne Gorsuch as the agency's head. The mother of Trump Supreme Court appointee Neil Gorsuch, she was, as her 2004 obituary in *The Washington Post* put it, "a firm believer that the federal government, and specifically the EPA, was too big, too wasteful and too restrictive of business." She slashed the EPA's budget by 22 percent, and, between the years of 1981 and 1983, stacked the agency's upper administration with people who'd devoted their professional lives to defending industry against regulation. It was under her watch that the EPA lowered its standards for an "acceptable" risk of cancer from one in a million to one in ten thousand, opening the door for permethrin's approval for home use by people like me.

———

In 1983, plainly frustrated union members belonging to the National Federation of Federal Employees (NFFE, Local 2050) argued that as government scientists they had "a duty and a right to perform our work in an ethical environment, and to see that our work is not distorted, misrepresented, stolen or lied about in devising false cover for Agency policies." They said their professional ethics were being undermined by the influence of "economically powerful industries that are doing things harmful to the environment."

The union blamed the EPA administration for allowing large companies and industry-sponsored organizations to corrupt science. According to Michelle Murphy, author of *Sick Building Syndrome and the Problem of Uncertainty: Environmental Politics, Technoscience, and Women Workers*:

> The presence of corporate interests in environmental science even extended to experimental design and practice at the EPA. As practitioners of toxicological studies, the scientists knew that tinkering with humidity levels, changing strains of mice, modifying forms, or using stationary, rather than body-mounted, air samplers could determine whether a chemical exposure was detected or remained invisible. They also knew that corporate scientists were expert at those manipulations.

———

And then came the day in April 1988 when the EPA deployed its Environmental Response Team—a corps of specialists usually assigned to chemical spills and toxic waste dumps—to test the air in its own building. Five months earlier, the government agency charged with "working for a cleaner, healthier environment for the American people" had begun renovating the poorly ventilated Waterside Mall, and as the renovations moved deeper and deeper into the mazelike passageways of the building, more and more people fell ill. Scientist Bobbie Lively-Diebold, who worked for the Superfund program, was one of them. She walked into her office one day and smelled a strong, acrid chemical odor. "Almost immediately," she later wrote, "I began coughing and felt dizzy and nauseated. My breathing became labored, and my lungs started to hurt. In addition, I was disoriented and lost my voice. I left the office and remained outside until my head was clear enough that I could drive home." Over eight hundred employees eventually suffered symptoms including burning eyes and lungs, fatigue, cognitive dysfunction, headaches, nausea, dizziness, and more.

How did the EPA administration respond to the tide of health complaints by its very own scientists, lawyers, administrative assistants, and other employees?

For a long time it denied the problem. And continued renovating.

———

The EPA received over a thousand complaints about the air quality at the Waterside Mall. Like replaceable parts in an enormous machine, when someone fell ill from the toxicants in a certain area, they were simply moved to an area that had not yet been renovated, or, in the worst cases, were allowed to work from home or in locations outside of the building. Then a new worker would be moved to the area without being notified of the symptoms suffered by the previous employee. Soon enough, the newly installed worker would get sick, and a replacement would be brought in to fill the space, and so on.

Those who got sick inside the EPA headquarters realized they would need to organize. Calling themselves the Committee of Poisoned Employees (COPE), they counted among their ranks toxicologists, analysts, lawyers, and regulators. They formed a coalition with the 1,200 members of their union (NFFE, Local 1200) and the union of the American Federation of Government Employees (AFGE, Local 331), which represented clerical workers and other nonprofessionals. The coalition organized a protest and circulated a flyer that detailed the rash of complaints. Reading that flyer was the first time many of those who had been struck ill made the connection between their symptoms and the building in which they were working. Some made dark jokes about their predicament, referring to themselves as EPA test animals.

What the EPA's Environmental Response Team found in April 1988, when it tested the air at Waterside Mall, was a wide variety of volatile organic compounds, but none of them at levels high enough for administrators to consider problematic based on the industrial standards normally applied to outdoor sites. Members of COPE and the two unions suspected corrupted results. After all, as Bobbie Lively-Diebold later pointed out in legislative testimony in support of the Indoor Air Quality Act of 1989, "Some [of the victims] have no problems visiting hazardous waste sites for a week at a time, but become ill after 15 minutes inside Waterside."

According to EPA attorney James Handley, who developed multiple chemical sensitivity as a result of the poor air quality at Waterside Mall, "During the test, the building's ventilation fans ran faster than we had ever heard them running before. For the first time, we noticed that papers were blowing off people's desks, and the air in the building had never been fresher." Another employee reported that chemical monitoring equipment was positioned directly beneath a fan, guaranteeing an inaccurate reading.

EPA investigators and employees later learned that the air exchange rates had indeed been increased and new filters had been put in the fans serving the areas tested. It's no wonder EPA management was unable to detect problems with their air samples.

Lively-Diebold was not far off the mark when she unfavorably compared the air at a Superfund site with the air at Waterside Mall. In a 1998 article in *Scientific American*, researchers Wayne Ott and John Roberts wrote that exposures to airborne toxicants at a Superfund site were negligible compared to those found in homes, cars, and offices. "The chief sources appeared to be ordinary consumer products such as air fresheners and cleaning compounds, and various building materials," they wrote.

Even as far back as June 1987, just four months before the Waterside Mall renovations began, a large-scale EPA-sponsored study about air quality came to unexpected conclusions. People had always thought of pollution as an outdoor problem; they did not think of pollution as inhabiting their own homes. But the Total Exposure Assessment Methodology (TEAM) study determined that even in the smoggiest areas of the country, *indoor* air pollution accounted for somewhere between 75 and 98 percent of total exposure to airborne toxicants, causing more cancer than smokestack emissions, water pollution, or toxic waste dumps.

The TEAM study may have been the first to put the term *sick building syndrome* in writing. As a result of these studies, in 1988, Congress added an indoor air division to the EPA.

But the EPA remained silent about the unhealthy air in its own building.

———

Because many of those affected were scientists, they were in a unique position to challenge the results they were given. They launched their own investigations, and the cumulative evidence was damning. The Local 2050's health and safety representatives found that 90 to 95 percent of the air circulating through the building's ventilation system was recycled indoor air that included air from twelve photocopy centers that operated almost continuously. In addition, the building management allowed outdoor paint to be used indoors, and rather than repair a leak, management ordered maintenance workers to divert rainwater into the ventilation system, where it festered in a dark brown pool, growing fungus that subsequently circulated throughout the building.

And then there was the carpet—27,000 square yards of it. In the words of James Handley, "Installing cheap and probably defective carpet that released solvents into a poorly ventilated building was a formula for a gas chamber." Among the chemicals employees were exposed to were dangerously high levels of several volatile organic compounds including 4-phenylcyclohexene (4-PCH), a potent neurotoxin.

The NFFE, Local 2050, and the members of COPE contacted Anderson Laboratories and asked if the lab would videotape an experiment demonstrating whether or not the Waterside Mall carpet was neurotoxic to mice.

Using a test originally developed for the Department of Defense to study the potency of nerve gases to be used by the U.S. Army during the Vietnam War, Dr. Rosalind Anderson, a toxicologist, placed a piece of the carpet in a glass chamber that collected its chemical emissions. She put mice in a separate glass chamber and flipped a switch that blew air from the carpet into their chamber. Then she had the mice run down a narrow track. The control mice—which were not exposed at all—navigated the track handily. Mice that were exposed to the carpet for an hour weaved like pub crawlers heading home at closing time, and took longer to cross the finish line than the controls. These mice did better, however, than the mice exposed to the carpet for two hours. Many of those fell off the track and didn't complete the run at all.

And the mice exposed for three hours? They were either comatose or dead.

Anderson later told Handley that the damage to the mice's brains was like a cumulative series of small strokes.

When the EPA was subsequently involved in an unrelated joint project with the Consumer Product Safety Commission (CPSC) to study carpet complaints, the union petitioned to protect consumers by testing and regulating carpet emissions. But management told the union "off the record" that because the petition could potentially cost the carpet industry billions of dollars, it would not be granted.

In the United States, a cost-benefit analysis is integral to the EPA's decision-making process. But since 2003 the European Union has based *its* decisions on the precautionary principle—the idea that when scientific investigation has found a plausible risk of harm, government and corporations have a social responsibility to protect the public unless further studies can find sound evidence of safety. Many of the chemicals found in products in the U.S. are banned in the E.U.

———

In May 1988, seven long months after people began suffering sick building symptoms, pressure from the unions finally halted the carpet installation and other renovations. EPA administrators, however, made plans to lay the unused carpet in other EPA buildings. In August of that year, while agreeing to a policy of not using carpet containing 4-phenylcyclohexine in its headquarters and accommodating chemically injured employees by providing space for them in a nearby building, the EPA officially denied that its employees were suffering from "real" injuries and claimed that the carpet posed no problems.

Here it was again: the social gaslighting of ill people by the very government agency that was supposed to protect them—and us.

Twenty people brought suit against Waterside Mall's owners and management company. Eventually, the law firm chose five of the most highly affected employees and one spouse to initiate the lawsuit.

In 1994, a jury awarded the plaintiffs damages amounting to what would now equal almost $2 million—but it was a pyrrhic victory. Experts for the defense had effectively argued that the plaintiffs were suffering from a somatization disorder. One expert for the defense, an EPA "risk management consultant" who wasn't even a health professional, testified over objections by the plaintiffs' lawyers that some employees who had reacted to what they "believed had been a toxic release . . . reflected the characteristics of mass psychogenic illness." Another even diagnosed hysteria.

The jury decided that just one of the plaintiffs suffered a physical injury. Susan Watkins was able to provide medical evidence of toxic encephalopathy (brain damage) after a battery of tests showed abnormal neurological functioning, impaired balance, decreased grip strength, memory loss, chronic inflammation of the mucous membrane, and episodic tremors in her upper extremities. The other four plaintiffs, the jury determined, were simply suffering from somatization disorders triggered by the renovations. Nonetheless, it found the building owners and the management company at fault for the somatization, and thus elected to award damages to all the plaintiffs.

As soon as the jury was dismissed, however, the defendants filed a judgment notwithstanding the verdict (JNOV), arguing that the plaintiffs had failed to prove either negligence or causation, that somatization disorder was not generally accepted in the medical community as an illness or injury, and that it was therefore not compensable. A JNOV allows a presiding judge to overrule or amend a jury's verdict. In 1995, a DC Superior Court judge did just that, overturning the damages on all but Susan Watkins. She was awarded today's equivalent of $440,000, and that sum was split between all twenty plaintiffs.

If a group of EPA employees couldn't get their disabling exposures to toxic chemicals taken seriously, what hope do the rest of us have?

As I continued my research, I uncovered the chilling story of a company protecting its bottom line even when a baby's health was at stake. Around the same time as the EPA sick building debacle, a ten-month-old baby named Christopher, lying on a newly laid carpet, suddenly tensed and trembled in what his mother later described as a "strange, seizure-like reaction." His mother, Jocelyn McIvers, a lawyer, rushed him to the hospital, but after a week of testing, doctors were only able to to offer the diagnosis of "tremors of unknown origin." Back at home, the episodes continued—forty to fifty times a day. Finally, Jocelyn's father, a building contractor, suggested that Christopher's symptoms were perhaps being triggered by the handsome new carpet that Jocelyn had so carefully chosen.

Her husband Kevin, a trial lawyer, called the manufacturer, described Christopher's symptoms, and asked a carefully worded question: "I don't want to know if the industry believes that carpet can cause problems, or if it's scientifically documented or anything like that. Just tell me, please, has anyone ever complained or claimed that they have had a neurological or neuromuscular reaction of any kind to carpet?"

The answer he got was "No. We've never heard of it." A month later, Kevin received a follow-up letter in the mail that stated unequivocally, "We have not heard of any reactions similar to what you describe."

On the advice of an indoor air consultant, the McIverses tried steam-cleaning the carpet several times and baking out the VOCs in the air while living for six weeks with Jocelyn's mother. Christopher's tremors decreased during this time, but returned when they moved back in.

A CBS *Street Stories* episode about the Anderson Laboratories carpet studies aired in October of that year, and after seeing it, the McIverses sent a swatch of their new carpet in for testing. "And sure enough," said Jocelyn, "the mice were rolling over and shaking just like our son did." They immediately removed the carpet and pad, baked the VOCs out again, and then aired their house out. When they returned, their son's tremors stopped. His immune system showed signs of damage, however, and antibodies to the myelin in his nervous system indicated nerve tissue damage. Whether the damage was permanent or not, only time would tell. "Looking back on all this," said Jocelyn, "we wished we had just ripped it out, but they [the manufacturer] assured us the carpet wasn't the cause and we just believed them—which was really stupid, but we did."

The McIverses later learned the manufacturer was being disingenuous when it told them that there had been no complaints about carpet. The company had people on the board of the Carpet and Rug Institute, which had received, at the very least, over a thousand complaints from the EPA workers who were made ill at Waterside Mall.

In "Carpet Concerns: Industry Strategizing Memorandum Comes to Light," Cindy Duehring, the now-deceased founder of the Chemical Injury Information Network (CIIN) and 1997 winner of the Right Livelihood Award, uncovered a November 1992 memorandum that reveals the culture of denial endemic in industry. The memorandum, written by Dallas A. Meneely, a Monsanto public communications representative, outlined recommendations from a public relations firm for dealing with the Anderson Laboratories findings. The thrust of the plan was twofold, he said: "to publicly refute Anderson's research and repair damage to the image of carpeting." The firm recommended efforts to "erode the credibility of the Anderson study," adding, "The key is to discredit her methodology, results and motives." Meneey added: "It may be necessary to publicly discredit and disgrace her."

Meneely also wrote: "At Monsanto we could initiate an employee awareness program and make our employees spokespeople for the safety of carpet." To that end, in December 1993, the Carpet and Rug Institute (CRI) distributed a question-and-answer sheet throughout the carpet and rug industry to guide sales representatives in responding to consumer concerns. To the question, "Haven't there been some tests with carpet that actually killed mice?" the CRI suggested this answer:

> One isolated laboratory purported last year to have killed mice with carpet emissions. Since then, the Environmental Protection Agency (EPA) and independent tests have been unable to duplicate the results. Scientists tell us that the isolated laboratory experimental tests were seriously flawed and irrelevant.

In response to this revelation, Congressman Bernie Sanders (I-VT) said, "We're disappointed but we're not surprised that when confronted with this serious health problem, they chose to undertake a comprehensive public relations campaign instead of a comprehensive effort to research the problem and make changes that would protect the consumers."

———

Although the EPA has since moved out of Waterside Mall to a cluster of buildings where the air is presumably healthier, its oversight of the chemical industry is more noxious than ever. In 2021 several whistleblowers provided *The Intercept* reporter Sharon Lerner with extensive documentation and behind-the-scenes details revealing a pernicious culture of corruption at the agency. The scientists described a coercive atmosphere where managers pressured them to change their risk assessments to make new chemicals appear less toxic than they actually were, with the consequences for refusal being downgraded performance ratings in annual reviews, reassignment to other offices, and bullying behaviors like shouting, name-calling, and denigration in front of coworkers. The whistleblowers also reported that their conclusions, when unfavorable to industry, were sometimes altered without their knowledge or permission.

In a recording of a November 2020 meeting, an EPA manager

asks information technology contractors to add a button to the new chemical review tracking system that would allow "an all-powerful person" to "override everything" in what are known at the agency as hair-on-fire situations—cases in which industry is exerting pressure, sometimes with the help of federal legislators, to expedite the approval process or minimize recommended restrictions. According to Lerner, it's unclear whether this button has materialized.

Performance ratings of managers in the New Chemicals Division are based in part on the number of chemicals they approve, and EPA employees who please the companies they're supposed to regulate often go on to take jobs at those very corporations.

One thing the chemical industry must find very pleasing is when the EPA decides to skip toxicity testing altogether. Between December 2011 and May 2018, the agency's Office of Pesticide Programs saved companies more than $300 million by waiving 972 toxicity tests that would have checked for risks of cancer, developmental neurotoxicity, and immune system damage. In September 2018, when that number hit 1,000, administrators threw a party.

There's no telling what harm those pesticides will do to humans and the environment in the generations to come. A 2019 study found that three years earlier, Americans dumped 322 million pounds of pesticides that were banned in other countries into the environment, a quantity that has almost certainly risen.

We now know that the EPA colluded with Monsanto to cover up the carcinogenic effects of glyphosate, the active ingredient in Roundup and other weed killers, and that the agency continues to downplay the cancer risks of malathion, the pesticide I once used to kill aphids in the house museum's perennial garden.

———

Here are just some of the harmful chemicals that are likely to be in the homes—and bodies—of anyone living in this country.

Phthalates [*thal*-eyts], which are hormone disrupters—chemicals that can mimic or interfere with the body's own hormones—are used in a wide range of products, including synthetic fragrances, air fresheners, personal care products, detergents, plastic wrap, vinyl flooring, automotive plastics, shower curtains, garden hoses, medical tubing, and even some children's toys. They leach out of plastic food containers (particularly when heated in the microwave) and water bottles. Because phthalates are stored in body fat, they're difficult to eliminate, and are particularly risky for women, who tend to have a higher percentage of body fat than men.

Prenatal exposure is linked to genital abnormalities in baby boys, and exposure in childhood is linked to asthma, allergies, and behavioral and cognitive issues. Phthalates have also been tied to lower sperm counts, breast cancer, and higher weight. Biomonitoring studies by the CDC have found that phthalate exposure is widespread in the U.S. population.

In 1973, before **polybrominated diphenyl ethers (PBDEs)** were widely used in domestic products, their levels in Americans' blood were undetectable. But then manufacturers started to add the purported fire retardant to furniture, curtains, carpet padding, electronics, and more, and by 2005 PBDEs had reached significant levels in human bodies. PBDEs are hormone disrupters with links to cancer, thyroid disruption, fetal defects, and reproductive problems. Evidence is mounting that PBDEs aren't even effective at slowing fires. In 2014 the California-based healthcare company Kaiser Permanente declared that all its new furniture purchases—a $30 million budget—would be free of flame retardants.

Bisphenol A (BPA) is another hormone disrupter, and in addition to plastics and cans, it's also found in checkout receipts. Even low doses of BPA are linked to breast and prostate cancer, higher weight, reproductive abnormalities, impaired brain development, and ADHD.

Formaldehyde, a known carcinogen, is found in carpets, kitchen countertops, and any furniture constructed with particleboard. As these products age, the formaldehyde evaporates into the home or workplace and accumulates in people's bodies. According to a 2009 survey by the California Energy Commission, almost all homes had formaldehyde concentrations exceeding the guidelines meant to protect people from cancer. Formaldehyde or formaldehyde-releasing ingredients are also common in cosmetics, nail polish, and other personal care products.

Over 9,000 synthetic chemicals belong to the family of **per- and polyfluoroalkyl substances, better known as PFAS**. First introduced in the form of Teflon—the nonstick coating on many frying pans and baking sheets—now these chemicals are found in water-repellent clothes, stain-resistant carpet, personal care products and cosmetics, fast-food wrappers, and more.

Upwards of 110 million people in the U.S. alone may be drinking PFAS-tainted water. The toxicants are in the blood of virtually every human in the world, even unborn babies. Known as forever chemicals, they represent another way that America's unfettered industrial capitalism colonizes our land, our water, and our bodies. Studies link the chemicals to several types of cancer, reproductive problems, low birth weight, weakened childhood immunity, and weight gain. It's in the deer and fish we eat; it's in whales, polar bears, and seabirds. In 2022, the EPA finally moved to add two PFAS chemicals (PFOA and PFOS) to its official list of hazardous substances.

———

Asthma, learning disabilities, Alzheimer's, Parkinson's, sterility, migraines, autoimmune diseases, and some cancers—all are on the rise. The chemicals that have become ubiquitous in homes, schools, and workplaces, on our land and in our food, are making more and more of us sick. How many of these illnesses are preventable?

The growing tide of people with multiple chemical sensitivity appears to be striking fear in the hearts of industry execs, who have gone on the offensive to protect their companies' bottom lines. Their goal, says Ann McCampbell, MD, in a paper published in the *Townsend Letter*, "is to create the illusion of controversy about MCS and cast doubt on its existence." To this end, in 1996, at a conference purportedly convened to study MCS and other environmental illnesses, a panel that included representatives from BASF (which bills itself as the largest chemical company in the world), Monsanto, Bayer, and Coca-Cola proposed that multiple chemical sensitivity be renamed idiopathic environmental intolerance, or IEI. *Idiopathic* simply means "of unknown etiology," but some workshop participants reported to the media and at scientific meetings that the *idiopathic* in IEI meant "self-originated." Either way, says McCampbell, "This would be analogous to the tobacco industry trying to change the name of 'smoker's cough' to 'idiopathic respiratory paroxysms.'"

Six years earlier, at the 1990 meeting of the American College of Allergy, Asthma & Immunology, Novartis—a company that sold pesticides like atrazine and diazinon (later divesting of its agrochemical arm in a deal with Syngenta) and psychotropic medications such as Anafranil, an antidepressant; Mellaril, an antipsychotic; and Ritalin for ADHD—planned a one-day workshop characterizing people with MCS as mentally ill. Clearly, Novartis had a stake in the matter of MCS and attempted to wield its influence over healthcare professionals. If MCS had been classified as a mental illness, then any potential lawsuits accusing the company of making people sick could be averted, and as an added bonus the company could entice more doctors to prescribe psychotropics to any patients who described themselves as chemically sensitive. Protesters, however, were successful in shutting the event down.

The Environmental Sensitivities Research Institute (ESRI), a corporate-funded nonprofit, paid a medical journal called *Regulatory Toxicology and Pharmacology* to publish proceedings of what McCampbell calls "an anti-MCS conference" in its supplement. One of the conference orchestrators was a consulting firm owned by Ronald E. Gots, MD, PhD, who also happened to be the founder and director of ESRI, and who once called MCS "a peculiar manifestation of our technophobic and chemophobic society." Gots's consulting firm, the National Medical Advice Service, provided expert witnesses to lawyers defending corporations in product liability lawsuits.

Later, the ESRI-funded papers were cited as references in materials submitted to the legislature by an industry lobbyist—sans any reference to ESRI, whose past board members included representatives or employees of Monsanto, Procter & Gamble, and the Cosmetic, Toiletry, and Fragrance Association (now the Personal Care Products Council). In 1996, ESRI sent literature to a state disability agency offering advice on how to avoid accommodating the needs of chemically sensitive employees, and Gots traveled to Santa Fe, New Mexico, to urge a Medicaid advisory committee to deny benefits for the diagnosis of chemical sensitivities.

———

In Alice James's time, the New York City editors of the *Medical Record* wrote a facetious editorial accusing their "interesting colleagues of Massachusetts" of promulgating arseniophobia—an irrational fear of arsenic. Many New York doctors viewed the arsenic scare as the latest "Boston fad." Eventually, however, the dangers of arsenic in domestic products were generally acknowledged, and gradually manufacturers removed the toxic element from their products.

Now big industry throws the word *chemophobia* around to discredit legitimate concerns about the dangers of synthetic chemicals. One nonprofit that describes itself as a "consumer education group," the

American Council on Science and Health (ACSH), even released a position paper called *Scared to Death: How Chemophobia Threatens Public Health*. The ACSH declares a mission "to add reason and balance to debates about public health issues and to bring common sense views to the public." But *Mother Jones* revealed in 2013 that the ACSH's donors and targeted potential donors "comprise a who's-who of energy, agriculture, cosmetics, food, soda, chemical, pharmaceutical, and tobacco corporations." The group's executive director, Dr. Gilbert Ross, did prison time for defrauding New York State's Medicaid program of roughly $8 million. Dr. Ronald E. Gots, founder of the Environmental Sensitivities Research Institute, is listed as an ACSH scientific advisor.

When we can't trust the corporations or the government to keep us safe, is it really irrational to be afraid?

PART III

The American Way of Stress

Americans are a queer people; they can't rest.

—Stephen Leacock, Canadian humorist,
"In Praise of the Americans," 1932

If into the life of a man whose powers are fully taxed we bring the elements of great anxiety or worry, or excessive haste, the whole machinery begins at once to work, as it were, with a dangerous amount of friction.

—S. Weir Mitchell, *Wear and Tear: Or, Hints for the Overworked,* 1871

NO TIME: the chronic complaint. No time to question the validity of the two-hour commute. No time to prepare a meal that isn't prepackaged. No time to nurture relationships, let alone a garden or an art. The army and religious cult leaders have long known the value of sleep deprivation in the indoctrination process. Physically and mentally weakened, deprived of time for reflection, are we more vulnerable to manipulation and control? Is the overworked society more susceptible to its own propaganda? Has leisure become radical?

—Deborah Campbell, "In Praise of
Radical Leisure (In Seven Parts),"
Adbusters (May/June 2003)

CHAPTER 9

Clockwork

The long, dim hallways and glass-doored offices in the 1920s building where I'd just signed a lease reminded me of old detective movies, but the lettering on the doors advertised hairdressers and artists and other therapists like me. I had just signed a lease and picked up my key, and I was doing my level best to act like a grown-up and not jump up and down and horse-gallop to my new office.

For four years I had worked at state-licensed agencies, passing several exams and accruing all the hours of experience, supervision, and training I needed to finally open my own private practice. I had worked so long for this. It felt like I was twenty-one again, and finally leaving home.

I'd been scouring Craigslist and the used furniture stores for a big desk and comfy couches and chairs. Frank had created a logo with monarch butterflies bursting into flight, built me a website, and designed business cards and a brochure. I wrote copy for the brochure and the website, set up an Excel spreadsheet to track my income and expenses, and created forms for progress notes and treatment plans and billing. I was busy filling out the paperwork to get credentialed with Aetna, Anthem, Harvard Pilgrim, United, Medicare, and some others I'd never even heard of.

Each company's paperwork was different, the questions sometimes unclear and bewildering. So then I would have to call and ask their customer service reps for clarification. If I made a mistake, it could mess everything up. And the people at the other end of the line said it could be up to ninety days before the credentialing went through. What would I do for income in the meantime?

It felt like a race against time. I would be moving into my new office in two weeks, I needed the income to start flowing, and I wanted everything to be just right.

I had no idea how much more stressful my life was about to get.

But I wasn't the only stressed-out American. It seemed like *everyone* was stressed. I was beginning to contemplate how America's unique form of capitalism impacts the health of those of us who live here, and the health of the nation itself.

———

I'd always wondered if the reason my mono turned into ME/CFS and MCS had something to do with stress. It made sense to me that a body under duress might not have enough reserves in store to fight off, say, the Epstein-Barr virus, and that a body encountering mononucleosis *combined* with stress might be a little like a pair of feet under a mud-stuck Flintstones car, scrambling but going nowhere.

Substantial evidence does indeed link stress with suppression of the immune response. Two separate meta-analyses covering decades of research revealed immune dysregulation in people under stress, as evidenced by total white blood cells, helper T cells, natural killer cells, and other markers.

In *Why Zebras Don't Get Ulcers*, neuroendocrinologist Robert Sapolsky reports that a series of studies found that people under higher levels of stress are about three times more likely to succumb to the common cold when exposed to the virus in a lab. In a passage that echoes statements made by George M. Beard and S. Weir

Mitchell, Sapolsky writes: "In order to gain a detailed, quantitative understanding of [the stress response], one must become something of an accountant—learning what the currency of energy is in the body and how much it costs to make all those deposits and withdrawals in the body's metabolic banks."

Sapolsky also notes that when confronted with something uncontrollable, people with "a strong internal locus of control . . . have far greater stress-responses than do those with external loci." In other words, people who are used to taking charge of their lives get *extra* stressed when faced with something beyond their control.

For a driven young woman exposed to a virus that stole her ability to take charge of her life, the body's stress response would likely be very high—and a never-ending loop of stress and illness might manifest.

—

Chronic stress is epidemic in America. In 2016, 25 percent of adults polled for the American Psychological Association's Stress in America survey reported that in the previous month they had felt fairly or very often that difficulties were piling so high they could not overcome them. As sociologist Juliet Schor, author of *The Overworked American: The Unexpected Decline of Leisure*, points out, "Millions of Americans have lost control over the basic rhythm of their daily lives. They work too much, eat too quickly, socialize too little, drive and sit in traffic for too many hours, don't get enough sleep, and feel harried too much of the time."

Since the annual Stress in America survey's launch in 2007, women have consistently reported higher average levels of stress than men. Adults whose household income was lower than $50,000 had an average stress level 5 percent greater than those with higher incomes. Stress was also notably higher for Black, Indigenous, and people of color (BIPOC), LGBTQIA+ folx, and people with disabilities. More than 60 percent of men and women rated both money and work as significant sources of stress.

———

People weren't always so busy. Before capitalism, Europe was largely "timeless," says Schor. People were task-oriented rather than time-oriented. When the first public clocks appeared in fourteenth-century Europe, they were called *Werkglocken*, or "work clocks," meant to increase productivity during an economic crisis in the textile industry. Quoting the English historian E. P. Thompson, Schor notes that time became "currency . . . not passed but spent." Eventually, she says, "workers came to perceive time, not as the milieu in which they lived their lives, but 'as an objective force within which [they] were imprisoned.'"

> As capitalism raised the "price" of time, people began to think of time as a scarce resource. Indeed, the ideology of the emerging market economy was filled with metaphors of time: saving time, using time wisely, admonitions against "passing" time. . . . When Benjamin Franklin preached that time is money, he meant that time should be used productively. . . . *Time itself had become a commodity.*

———

In contemporary America, time feels scarce, and the dearth of it constricting and stressful. For those felled by a fatiguing illness, however, time is long, each moment an infinite void. And that void can be a stressor, too. There's no escape from the disquieting existential questions that arise, the confounding thoughts and emotions.

So Alice's stressors were internal, secret. The stress of not having a voice, of not being allowed a vocation, of a confusing relationship with family. The stress of not knowing if she would ever find love in a city where, post–Civil War, women outnumbered men by 66,000; and the stress, possibly, of being a woman attracted to women—or at least one particular woman, Katharine Peabody Loring, with whom Alice had once taught at the Society to Encourage Studies at Home—in a homophobic culture: the stress of bearing a secret. The illness itself was a stressor. Would she be able to walk today? Would the pain engulf her as it had the day before?

In July, a little over a year after her collapse, the "two virgins of thirty summers," as Alice put it in her letter to Sara, spent two weeks at a cabin in the Adirondacks that Alice described as "William's panacea for all ills." In other words, although she only got as far west as Upstate New York, Alice made an attempt at the West Cure.

She did not take well to the woods, but not for lack of trying. "We perched ourselves on the sharpest stones we could find and religiously spent endless hours in listening to the babbling water, the gentle hum of the mosquito, giving j'oy [sic] untold to the sportive midge who found me quite the loveliest production civilization had yet sent to him," she wrote to Sara. In the end, "the bosom of nature was just about as much of a humbug as I always knew it was." They left early.

Two years later, on May 21, 1881, Alice and Katharine set sail for a three-month tour of England and Scotland. When they met up with Henry in London that July, he found Alice "rather weaker in body than I expected, but stronger in spirits, cheerfulness, &c."

Their travels were curtailed, however, when Alice relapsed on a visit with Katharine's aunt and uncle. After two weeks' convalescence, they settled into rooms near Henry's apartment in Piccadilly. Alice still had all the waking hours of a day to fill, but now she was well enough to shop, attend the theater, and take long walks with Katharine.

In other words, she had regained enough health to fill time.

———

Until 1883, in the United States there was no standardized time. Each town kept its own time based on the sun. People traveling across the country by train consulted elaborate timetables to make their connections. But with the driving of the golden spike that in 1869 united the nation's East-West economies, the needs of America's burgeoning industrialization took on a new urgency and the railroads adopted a standardized system called "Railroad and Telegraph Time." As Rebecca Solnit puts it in *River of Shadows: Eadweard Muybridge and the Technological Wild West*, "In the course of the nineteenth century, time ceased to be a phenomenon that linked humans to the cosmos and became one administered by technicians to link industrial activities to each other. . . . The railroad had eclipsed the sun."

————

And so had the lightbulb.

Its inventor, Thomas Edison, claimed to sleep just three to four hours a night. He declared it a virtue. "The person who sleeps eight or ten hours a night," he proclaimed, "is never fully asleep and never fully awake. He only has different degrees of doze through the 24 hours." Too much sleep, he said, made a person "unhealthy and inefficient." Never mind that he was an inveterate napper who would fall asleep at his laboratory workbench. "Life, in his eyes," writes David K. Randall, author of *Dreamland: Adventures in the Strange Science of Sleep*, "was like an assembly line where any downtime could be only wasteful." Who but such a man would invent the filament lightbulb? His goal, says Randall, was "to domesticate light." And so he did.

With the invention of artificial lighting, the working day would stretch deep into the night. By 1900, with lightbulbs illuminating factories and mills all over the country, the twenty-four-hour workforce was born.

In medieval Europe, time wasn't measured by minutes and hours but instead was marked by day and night. A typical working day in the Middle Ages spanned from dawn to dusk—sixteen hours in the summer, eight in the winter—but the tempo of life was slow: people paused work for breakfast and then lunch and a nap, and stopped again for dinner, turning in for the night when the sun went down. Some places also had midmorning and midafternoon breaks, and the months were punctuated with many holidays—far more than we celebrate now. According to Schor, holiday breaks in medieval England amounted to about a third of the year. "Our ancestors may not have been rich, but they had an abundance of leisure," she writes. "In the absence of a culture of consumption, there was no need to work longer hours."

Here in the New World, as Europe transitioned from feudalism to capitalism, settlers forged a nation out of the raw material of its natural resources. What they saw when they landed was a vast and treacherous frontier. They could triumph or they could die. The perception of the earth as a nurturing mother—subsumed as it was by the Cartesian values of rationality and mechanization—gave way to a different view: nature as disorder, and the imperative to reign over it. And now here they stood, poised at the edge of what was to them an uncharted frontier, excited, afraid, determined to survive. They would create order out of chaos through hard, ceaseless labor.

By the time industrial capitalism hit America in the late 1700s, workers toiled twelve, fourteen, and even sixteen hours a day. In the U.S., unionized male artisans and craftsmen began the long fight to reduce their workdays to ten hours, an unthinkable prospect for most workers at that time and for decades to come. In 1827, Philadelphia journeyman carpenters resolved that "all men have a just right . . . to have sufficient time each day for the cultivation of their mind and for self improvement." In the 1830s and '40s, female textile workers—who labored for up to fifteen hours a day—became major players in the struggle. But industrialists fought the campaign . . . and so did moralists. A Unitarian minister named Jonathan Baxter Harrison, in an 1880 book called *Certain Dangerous Tendencies in American Life,* illustrated the prevailing class and race bias when he wrote that by being kept busy, factory workers had "little leisure for vicious thoughts, for nourishing mischievous and profligate desires," and concluded that it was better for workers to toil for longer hours "in order to keep down and utilize the forces of the animal nature and passions."

––––––

It took decades of protest before the eight-hour day was finally legislated under the Fair Labor Standards Act of 1938, part of President Franklin D. Roosevelt's New Deal. By 1973, Americans worked fewer than forty hours a week. That same year, wages peaked for hourly employees (who made up the majority of U.S. workers, as they still do). Thereafter Americans began working harder and longer for less money and fewer benefits.

For that, we can thank the oil crises of 1973 and 1979, the resulting 1981 recession, and the ensuing Reagan years. A cutthroat business culture and mass layoffs pressured white-collar workers to invest more time and energy in their jobs. Meanwhile, blue-collar workers were dealt a massive blow in August 1981 when Reagan fired over 11,000 striking air traffic controllers, signaling to unions all over the country that their days were numbered.

On average, union members earn 13 percent more than nonunion workers in similar jobs, and a strong union presence in a community helps to raise the pay scales even for non-union jobs. In 1973, almost a quarter of U.S. workers were unionized. That figure has now dropped to just 10 percent, and the number of major strikes and lockouts has plummeted from 317 that year to just 16 in 2021. Meanwhile, in

Iceland 90 percent of wage and salary workers belong to trade unions, in Italy 34 percent do, and in Canada 25 percent are empowered by unionization to fight for living wages and fair working conditions.

The decline of unions in the U.S. has played a significant role in wage stagnation and loss of benefits—including health insurance and vacation time—not to mention the widening chasm between rich and poor.

Today the United States is the only industrialized country that hasn't legislated guaranteed paid vacation days, and nearly a quarter of Americans in the private-sector workforce—some 26 million workers—aren't offered any paid time off at all. Americans with full-time jobs are guaranteed just ten holidays, a paltry sum when compared to the combined holidays and vacations adding up to thirty-six to thirty-seven days a year for workers in France, Spain, and the United Kingdom.

The per capita gross domestic product (GDP) in countries like Norway, France, and Ireland is nonetheless similar to or *higher* than America's. In other words, although Americans are working much harder than Europeans, we are generally not more productive. According to the Center for Economic and Policy Research, Americans "work an unusually high number of hours for the country's level of productivity." After a certain point, we're just rats on a treadmill.

———

This lifestyle difference between the United States and England was apparent to Alice even in the nineteenth century. Three years before her death, when she was living in England, she remarked in her diary,

> It's rather strange that here, among this robust and sanguine people, I feel not the least shame or degradation at being ill, as I used to at home among the anaemic and the fagged. It comes of course in one way from the conditions being so easy, from the

sense of leisure, work reduced to a minimum and the god *Holiday* worshipped so perpetually and effectually by all classes.

The difference was something she could *feel* in her body.

In May 1890, hundreds of workers assembled in London's Hyde Park to rally for the eight-hour workday; Alice cheered them on in her journal. She was, says Strouse, "fervently radical" and "opposed to all forms of social oppression."

———

By 2015, the average American worker was putting in 124 more hours per year than in 1979. Forty percent of Americans work 50 hours or more a week. Eighteen percent work over 60. Americans between the ages of twenty-five and fifty-four work almost 8 percent more hours than they did forty years ago. And now that we have email and cell phones, people remain connected to their jobs even when they're not officially on duty.

American workers passed up 212 million paid vacation days in 2017—a $62.2 billion bonanza to the companies that employ them.

———

In a rabidly capitalist culture like America's, it's not surprising that an illness like ME/CFS has been scorned and dismissed. People with the illness don't have any place in the American cult of productivity. In a 2016 interview, Marissa Mayer, the former chief executive of Yahoo!, said that working 130 hours a week was possible "if you're strategic about when you sleep, when you shower, and how often you go to the bathroom." Two years later, PayPal cofounder Elon Musk, CEO of Tesla, tweeted that there are easier places to work than his automotive and energy company, "but nobody ever changed the world on 40 hours a week." He went on to say that the correct number of hours "varies per person," but is "about 80 sustained, peaking about 100 at times." But in fact, a 2014 study for the Institute for the Study of Labor (now the Institute of Labor Economics), an international research nonprofit, found that people working 70 hours a week produced little more than those working 55.

As Erin Griffith pointed out in a 2019 piece for *The New York Times*, such "hymns to the virtues of relentless work" tend to be the rallying cries of those who would benefit most from workers' participation in their own exploitation—the managers, financiers, and owners.

Aidan Harper, creator of the 4 Day Week campaign in Europe, told Griffith that this corporate drumbeat "creates the assumption that the only value we have as human beings is our productivity capability—our ability to work, rather than our humanity." At a time when participation in organized religion is dropping, Griffith describes those seduced by this message, rooted as it is in the Protestant work ethic, as "congregants of the Cathedral of Perpetual Hustle," worshipping, as Harper says, "at the altar of work."

In a 2004 essay about the virtues of idleness, the novelist Mark Slouka asked, "Could the Church of Work—which today has Americans aspiring to sleep deprivation the way they once aspired to a personal knowledge of God—be, at base, an antidemocratic force?"

———

Advertising helps to propel the hustle.

With all the technological advances of the Industrial Revolution, by the early 1920s corporations were producing more than they could sell. According to historian Ben Hunnicutt, economists and business owners worried that the economy would stop growing because people had everything they needed. At the same time, the new assembly lines were fragmenting labor, depriving workers of the satisfaction of craftsmanship. It's hard to realize a sense of meaning, empowerment, worth, or wholeness when you know you're just a cog in a machine.

Into this void stepped the advertisers. They could, as Hunnicutt put it, "convince people to buy things they never needed before." Through a little bit of corporate sleight of hand, advertising could distract workers from the real source of their discontent and convince them that the void could be filled if only they had the latest Model T or a vacuum cleaner or the trendy new ready-to-wear fashions. Through consumption, people began to try to reclaim their sense of identity and power. By the mid-1920s, advertising had become a major industry.

In his 1928 book, provocatively entitled *Propaganda*, public relations pioneer (and Freud's nephew) Edward Bernays made a disturbing claim, declaring that "the conscious and intelligent manipulation of the organized habits and opinions of the masses is an important element in democratic society. Those who manipulate this unseen mechanism of society constitute an invisible government which is the true ruling power of our country." He came to call this "the engineering of consent," and learned its precepts while working for the Committee on Public Information—a government agency established to disseminate propaganda that would build enthusiasm for World War I—and exploited them for the duration of his long and influential career as a consultant for corporate America.

To that end, in addition to moving inventory, advertising sells a standard of normalcy, curating American desire, homogenizing American taste and culture, and selling a way of life that profits the corporations and distracts people from the high social cost of industrial capitalism. And because advertiser dollars are the engine that powers the mass media, our primary sources of information must to some degree cater to the ideologies of corporate America. Advertising has inculcated in us the belief that consumption offers the most direct route to our constitutional right to the pursuit of happiness. But the more we buy, the more we have to work.

Since 1973, free time in America has dropped by almost 40 percent, from a median of twenty-six hours a week to sixteen. But some Americans are finding ways to get their time back. New Dream, a nonprofit whose motto is "More fun, less stuff . . . More joy, less stress . . . More love, less waste," found in a 2004 survey of people who had deliberately cut back their hours that 23 percent said they were happier and didn't miss the money. Sixty percent reported being happier but did miss the money to varying degrees. Just 10 percent regretted the change.

A 2015 Swedish study found that households that decrease their work hours by 1 percent may reduce their energy use by 0.7 percent and their greenhouse gas emissions by 0.8 percent, largely due to reductions in consumption. When people have more time, they can reduce their carbon footprint by using public transportation or riding their bikes to work, hanging their clothes on the line rather than running the electric dryer, cultivating vegetable gardens, cooking their meals rather than relying on processed foods. They spend less money not only because they have less money to spend, but also because they no longer feel the same need to reward themselves for getting through another workweek. And people with less money buy smaller houses that require fewer natural resources to heat and light. When people prioritize leisure over earnings, they consume less. When people are more integrated with life, life becomes its own reward.

A 2006 study conducted by the Center for Economic and Policy Research estimated that if Americans pared back work hours to match those of Western European countries, workers would find themselves with an additional seven weeks off per year and U.S. energy consumption would decline by about 20 percent. The authors also calculated that if that energy savings were directly translated into lower carbon emissions, then the United States in 2003 would have emitted 3 percent less carbon dioxide than it did in 1990.

Juliet Schor and her colleagues, in their 2013 paper, looked at all industrialized countries over a period of fifty years and found that those with shorter working hours had "considerably smaller ecological and carbon footprints."

———

Of course, some low-wage earners are working two or three jobs because there's no other way to meet their basic subsistence needs. At $7.25 an hour, the federal minimum wage has not budged since 2009 despite strong public support for increases. It has lost more than 27 percent of its buying power since that time due to inflation. Raising the minimum wage helps to push up wages for workers whose pay is a little above the minimum, improving the standard of living for many low-wage workers, whose money gets pumped back into the economy as they spend their paychecks on goods and services. While many cities and states are proactively raising the minimum wage in their communities, the federal government is lagging.

———

In 1930, the economist John Maynard Keynes predicted that due to technological advances, people would be working as few as fifteen hours a week by 2030. Now that we're inching closer to that date and working harder than ever, this prediction sounds absurd.

The average productivity per American worker has increased 430 percent since 1950, which means that in fact we *should* be able to afford the same standard of living as a 1950 worker by working just 10 hours a week. But wages haven't kept up with productivity. If the median hourly compensation had kept pace with the productivity since 1979, the median worker would now be earning nine dollars more per hour, or about $19,000 more per year. Americans are busier now than ever, working more and vacationing less than any other industrialized country, all while we get less in unemployment, disability, and retirement benefits, and retire later than people in similarly wealthy countries.

In a 2018 Gallop poll, 55 percent of American adults said that on the previous day they had experienced stress "a lot of the day." This figure was 20 percent higher than the global average. As Nobel prize–winning economist Joseph Stiglitz puts it, "In America the consequences of not being at the top are so dramatic that the rat race is exacerbated. In a winner-takes-all society you would expect this time crunch."

All of this job-related stress is estimated to cost American companies more than $300 billion per year in health costs, absenteeism, and poor performance. In *The Great Acceleration: How the World Is Getting Faster, Faster*, Robert Colvile notes that "while our bodies are designed for brief periods of stress and sudden bursts of activity, the modern workplace, with its demands for nonstop attention and decisions, pushes our fight-or-flight response to the limit, leading to burnout." The National Institute for Occupational Safety and Health (NIOSH) found that healthcare expenditures are nearly 50 percent greater for workers who report high levels of stress. Unsurprisingly, when workers are healthy and enjoying their lives, they actually perform better.

———

One day, rushing back to my office after running an errand on my lunch break, I crossed paths with an acquaintance who asked how I was doing. When I answered breathlessly, "Busy! Too busy!" he replied, "Ahh, the American propensity for busyness. It makes us all feel so important."

We do live in a culture that promotes the belief that if we're not stressed out, we're not working hard enough. But what my acquaintance failed to account for was that what's keeping us so busy is runaway capitalism.

I'm reminded of the widespread suggestion that neurasthenia was a "fashionable" illness—a signal of the leisure and prosperity of the upper classes. Now, some say, Americans signal our prosperity and social status through busyness and stress. But when a poll taken the year I fell ill asked people which of two full-time career paths they would prefer—one that allowed them to schedule their own work hours and give more attention to their families, but with slower career advancement, or one with rigid work hours and less time for family but faster career advancement—almost eight out of ten chose the path with more free time. We don't seem to know how to escape this maze.

———

And women are hardest hit. While we've made many advances since Mary Wollstonecraft's groundbreaking 1792 treatise *A Vindication of the Rights of Woman*, including the freedom to choose careers and earn our own money (albeit, just 84 cents to every man's dollar), women still do three times as much housework as men, spend more than twice the amount of time preparing meals, and do nearly twice as much child care. As a result, men get nearly a full hour more per day for leisure activities.

In Alice's time, the quintessential woman was known as the "angel in the house"—a passive and self-sacrificing woman much like Alice's mother, Mary, who devoted herself to caring for her children and creating a sanctuary for her husband. During this time, says Juliet Schor, "a class of experts in homemaking and child rearing . . . imposed ever-more exacting practices on American women." Reformers like Harriet Beecher Stowe and her sister Catharine Beecher aimed to "professionalize housework," writes Schor, creating a new "'domestic science' and a home economics movement which spread their gospel into homes, schools, and the media," urging "scientific" cooking and a new war on germs.

A century later, the technological revolution of the 1950s brought labor-saving appliances such as automatic washing machines and dryers, the electric iron, and affordable vacuum cleaners into the home. An industrial engineer named Lillian Gilbreth, translating Frederick Winslow's principles of scientific management for the home, analyzed motions to find more efficient ways to do dishes and worked at General Electric to improve kitchen designs. (She also invented the foot-pedal trash can.)

Women were barraged with television, radio, and magazine ads designed to amp up social pressure and sell more products, says Schor: "Housework was functional for capitalism." Ads warned women of the perils of germs and promulgated heightened standards of cleanliness. In one sinister ad Schor unearthed, a floor polish company warned, "By Their Floors Shall Ye Judge Them. . . . It is written that floors are like unto a mirror, reflecting the character of the housewife."

By the 1990s dishwashers and microwaves had joined our growing arsenal of timesaving devices. Yet, says Schor, "with all these labor-saving innovations, no labor has been saved. Instead, housework expanded to fill the available time. Norms of cleanliness rose."

As Barbara Ehrenreich and Deirdre English put it in *For Her Own Good: 150 Years of the Experts' Advice to Women*:

> Washing machines permit you to do daily, instead of weekly, laundries. Vacuum cleaners and rug shampooers remind you that you do not have to live with dust or countenance a stain on the carpet. Each of them—the dishwasher, the roll warmer, the freezer, the blender—is the material embodiment of a task, a silent imperative to *work*.

———

Because the fight for fewer work hours was associated with socialism, the movement was stymied by the anticommunist frenzy of the McCarthy years and its aftermath. But some companies have discovered that six-hour days or four-day workweeks can actually *boost* efficiency. When a Toyota service center in Gothenburg, Sweden, transitioned its mechanics to a thirty-hour workweek over ten years ago, it found happier employees, greater customer satisfaction, and a boost in profits. A Swedish nursing home that cut hours from forty to thirty per week discovered that its nurses were more productive, took fewer sick days, experienced less neck and back pain, and felt happier. City workers in Reykjavík, Iceland, maintained productivity and took fewer sick days when their workweeks were cut by four to five hours. And in 2021 the entire nation of Spain became the first European country to implement a four-day workweek.

As Juliet Schor notes, "Historically, the working day has been 'too long' in the sense that fatigue impaired effectiveness. Each time the workday was reduced—first to ten hours and then to eight—productivity rose."

———

There are other ways employers could help their employees be happier and healthier. Transforming overtime into "comp time" would allow workers to bank overtime to invest in extra days off, longer vacations, or even sabbaticals. Permitting full-time workers to switch to part time, with prorated benefits like health insurance and pension plans, would be another way to allow workers more control over their time without loss of security.

What would people do if they had more time? Maybe they'd sleep more, which would be good, as 40 percent of Americans get six or fewer hours of sleep per night, notably less than the seven to nine hours experts recommend for optimal health (thus increasing their risk of developing high blood pressure and mental health issues as well as chronic conditions like heart disease, stroke, and diabetes). Maybe they would take their kids for hikes in the woods. Maybe they'd join a softball team or take dance classes, perform in community theater, write poetry or learn to play ukulele. Maybe they'd run for city council or drive the elderly to their medical appointments or volunteer to get out the vote. Maybe they'd have more time to fight for new laws that would protect them from harm, laws that would protect us all.

―――――

"The basic premise of conflict theory," said Steve, my social work professor back in that classroom in 1998, "is that resources are limited, and those with wealth and power do everything they can to hold on to their wealth and power, and they do this by suppressing the poor and the powerless in order to maintain their own domination."

There were eighteen of us in the class, our desks arranged in a circle. We scribbled in our notebooks. Steve set one elbow on his desk. "Karl Marx said that in this system, workers are commodities, and dispensable. And so industry doesn't actually *want* 100 percent employment. Because if everyone was employed and no one was standing at the gate looking for a job, workers would be empowered to demand better wages and benefits. But at the same time, the powers that be don't want too much *unemployment*, because that would lead to revolt. So instead, we tread a thin line between these two places, always afraid that the person behind us is going to take our job and our security."

Steve looked around the room. "It's an inherently dehumanizing and disconnecting system." And then, almost as an afterthought, he added, "Think about this mad race we're all running. It keeps people just busy enough that they don't have any time to *organize*. Imagine the trouble people could stir up if they just had more *time*."

―――――

Slowly, over two years, I prepared a policy manual and all the paperwork necessary to transform my private practice into a state-licensed

agency without walls, and then in 2011, I brought on my first affiliate—
an independent contractor who billed through my agency—and
then another, and another, until there were six of us. Each time I
took on someone new I did all the insurance credentialing and filled
out forms for the state so that the practitioner could get reimbursed
by Medicaid, and I kept track of all the incoming payments. The affiliates had their own offices all over the city, and twice a month we came
together for supervision. I took all the calls and emails from prospective
clients and helped match them to the right therapist. The paperwork
was never-ending. I was always behind. I saw my first client at eleven
A.M., typed progress notes at my computer through lunch, and forced
myself to leave the office at eight P.M., or maybe a little bit after, even
though there was more to do, more to do, always more to do.

Neurobiologist Robert Sapolsky, in *Why Zebras Don't Get Ulcers*,
says that stress is the unifying element that pulls together the seemingly disparate disciplines of biology and psychology. Our stress
response system evolved to help us respond to immediate physical
threats such as an attack by a cougar. However, those of us living in
industrialized countries rarely face immediate threats to survival—
nor did the "brain workers" and others of the nineteenth century.
But that doesn't stop our hypothalamic-pituitary-adrenal (HPA) axis
from being activated. In fact, for many Americans these systems are
chronically *overactive*.

When we are exposed to a stressor, our hearts beat faster, our
breathing gets quick and shallow, blood pressure rises, glucose floods
our bloodstream, and adrenaline rushes through our body, making
us stronger and faster than we ever thought possible, and together all
these adaptations help us to fight or flee until the threat passes.

But I was sitting in my office. There *was* no cougar. Or the cougar
had morphed into the many piles of papers on my desk and the clock on
my wall and the night falling before all the papers had been processed.
I had a constant sense of urgency—as if my very survival was at stake.

CHAPTER 10

Load

Meanwhile, I was squeezing in weekly healthcare appointments and sessions with a therapist in my ongoing efforts to reclaim my health. I prepared at least two meals a day, eating lots of protein and vegetables, avoiding grains and sweeteners because they now made me tired and itchy, avoiding foods from the evening nightshade family (like potatoes and tomatoes) because they now made my joints ache, avoiding dairy because it now upset my stomach. Like Alice, I seemed to have made what she sardonically described as a "life-long occupation of 'improving.'" I tried rigorous candida treatment, detox footbaths, and after two separate doctors told me that based on my test results and their clinical judgment they believed I had Lyme disease, a lengthy—and decisively unsuccessful—antibiotic protocol. And I still needed periods of intensive rest.

My illness was my second career—a part-time job at least, but not a lucrative one. In fact, since Medicare covered only mainstream treatments, my illness career was costing me everything I had. But I kept going. I ran my small agency and saw just fourteen clients a week, a little more than a half-time caseload, but that combined with my career as a sick person made me pretty much a full-timer.

———

Long-term stress can cause tension headaches, indigestion, insomnia, shortness of breath, high blood pressure, high blood sugar (increasing the risk of diabetes), a pounding heart, an increased risk of heart attack, stomachache, fertility problems, erectile dysfunction, low sex drive, missed periods, and tense muscles.

The American Psychological Association's annual Stress in America survey found in 2016 that significant numbers of adults experienced mental health symptoms as a result of stress in the previous month. Forty-two percent reported feeling nervous or anxious, 37 percent reported feeling depressed or sad, 33 percent reported constant worrying, and 37 percent reported irritability or anger due to stress. Americans make up 5 percent of the world's population and consume 65 percent of the world's psychotropic drugs, including tranquilizers and antidepressants.

———

As is true of many Americans—overwhelmed by debt, by demanding jobs, by the effort to balance work and chores and time for family— my stress response stayed switched on. I'd been slowly recovering from a chronic condition for almost twenty years, and I knew that my constant revved-up feeling wasn't good for me, but I couldn't stop.

The hypothalamic-pituitary-adrenal (HPA) axis is a complex hormonal response system that mediates our body's reaction to stress and regulates many body processes, including digestion, sexuality, mood and emotions, energy storage and expenditure, and immunity. When faced with a stressor, the hypothalamus stimulates the pituitary gland to secrete adrenocorticotropic hormone (ACTH), which triggers the adrenal gland to produce cortisol, a steroid hormone that floods the system with glucose, which temporarily increases energy production to enable the fight-or-flight function to kick in. At the same time, the adrenals secrete the hormone adrenaline. Cortisol narrows the arteries while adrenaline increases the heart rate, both of which force blood to pump harder and faster, thus transporting nutrients and oxygen at greater rates, and this helps us to fight or flee the stressor with more strength and speed than we otherwise could. When you're stressed, the muscles that help you breathe tense up, which can leave you short of breath. This explains why during the most frenzied times at the office I could not catch a breath that went all the way down to the bottom of my lungs.

Robert Sapolsky points out that in a stress emergency, "it makes sense that your body halts long-term, expensive building projects" having to do with digestion, growth, and reproduction. Additionally, because all the body's energy is being invested in the stress response, the immune system is inhibited. As Sapolsky puts it, "The immune system . . . is ideal for spotting the tumor cell that will kill you in a year, or making enough antibodies to protect you in a few weeks, but is it really needed this instant? The logic here seems to be the same—look for tumors some other time; expend the energy more wisely now."

So while the stress response system is excellent for helping us through short-term crises, it's really not set up to manage chronic stress. And this is what leads to problems. Research confirms that stress makes it harder to fight illness, makes symptoms worse when we do get sick, and even slows the ability to heal wounds. Sapolsky notes that "if you constantly mobilize energy at the cost of energy storage, you will never store any surplus energy," and fatigue can result.

When stress is unrelenting, as it is for many Americans, eventually the adrenals can get overwhelmed and are no longer able to do their job adequately. Cortisol production declines, causing instability in the body's internal systems. This is called *allostatic overload*. The constant state of arousal, like the gunning of a car's engine, wears us down over time, increasing our risk of disease. Interestingly, in his 2005 paper about allostasis, neuroendocrinologist Bruce S. McEwen uses chronic fatigue syndrome as an example of an allostatic state of imbalance resulting in excessive production of some immune system mediators and inadequate production of others. In the case of chronic fatigue syndrome, he describes the chronic elevation of inflammatory cytokines—which are responsible for switching the immune system on and off—accompanied by low cortisol.

Perhaps, as Strouse suggested, Alice *did* collapse as a result of William's impending engagement to the other Alice. But if so, rather than its being a manipulation, perhaps the emotional stress took a physiologic toll on an already compromised body.

———

I awoke with a start. Staggered to the bathroom in the dim predawn light, skimming my hand against the wall for support, sat down on the toilet and peed in the dark with my eyes closed, then climbed back into bed and pulled up the covers. And then I thought of the client whose family was in the process of being evicted for getting behind on the rent. *Where would they go? How would they be okay?* Then I remembered that I had forgotten to fill out a form that needed to be sent out in order for a new affiliate to get paid, and then, there in the dark, I began mentally scanning that day's list of things to do, and then I was awake and there was no getting back to sleep. It was four A.M. I switched on a light and opened a book.

I slept with earplugs and a white noise machine, closed my shades every night before bed, and took melatonin, and eventually Ambien, too, but nothing worked. Every morning I awoke at four and fought to get back to sleep, and sometimes it worked and sometimes it didn't. More than ever, I had to refer to my notes when sitting with clients so I could keep track of the threads of their thoughts. I was in a fog, forgetful, groping around for words, closed in on myself, grouchy

with Frank. I felt an urgency in my belly all the time. It was a panicked feeling, a rushing feeling, like I had been dumped off a raft into
swirling rapids and was scrabbling to get back on.

And money was always an issue. I was always scraping by, worrying each month about how I would pay the bills. Even though my
entire life I'd railed against the idea that one's income equals one's
value, as a businesswoman I felt I needed to maintain the appearance
that I was financially doing okay.

But the truth was, I was never doing okay. And I didn't feel like
a businesswoman. I felt like a person drowning. I felt, I suppose, like
an impostor. And I felt that way mostly because I was broke. So I had
to keep on flailing.

———

Self-care, self-care, self-care. The buzzword of the therapy world. My
colleagues and I taught it to our clients; we admonished one another
to do more of it.

Here is a brief summary of my evolving self-care protocol:

I decided to spread my clients' appointments further apart so I
    had twenty-five minutes between each one. I limited myself
    to five clients a day.

I squeezed all my clients into three weeks so that I could take
    one week of every month away from my work as a therapist
    and have uninterrupted time to write.

In that writing week, I also tried to catch up on my sleep, since
    I didn't have to get up at seven A.M.

I ate healthy meals.

I took multiple nutritional supplements.

I walked my dog. I walked to work. I cuddled with my cats.

I laughed with Frank.

Somebody recommended yoga, so I tried it. I did *Yoga with Adriene* online for a full thirty days. Then I stopped. The mild positive effects were negated by the stress of the time lost.

I tried meditation. It made me antsy.

I learned how to dance the tango. I loved the chest-to-chest connection. Here I had to decide nothing. My only job was to connect and to listen to my partner's body.

I used a light box in winter.

I made sure to spend at least a week somewhere warmer than Maine in the dead of February, even though I couldn't really afford it.

I did it all, but it was never enough. Because enough wasn't possible. I was always overwhelmed, always broke, always stressed. At first I blamed myself. But then I looked around at everyone else and I began to think it wasn't me that was the problem.

———

When it comes to managing their stress, 63 percent of people say they feel they are doing enough; 21 percent say they're not. The question is: How much is enough? It seems to be that the *stress management* imperative can become yet another gaping maw of demands.

I didn't have any *time* to add more self-care. I was already getting just six or seven hours of sleep a night—less when insomnia woke me up at four A.M. How could I possibly squeeze in time for *more self-care*?

———

It's not only impossible to adjust to certain stressors, but it would actually be unhealthy—and bad for self and society—to do so. For instance, should a minimum-wage single parent with two kids "just stop being stressed"? Would all the yoga in the world work for *that*? Or for structural racism? Or anxiety about the climate crisis? And *should* it?

There's a tremendous amount of pressure on people to calm their own stress with self-care. But what if the best way to fix a stress problem is to *fix the actual source of the problem*? At what point is the self-care imperative a form of propaganda meant to keep us focused on our individual shortcomings rather than on the failings of our country?

———

Stress doesn't just impact adults, but until relatively recently we had no idea the long-term physiological effects of childhood stress. In the late 1990s, Vincent Felitti, head of Kaiser Permanente's Department of Preventive Medicine in San Diego, and Robert Anda, an epidemiologist from the Centers for Disease Control and Prevention (CDC), made an astonishing discovery. In their groundbreaking Adverse Childhood Experiences (ACE) study, they found that the number of stressors endured as a child has a cumulative effect on that child's risk of disease as an adult, even when accounting for unhealthy adaptive behaviors such as smoking, drinking, and junk-food diets.

The researchers developed a simple ten-point questionnaire covering circumstances of neglect and domestic violence, as well as physical, emotional, verbal, or sexual abuse, plus physical or emotional absence of a parent due to death, divorce, prison, substance use disorder, or mental illness. For each yes response, one point was added to the respondent's score. Subsequent research has shown that people with an ACE score of 4 are twice as likely to be diagnosed with cancer than those who have not faced any childhood adversity. The chance of being hospitalized for an autoimmune disease rises by 20 percent for every point. And the risk of depression is 460 percent higher for someone with an ACE score of 4 compared to someone with a score of 0. The higher the ACE score, the higher the probability of developing heart disease, bowel disorders, and other health problems. An ACE score of 6 or higher slashes almost twenty years from a person's lifespan.

In fact, studies have found that a history of adverse childhood experiences is associated with a three- to eightfold increased risk for ME/CFS. One of these, published in 2009, argues that "evidence from developmental neuroscience suggests that early experience programs the development of regulatory systems that are implicated in the pathophysiology of CFS, including the hypothalamic-pituitary-adrenal axis," and concludes:

> our results confirm childhood trauma as an important risk factor of CFS. In addition, neuroendocrine dysfunction, a hallmark feature of CFS, appears to be associated with childhood trauma. This possibly reflects a biological correlate of vulnerability due to early developmental insults.

In 2012 the American Academy of Pediatrics released a landmark statement warning that "toxic stress" in childhood "can leave a lasting signature on the genetic predispositions that affect emerging brain architecture and long-term health." According to the report, "advances in fields of inquiry as diverse as neuroscience, molecular biology, genomics, developmental psychology, epidemiology, sociology, and economics are catalyzing an important paradigm shift in our understanding of health and disease across the lifespan," suggesting "that many adult diseases should be viewed as developmental disorders that begin early in life."

In other words, even experiences we've historically thought of as only psychological have long-term impacts on the body. As Donna Jackson Nakazawa declares in her 2015 *Aeon* piece about ACEs, "The correlation between childhood trauma, brain architecture and adult wellbeing is the newest, and perhaps our most important, psycho-biological theory of everything."

Adverse childhood experiences impact not only the child's immedi-ate emotional and physical well-being but also embed themselves in the child's brain chemistry, with long-term consequences for the immune system. In an article for the *Journal of Restorative Medicine*, physician and author Gabor Maté explains how this happens. "Happy, attuned emotional interactions with parents stimulate a release of natural opi-oids in an infant's brain," enhancing the attachment relationship and the development of receptors and circuitry for the further production and distribution of natural opioids, dopamine, norepinephrine and oxytocin, all chemicals that help create an emotional buffer against external stressors. But adverse childhood experiences, including un-predictable or absent parental attunement, inhibit this development, establishing a lower "set point" for a child's internal stress system, which increases the child's sensitivity to stressors even into adulthood.

What the ACE studies show is that medicine's false dichotomy between mind and body is failing patients. But doctors aren't trained to incorporate emotions or psychosocial histories into their interviews or interventions. As Vincent Felitti told one interviewer,

> When I was first in practice, I wouldn't have wanted to go near any of this with a pole because I would have felt incompetent. What am I going to do? There's no prescription for this, there's no operation, there's no injection for this, etc. And it took so long to realize that one didn't always need to do something. Indeed that asking and listening . . . was itself a very powerful form of doing.

His research changed his office visits. Felitti began asking his patients, "Can you tell me how this adverse childhood experience has affected you later in your life?" and giving them a little time to talk. In the year following these discussions, his patients' doctor vis-its decreased by 35 percent; their emergency room visits dropped by

11 percent. If this intervention had been a pharmaceutical, it would have been hailed as a miracle drug.

———

Another stressor associated with susceptibility to disease is low socio-economic status. Forty years ago, the United States was one of the most egalitarian countries in the world. Now the disparity between rich and poor is greater than in any other industrialized nation. As Robert Sapolsky points out, the diseases that correlate most strongly with low socioeconomic status are those "with the greatest sensitivity to stress." These include heart disease, rheumatoid disorders, and diabetes. Epidemiologist Richard Wilkinson of the University of Nottingham in England found in a series of studies that the greater a country's income inequality, the worse its health and mortality rates. Remarkably, he found that not only the poor but the wealthy, too, are healthier in more egalitarian countries than in less equal societies with similar average incomes.

———

In my therapy practice, my clients were low-income or middle class, so I saw firsthand the impact of the disparity. My poorest clients were covered by Medicare because they were disabled by one or more dis-orders, including PTSD, depression, anxiety, bipolar disorder, brain injuries, chronic Lyme disease, ME/CFS, fibromyalgia, multiple chemical sensitivity, Ménière's disease, arthritis, asthma, and COPD. And they were covered by Medicaid because they were poor. I never had a Medicare/Medicaid client who wasn't a trauma survivor.

And not only that, but their cars frequently broke down or they didn't own cars and had to rely on a government-contracted company that picked them up either an hour early or so late that they'd miss their appointments. Often the companies left them standing by the road after their appointments, waiting and wondering if their ride would ever show up. Sometimes it didn't. Their phones got disconnected because they couldn't pay their bill, or their power got shut off, or they got evicted and had to move again. They ran out of food at the end of the month because their food stamps weren't enough to get them through. They couldn't afford dental care because the only thing their insurance would cover was pulling an abscessed tooth. They couldn't afford child care and had to rely on family members, and if that fell through, they had to cancel their appointment or maybe bring their kid with them if the child was old enough to sit in the waiting room. I couldn't recommend acupuncture or massage or dance classes or a night out or a Florida vacation because there was no money for any of these things.

Over a decade of sitting across from clients who were living with the effects of so much trauma and injustice had begun to wear me down. The problem, in so many cases, wasn't my clients: it was the system that was failing them, failing all of us.

———

My clinical consultant, Rona, had gray shoulder-length hair and a warm smile and the round, full body of an earth goddess, and I always left our appointments feeling grounded and fortified. Here, in Rona's cozy office, I settled into my chair.

"I've got this client with chronic Lyme," I said. "She's a wonderful person—smart and creative, and even though she's up against a lot she often tells me things she's grateful for, even if it's the rice crackers she brought with her or the nice conversation she had with her driver on the way in or the extra effort her case manager put in . . . or me. But she's *really*, really sick." I told Rona that my client was so fatigued that she often couldn't get out of bed, and she was in pain every day and deeply depressed, and lately it seemed like all of it was getting worse. She was too sick to make friends. She survived trauma as a child, got out of an abusive marriage, and a year after we started working together was homeless for several days before she got into a halfway house and then finally subsidized housing. She had a treatable disease, but she couldn't get treatment.

"She had a wonderful doctor, but that doctor moved away. We've been looking and looking for another Lyme-literate doctor who takes her insurance, and we can't find *anyone*. Well, that's not true. I found *one* doctor who takes Medicare and she scheduled an appointment with him but then the receptionist called back and *canceled*, and so with the client's permission *I* called, and first the receptionist told me it was because her Medicaid was *primary*, and I told her that was not true, the *Medicare* is primary, and *then* the receptionist told me that they wouldn't see her anyway because she wouldn't be able to afford the out-of-pocket treatments."

I heaved a big sigh, and then another, and the second one came out jagged, and I put my face in my hands and started to sob.

"It's hard to feel so helpless," said Rona.

"It *is*." I felt the fury rise up and looked her in the eye. "It's just *so . . . fucked*." I pulled two tissues out of the box and wiped at my eyes.

Rona's eyes were warm and gentle. "You help her not be so alone," she said.

"It's not enough."

———

In my next appointment I told Rona how depleted I'd been, and she gave me a knowing look. "Sounds like you may be dealing with vicarious trauma," she said.

"Really?"

"It's a professional hazard."

"Yeah, but I work so hard on my self-care." I listed all that I was already doing. "I mean, how much more can I do? I'd have to quit my job completely to make time for any more."

"Well, you've got a point there," said Rona.

———

One steamy summer day, a friend took me to his secret swimming hole two towns over. I grew up on a river, but I hadn't swum much at all in years. I didn't know of any nearby bodies of water other than the icy ocean, and I'd stopped swimming in pools because I was afraid that with regular chlorine exposure, I'd develop an additional sensitivity that would constrict my life even more.

In the river, the water surrounded and held me, just as it always had when I was a girl. Above me, the blue sky. All around, trees. The mussels embedded in the sand below me. The quiet trickling sound of the water as I dipped and breathed, dipped and breathed, right arm, left arm, kick, kick, kick. We swam across the river and back and it felt so good to be in my body.

When we were finished, I noticed that my breathing was deep and calm. I wondered what would happen if I swam in that river every chance I could all summer long. What would happen to my anxiety? My insomnia? I decided to find out.

I did my best to squeeze all my clients in by five P.M. twice a week so I could get out of work at six instead of eight, and on these days I rushed home, an eight-minute walk, then threw on my bathing suit and grabbed my goggles and towel. I sped to get to the river before dark, a twenty-five-minute drive, then swam across the river and back, twenty minutes, then drove home, changed clothes, cooked and ate dinner, climbed into bed and did some more administrative work, set my alarm for seven A.M., read a page or two of nonfiction and another page or two of fiction, and turned the lights out around midnight.

All summer long I swam. I swam once or twice on weekdays and once or twice weekends, three times a week until the water was cold enough to make my teeth chatter, and then I decided to keep swimming, chlorine be damned, at the community pool.

I felt calm after a swim, embodied. I could breathe. My new routine didn't cure me, but it did help to ratchet the anxiety down a notch. I still had to dose myself with melatonin and Ambien staggered throughout the night to get me through till morning, but now it generally worked.

In the water I didn't feel like I was underwater. In the water I didn't feel like I was drowning, like I was sinking. In the water I could float.

———

After several years, Frank and I decided to move in together. We wanted to buy a house, but even with our combined incomes, it seemed completely out of reach. On our drive to the dog park every weekend, I gawked at all the homes we couldn't have.

"When we get a house, can it have a red door?" I asked. "Can we get a house with a yard . . . for chickens?" "When we get a house, can we plant sunflowers and morning glories?"

"Sure," said Frank each time, humoring me.

We found a mortgage broker who ran the numbers, and we started looking. There was a house we could afford next to the highway on-ramp. And by the railroad tracks near the jail, one that stank of air freshener, probably to hide the smell of mold. And one with asbestos siding and a furnace in the kitchen. "I don't think that's quite to code," said our Realtor with a wry smile.

We were in our mid-forties, we worked hard, and we couldn't afford a house we could safely and peacefully live in.

John, our Realtor, told us we could open up our options if we considered a duplex, and so our mortgage broker ran the numbers again, and John took us around to see some other places and then we found a sweet little duplex with a tiny front garden and a picket fence and a little backyard, big enough for a chicken pen.

When we climbed the front steps, I tugged at Frank's sleeve. "Look!" I whispered. "It has a red door!"

And so we bought the house with the red door. Frank built a coop for the chickens, which came in a peeping box via U.S. Mail, and three years later, in 2013, we got married.

———

But I could feel the cougar following me as I walked home from work in the dark. It slipped into the house with me, watched me while I ate my dinner, sat vigilant after I switched off the light and tried to fall asleep.

My cougar told me it wouldn't leave until all those piles were gone. And so every weekday, three weeks out of the month, I kept processing the papers, kept trying to dwindle the piles, but then more papers arrived, and so the cougar stayed.

CHAPTER 11

Gilt

When Donald Trump moved into the White House, he put in a request with the Guggenheim to borrow Van Gogh's *Landscape with Snow* for his private living quarters, but curator Nancy Spector told him the painting was unavailable. She offered him an 18-karat golden toilet instead. The artist, Maurizio Cattelan, had proposed the installation—a functioning toilet in a private stall—just after the billionaire business magnate and reality TV star announced his bid for presidency in mid-2015. Describing the piece as "one-percent art for the ninety-nine percent," Cattelan invoked the catalyzing 2011 Occupy Wall Street catchphrase that critiqued the inequitable distribution of wealth and power in the United States. He called his piece *"America."* At the time, few people imagined that the man with a well-documented penchant for gilded fixtures would soon be a fixture in the White House.

Alice James lived in America's first Gilded Age: now we're in another.

———

During the first Gilded Age, former president Rutherford B. Hayes lamented in his journal that America's government for the people was becoming "government of the corporation, by the corporation, and for the corporation." Industrialists lived by their own rules, using the emerging tenets of Social Darwinism—which assured the rich that the poor were impoverished due to inherent evolutionary shortcomings—to justify laissez-faire capitalism, ruthless competition, and social stratification. Between 1860 and 1900 the top 2 percent owned more than a third of the nation's wealth. Since the government hadn't caught up yet with all the technological innovations, a dearth of regulations left the door open for robber barons like John D. Rockefeller, Cornelius Vanderbilt, Andrew Carnegie, J. P. Morgan, and others to amass their fortunes in the fledgling industries of railroads, oil, steel, and finance.

Rockefeller, the owner of Standard Oil, conspired with railroad magnate Cornelius Vanderbilt to artificially ratchet up the price charged to competing oil companies for railroad shipping. Then when profits foundered, he bought the failing businesses for a fraction of what they were worth and formed a monopoly. J. P. Morgan took a similar tack, monopolizing the railroad industry by buying up smaller companies and dropping prices until the remaining rivals went bankrupt trying to compete, then buying out his competitors, cutting wages, and slashing the workforce. Carnegie closed his Pennsylvania steelworks in order to crush the union and bully his workers into accepting a substantial cut in pay.

The Sherman Antitrust Act of 1890 was written in response to unscrupulous market manipulations of this ilk. It prevented price-fixing by restricting the formation of cartels such as the one schemed by Rockefeller and Vanderbilt. As Senator John Sherman argued, calling forth America's very foundations in defense of the act he authored, "If we will not endure a king as a political power we should not endure a king over the production, transportation, and sale of any of the necessaries of life."

In 1904, President Theodore Roosevelt ordered the U.S. Department of Justice to break up Morgan's railroad monopoly, a decision upheld by the Supreme Court. Seven years later, a SCOTUS ruling finally dismantled Rockefeller's Standard Oil, splitting it into over thirty individual companies.

In 1913, a federal committee concluded that J. P. Morgan and two other financiers headed an illegal cartel of bankers and insurance firms known as the money trust, which controlled the U.S. economy, monetary system, and financial industry via manipulative control of the New York Stock Exchange and evasion of interstate trade laws. Clearly, the Sherman Act had failed to effectively curb the power of corporations to create trusts and monopolies. So President Woodrow Wilson signed the stronger Clayton Antitrust Act into law in 1914. The act also declared boycotts, labor unions, and strikes legal under federal law.

These rulings were made in order to regulate businesses; now, however, these very laws are used *against* unions. In 1954, Supreme Court Justice William O. Douglas criticized the judiciary for the lopsided ways that it interpreted and enforced antitrust law: "From the beginning it has been applied by judges hostile to its purposes, friendly to the empire builders who wanted it emasculated . . . trusts that were dissolved reintegrated in new forms. . . . It is ironic that the Sherman Act was truly effective in only one respect, and that was when it was applied to labor unions. Then the courts read it with a literalness that never appeared in their other decisions."

I once called up a therapist colleague to discuss organizing for better reimbursement rates from certain insurance companies notorious for paying egregiously low fees, but he informed me that due to antitrust laws we could get into legal hot water if we did so. I couldn't fathom it at the time. Now I understand.

———

Just a few months before the first Occupy Wall Street protesters set up camp in Zuccotti Park in 2011, economist Joseph Stiglitz published a piece in *Vanity Fair* called "Of the 1%, by the 1%, for the 1%." Remarking that "monopolies and near monopolies have always been a source of economic power—from John D. Rockefeller at the beginning of the last century to Bill Gates at the end," Stiglitz added that "lax enforcement of anti-trust laws, especially during Republican administrations, has been a godsend to the 1 percent."

He went on to say that when the 2010 Supreme Court *Citizens United* decision removed limitations on campaign spending, it "enshrined the right of corporations to buy government." And tax cuts have favored the rich: the Reagan tax cuts of 1981, the Bush tax cuts of 2001 and 2003, and the Trump tax cuts of 2017 dramatically reduced taxes for wealthy Americans. In July 2018, *The New York Times* reported that as a result of all those cuts, the top 1 percent would pay $111 billion less in federal taxes that year than they would have if the 2000 tax laws had remained untouched.

"Virtually all U.S. senators, and most of the representatives in the House," wrote Stiglitz, "are members of the top 1 percent when they arrive, are kept in office by money from the top 1 percent, and know that if they serve the top 1 percent well they will be rewarded by the top 1 percent when they leave office." So our representatives are not representing 99 percent of their constituents. And this has had a big impact on our so-called land of opportunity. "America has long prided itself on being a fair society, where everyone has an equal chance of getting ahead," wrote Stiglitz, "but the statistics suggest otherwise: the chances of a poor citizen, or even a middle-class citizen, making it to the top in America are smaller than in many countries of Europe."

Income inequality has swelled since the 1970s. While the average income of the top 1 percent has shot up by 240 percent, average wages for regular Americans have stagnated. Nearly 80 percent of Americans live paycheck to paycheck. America's top 1 percent take home about 19 percent of the income, while the country's bottom 90 percent owe about three-quarters of the country's record-high $13.5 trillion in household debt.

No wonder a Harvard study found that 51 percent of young adults between eighteen and twenty-nine disagree with the principles of capitalism, three-quarters have a favorable view of unions, and 33 percent support socialism. America's runaway capitalism isn't working.

Unchecked economic growth is like a cancer. If unstopped, it eventually kills the body it inhabits.

The corrupt cell at the epicenter of America's malignant form of capitalism is slavery. Sociologist Matthew Desmond made this abundantly clear in his essay for *The New York Times Magazine's* 1619 Project, where he revealed how slavery has been encoded in our founding documents, our laws governing private property and financial regulation, and even our legislative structure all the way down to the electoral college, which ensured that slaveholding states held disproportionate political power in congressional and presidential elections.

On the plantations, owners assessed each worker's productivity using spreadsheets from Thomas Affleck's *Cotton Plantation Record and Account Book*, first published around 1850, which also taught them how to calculate depreciation, a new accounting tool, which assessed the market value of enslaved people according to age, strength, gender, etc.

The White House was built by enslaved workers, and as Tiya Miles points out in another 1619 Project essay, "the original wall for which Wall Street is named was built by the enslaved at a site that served as the city's first organized slave auction."

In 1881, robber baron Leland Stanford, owner of the Southern Pacific Railroad Company, balked at a special tax and took his complaint to court, co-opting the Fourteenth Amendment—which was ratified after the Civil War to grant citizenship and civil rights to enslaved people who had been emancipated after the war—to argue that the tax was an unconstitutional act of discrimination. The case went all the way to the Supreme Court.

According to Adam Winkler, author of *We the Corporations: How American Businesses Won Their Civil Rights*, Stanford's lawyer, Roscoe Conkling, had as a young congressman served on the committee responsible for writing the Fourteenth Amendment. Now the last surviving member of the committee, Conkling argued in court that the drafters had changed the wording of the amendment, replacing "citizens" with "persons" so that corporations could be covered, too. Holding up for evidence an old journal that he claimed was a previously unpublished record of the drafting committee's deliberations, Conkling argued that laws referring to "persons" had "by long and constant acceptance . . . been held to embrace artificial persons as well as natural persons."

Over fifty years later, a deaf law librarian named Howard Jay Graham, who became the country's leading expert on the Fourteenth Amendment, made a pivotal discovery. Although the journal was indeed a record of the congressional committee's deliberations, the language of the equal-protection clause was never in fact changed from "citizen" to "person" and the journal contained no evidence whatsoever that the drafters intended to protect corporations.

The case wound up being settled without a decision being issued, and in a similar case with Southern Pacific, the justices declined to decide on corporate personhood. However, a former president of a different railroad company, J. C. Bancroft Davis, whose job as "reporter of decisions" was to write the summary of the court's opinion, falsely wrote that the court had ruled that "corporations are persons within . . . the Fourteenth Amendment." Later one of the court justices, Stephen J. Field, who knew this was not true, nonetheless proclaimed in an opinion on an unrelated case that "corporations are persons within the meaning" of the Fourteenth Amendment: "It was so held in *Santa Clara County v. Southern Pacific Railroad.*"

And so it began. With that, Field declared legal precedent where none existed. The case would be cited over and over by courts across the country, even by the Supreme Court itself, in order to justify striking down regulatory and labor laws. Over a century later, it's still used as the grounds for corporations to successfully argue that campaign donations are a form of free speech.

And that is how an amendment to protect the rights of Black Americans—ratified when Alice was nineteen years old—came to be used to endow corporations with the rights of people.

———

Not unlike railroads, the internet creates networks that connect people and goods—and for a few ruthless capitalists affords great opportunity for wealth. In a November 2018 interview in *The Sun*, Stacy Mitchell, co-executive director of the Institute for Local Self-Reliance and author of *Big-Box Swindle: The True Cost of Mega-Retailers and the Fight for America's Independent Businesses*, characterized the current CEOs of Amazon, Google, and Facebook (now Meta) as the robber barons of our day: "It's striking how similar this history is to what Amazon has done: a new technology comes along that gives people a novel way to bring their wares to market, but a single company gains control over it and uses that power to undermine competitors and create a monopoly."

Taking a page from John D. Rockefeller's book and flouting the antitrust laws that were put in place toward the end of the first Gilded Age, Amazon's Jeff Bezos—the fourth-richest person in the world—endeavors to buy out successful online retailers, and if they won't sell, markets their product for less than Amazon pays for it, taking losses in the millions so that the other company can't compete and is forced to sell. This is called predatory pricing, and it's precisely what happened to Diapers.com and online shoe retailer Zappos.

In 2018, Amazon racked up more than $11 billion in profits, paid

$0 in U.S. federal income tax, and received a $129 million federal tax rebate. All done legally, thanks to tax laws that favor corporations over workers.

"In the 1970s," said Mitchell, "a group of legal and economic scholars . . . argued that corporate consolidation should be allowed to go unchecked as long as consumer prices stayed low. The Reagan administration embraced this view. . . . Subsequent administrations, including Democrats, followed suit."

The U.S. has done little to limit the power of megacorporations like these. In 2017, the European Commission slapped Google with a record $2.7 billion antitrust fine after determining that by using its search engine to unfairly drive consumers to its own shopping platform the tech monolith had denied people "a genuine choice." But four years earlier in the United States, the Federal Trade Commission made the opposite determination in a similar case against Google. And after Facebook acquired Instagram and WhatsApp, more than forty state attorneys general took the corporation to court for antitrust violations, but a judge threw the case out.

In 2020, however, the House Judiciary subcommittee on antitrust released a report accusing Amazon, Google, Facebook, and Apple of monopolizing the marketplace in ways that do harm to the business climate and to consumers. The report recommended strengthening antitrust laws and enforcement.

———

Of course, the way monopolies keep prices low is by paying workers less. And when there's little competition, there are fewer employment alternatives, making it harder for people to negotiate for better wages and working conditions.

Amazon's warehouse workers are heavily monitored, says Mitchell. "Because the warehouses are so automated, the workers are in service to the machines, instead of the other way around. They have devices that tell them what item to pull from the shelves and count down the seconds they have to do it. It's difficult to take a break" and "injuries are common." Amazon has fought hard to fend off unionization, but after former rapper Chris Smalls staged a March 2020 walkout to demand better COVID-19 protections at the Staten Island warehouse where he worked—an act that got him fired—he tapped into his social justice values, his facility with language, and his creativity to lead the first successful campaign to unionize the company in the United States.

American approval of unions is the highest it's been since 1965, and the number of union filings in the first six months of fiscal year 2022 was 57 percent higher than the year before. First-ever unions have now formed at Starbucks, Google, Apple, Microsoft, and Trader Joe's, among others.

———

Because of their mandate to maximize shareholder wealth, corporate executives bemoan government regulations, contending that corporations should be entrusted with regulating themselves. To that end, in the early 1970s—reacting to an increase in government regulations protecting consumer and worker safety, human rights, and the environment—corporations started to post lobbyists in their own Washington, DC, offices. Until that time, says William Niskanen, chairman of the Cato Institute, a libertarian think tank, "relatively few corporations had much of a public role in federal politics." Now, however, all major corporations have lobbyists in Washington. I don't think it's an accident that worker pay stagnated in 1973.

Thanks to the 2010 *Citizens United* ruling, corporations now hold a great deal of influence over political decision-making through the donations they shower upon legislators. In the words of Anne Wexler, then one of the top corporate lobbyists in DC, "corporations essentially feel they're partners with government. . . . Essentially, the business/government relationship is a symbiotic relationship."

In his 2004 book *The Corporation: The Pathological Pursuit of Profit and Power*, corporate law professor Joel Bakan describes the ties between regulatory agencies and the corporations they are charged with regulating. "In addition to lobbying, corporations enjoy direct representation in government . . . certainly to a much greater degree than any other group in society, by virtue of the disproportionate number of high-ranking government officials who were formerly top executives."

Most notoriously, before he was Trump's pick to head the EPA (he was forced to resign due to ethical violations), Scott Pruitt, as Oklahoma's attorney general, worked closely with fossil fuel companies to fight federal environmental regulations. His successor, Andrew Wheeler, was a former coal industry lobbyist.

Erik Baptist, formerly a lobbyist and lawyer with the American Petroleum Institute, served as the EPA's deputy assistant administrator of the Office of Chemical Safety and Pollution Prevention from 2018–19. And Michael R. Taylor, deputy commissioner for foods at the FDA from 2010 to 2016, was previously Monsanto's vice president for public policy.

In 2018, there were over 160 former lobbyists serving under the Trump administration, and by the time he left office in 2021, over a hundred environmental rollbacks had been enacted, enough to "significantly increase greenhouse gas emissions over the next decade," according to *The New York Times*, "and lead to thousands of extra deaths from poor air quality each year."

———

America was founded on the principle that all people are created equal (well, except for Black, Indigenous, and people of color, and of course, women), and their rights and dreams matter. But when we gave corporations the rights of individuals, we took this ethos too far. As historian Howard Zinn said in Joel Bakan's companion to his book, the 2003 documentary *The Corporation*, "Corporations are given the rights of persons but they are persons with no moral conscience—designed by law to be concerned only with their stockholders," and not with stakeholders like workers, community members, or the environment. *Corpocracy* author Robert Monks added that "corporations have no soul to save and they have no *body* to incarcerate."

Consider the 2002 case of *Anderson v. General Motors Corp.*

On Christmas Eve in 1993, a drunk driver plowed into the rear end of Patricia Anderson's 1979 Chevy Malibu, which burst into flames, inflicting second- and third-degree burns on Anderson and her four children. Her five-year-old daughter's hand had to be amputated as a result of the accident, and the girl's face was permanently scarred.

The car ignited due to a cost-saving decision made by General Motors: the fuel tank was situated just eleven inches from the rear bumper, six inches closer than recommended.

Court proceedings revealed that General Motors had done a cost-benefit analysis before making this design change. The company had estimated that putting the fuel tanks at the recommended seventeen inches from the bumper would cost $8.59 per car. That was more than they wanted to pay, so they asked a GM analyst to use data to predict how many fuel-fed fire-related fatalities would occur if they instead put the fuel tanks where they wanted. The analyst did a calculation and multiplied that figure by an estimated $20,000 legal payout per fatality, and then divided that by the number of GM cars operating on U.S. highways at the time, concluding that each fuel-fed fire fatality would cost GM just $2.40 in payouts per vehicle sold. Even accounting for the predicted legal expenses, executives determined the company could thus save $6.19 per car by disregarding the recommendation, and made the decision to do so knowing that the new design would cause an increase in injuries and deaths.

GM was ultimately ordered to pay a $1.2 billion settlement—literally more than they'd bargained for.

The U.S. Chamber of Commerce came out on the side of GM, releasing a statement in support of such cost-benefit calculations. Because a corporation's primary function is to ensure the greatest possible profits for its shareholders, said the Chamber, abiding by such cost-benefit analyses is a "hallmark of good corporate behavior" and asserted that the logic underlying them is "unimpeachable."

In what world is making calculated choices to harm others "unimpeachable" behavior?

The corporate term for the trauma suffered by Patricia Anderson and her children is *externality*. In Bakan's documentary, economist Milton Friedman defines an externality against a backdrop of the classic pie fight scene from Laurel and Hardy, in which a woman throws a pie at a man who ducks, and the pie instead hits an innocent bystander leaning against the counter behind him: "An externality is the effect of a transaction . . . on a third party who has not consented to or played any role in the carrying out of that transaction."

Also in the documentary, Harvard political economist Elaine Bernard offers some clarifying examples of corporate externalities when she describes how deregulation shifts costs from corporations onto individuals and society:

> If a factory is polluting, it's saving money. Why? Because it's using worse technology. It's using resources that it's not paying for, and it's putting the cost of that waste onto the community as a whole. So in the company's books it looks very good. In society's books it's running a big deficit. . . . And today I think that corporations are externalizing a lot of costs onto the community, whether it's the cost of burning out employees by increasing the work time, by working them for a few years and then throwing them out, by not paying the full cost of the labor that employees give to a firm, by coming into a community, getting all sorts of grants, and then

turning around and leaving it in worse shape than they entered. All of those things externalize the cost onto the community of the corporation.

Bakan consulted the psychologist Robert Hare, the internationally renowned expert behind the Hare Psychopathy Checklist, who confirmed that if corporations were *actually* people, they would fulfill many of the criteria to be diagnosed as psychopaths.

First, because they are *not* actually people, corporations are literally *incapable of feeling empathy*. Like many psychopaths, they are prone to *grandiose* bragging about their accomplishments, perhaps most particularly in their annual reports to their shareholders, and their advertising campaigns give them a *superficial charm. Endlessly in need of stimulation*, corporations are always doing new and different things. Such as building a smaller Chevy with the fuel tank closer to the bumper. *They intentionally manipulate and exploit others* for financial gain, *lie* when they must to protect the bottom line, and *fail to accept responsibility for their actions*.

Sometimes they *take pride in getting away with* cost-saving or profit-making crimes—such as releasing toxic chemicals into a river to save the cost of properly disposing of them or hiding the dangers to fetuses of chlorpyrifos, a common ingredient in flea bombs, from the EPA or lying to physicians about the addictiveness of OxyContin. Corporations are *cunning* and *ruthless* in their pursuit of profit. As Bakan points out in his book,

> No one would seriously suggest that individuals should regulate themselves, that laws against murder, assault, and theft are unnecessary because people are socially responsible. Yet oddly, we are asked to believe that corporate persons—institutional psychopaths who lack any sense of moral conviction and have the power and motivation to cause harm and devastation in the world—should be left free to govern themselves.

The corporation and the state are not "partners," says Bakan. The state signs corporations into existence, and the state must take charge of keeping them in line. Our lives depend on it, and something more: our ability to live a good life depends on it, too.

———

To most people, the American dream is the idea that anyone who works hard can achieve success in this country because we don't have a rigid class system and everyone is afforded equal opportunity. But literary scholar Sarah Churchwell, author of *Behold, America: The Entangled History of "America First" and "The American Dream,"* says that the common association of the American dream with "gritty individual achievement" is a deviation from its original meaning. The term was first regularly used, she says, in response to monopoly capitalism.

In a 2019 interview in *Pacific Standard*, Churchwell explained that she found the earliest references to the term in the Gilded Age media.

There was . . . this new thing called a multimillionaire that America had never seen before. And people on the left said that if this multimillionaire is allowed to take hold of American society, it will mean the death of the American dream. One newspaper called it an *un*-American dream, because the American dream is of egalitarianism. It's of equality, of opportunity for all, not just for the privileged few.

And they saw very quickly that if you allow that kind of private wealth to consolidate and establish itself, you're going to replicate an aristocracy, which is exactly what the American government was designed to resist.

Those who first wrote of the American dream knew that the

wealthiest Americans would be able to control government interests and wanted to remind people of the values envisioned by the country's founders. "You'll hear right-wing pundits say that the American dream is antithetical to any kind of welfare state, to any kind of social democratic impulse," said Churchwell. "But it turns out that the phrase was coined to argue for exactly those kinds of social safety nets, and to argue against the privatization of wealth."

In the 1950s the American dream was repackaged for postwar America to bolster a message of consumption. The American dream began to have something to do with a new car in the driveway, tidy flower beds, a white picket fence, and the belief that these commodities—symbols, really—are acquired as a result of independence, honest labor, and good character. Those who fail to achieve this picture of the American dream are thus seen as lacking these qualities.

Our misguided approach to the pursuit of happiness has led us astray. Despite all that we own, despite living in the wealthiest nation in the world, America only ranks sixteenth on the United Nations' World Happiness Report. The top ten are mostly Nordic countries with strong social welfare systems and an emphasis on equality. The United States is the only country of the top twenty scorers that doesn't offer some form of universal healthcare.

———

While research verifies that money does indeed buy happiness, it also shows that once a person's individual income exceeds a certain amount, happiness starts to decline. A 2018 study found that on average, Americans who earned between $65,000 and $95,000 were happiest. This was enough for people in most of the country to adequately meet basic needs for food, housing, and medical care, with a little left over for vacations, meals out, and purchases. Rich experiences and interpersonal connection bring more lasting satisfaction than conspicuous consumption.

This happiness quotient holds true for nations, too. Evidence shows that happiness increased in countries like India, Mexico, and Brazil as they rose from poverty and began to experience economic growth. But once countries hit a certain economic threshold, happiness doesn't go up. In the United States, happiness has stagnated since 1975.

———

In the 1970s, in a rare interview with a reporter, the young king of the Himalayan country of Bhutan made a revolutionary statement. When the reporter asked, "What is your gross national product?" King Jigme Singye Wangchuck replied, "We do not believe in Gross National Product, because Gross National Happiness is more important." Recognizing that a Western-style pursuit of wealth and unlimited growth is harmful to communities and ecosystems, during the three decades of his reign, he set about defining a measurement of happiness that included health and psychological well-being, education, work-life balance, living standards, community vitality, cultural diversity, ecological resilience, and good governance. While the country's Gross National Happiness index does not reject material and economic progress, it does reject the pursuit of economic prosperity and growth as an end in itself without regard to other aspects of well-being. The king began implementing policies based on these ideals, ultimately introducing a form of parliamentary democracy.

The new government built into its constitution a commitment to preserve at least 60 percent of its territory as forest, and it's the first carbon-neutral country in the world. Its food production is 100 percent organic, and the country even has universal healthcare.

The head of Bhutan's Ministry of Information and Communication, Kinley Dorji, echoing the U.S. Declaration of Independence with its claims for the right to life, liberty, and the pursuit of happiness, told a *New York Times* reporter: "Happiness itself is an individual pursuit. Gross National Happiness then becomes a responsibility of the state, to create an environment where citizens can pursue happiness. It's not a guarantee of happiness by the government. . . . But there is a responsibility to, you know, create the conditions for happiness." He added, "When we say 'happiness,' we have to be very clear that it's not fun, pleasure, thrill, excitement, all the temporary fleeting senses. It is permanent contentment—with life, with what you have. That lies within the self. Because the bigger house, the faster car, the nicer clothes, they don't give you that contentment." In other words, the Bhutan government is responsible for creating the conditions for happiness based on the principles of Gross National Happiness, and happiness isn't found through consumption.

———

Of course, there's no such thing as Shangri-la, especially when television enters the picture. A few years after Bhutan became the last country in the world to get TV (in 1999), a group of Bhutanese academics conducted a study about its impact on the culture. They found "dramatic changes" to society, with increases in crime and corruption, and a high demand for Western products. Schools were faced with new discipline issues, including substance use, violence, and greed. The authors of a 2003 piece in *The Guardian* wrote: "Cable TV has created, with acute speed, a nation of hungry consumers from a kingdom that once acted collectively and spiritually." Now, more than 35 percent of parents would rather watch TV than talk to their children. Suicide rates have also risen.

Nonetheless, King Jigme Singye Wangchuck's brainchild has left an indelible legacy. In 2011, the United Nations unanimously adopted a General Assembly resolution, introduced by Bhutan with support from sixty-eight member states, calling for a "holistic approach to development" that promoted sustainable happiness and well-being. This was followed in April 2012 by a UN High-Level Meeting that brought together hundreds of government and business representatives, economists, scholars, and spiritual leaders to develop a new economic paradigm based on sustainability and well-being. The first World Happiness Report was released in 2012.

In 2011, researchers at the Faculty of Applied Health Sciences at the University of Waterloo in Ontario designed the Canadian Index of Wellbeing, which has been helping to drive change in municipal, provincial, and federal governments.

And in 2019 New Zealand became the first major country to institute a national budget that explicitly prioritizes well-being.

In the United States, there has been a movement afoot since 2003 to implement a well-being measure that is currently called a Key National Indicator System—a decidedly uninspiring name—but so far this has not come to fruition.

———

By thirty-eight, Alice had come to some peace with her illness and understood it within the wider context of the suffering and inequity in the world. In a letter to William she wrote: "Amidst the horrors of which I hear and read my woes seem of a very pale tint." She followed politics closely because she knew that elections and court decisions and strikes and protests all have repercussions that impact people's well-being, and she was emotionally invested in the stakes. In an 1888 letter from England to William and his wife in America, Alice referred to the upcoming U.S. presidential election and wrote that her insides "cramp themselves so convulsively over every little public event here." Our frailties are as collective as our well-being. This, Alice understood.

———

In "Are We on the Road to Civilisation Collapse?" Luke Kemp, PhD, a researcher at the Centre for the Study of Existential Risk at the University of Cambridge, writes that collapse "is a tipping point phenomena, when compounding stressors overrun societal coping capacity." Kemp lists several stressors that researchers have found to be historically associated with empire collapse, including environmental degradation, climatic change, and inequality and oligarchy.

The ecological collapse theory, says Kemp, suggests that "collapse can occur when societies overshoot the carrying capacity of their environment." Excessive deforestation, water pollution, soil degradation, and the loss of biodiversity can precipitate collapse, and of course, all of these are already worldwide issues. In addition, we're running out of oil. Kemp references a 2011 paper published in the *Annals of the New York Academy of Sciences*, which states that the depletion of conventional crude oil "may pose a problem for continued economic growth."

The collapse of the Mayan and Roman empires, among many others, coincided with abrupt climate changes, says Kemp—usually droughts. Now we face a global climate crisis. On a graph, the towering spike in carbon dioxide (CO_2) begins its steep ascent during the Industrial Revolution, when CO_2 was around 280 parts per million (ppm); in January 2022, the CO_2 in our atmosphere cleared 417 ppm.

America is the biggest producer of greenhouse gases after China; its cumulative emissions since 1750, however, make it far and away the all-time leading producer of greenhouse gases and thus the country that bears the greatest responsibility for climate change. Global temperatures are climbing, oceans are warming, glaciers melting, sea levels rising, the ocean acidifying, and the number of record temperatures, intense weather events, and out-of-control forest fires growing.

Inequality is another central driver of collapse, says Kemp, not only because it causes social distress, but also because it impedes a society's ability to respond adequately to ecological, social, and economic problems. He cites anthropologist Kevin MacKay, author of *Radical Transformation: Oligarchy, Collapse, and the Crisis of Civilization*, who points out that in an oligarchy, "a numerically small, self-interested elite" makes decisions in its own interests, at the expense of the best interests of society as a whole.

I wonder if an empire collapses the way a body does: slowly and then suddenly, an accretion of minor insults finally overwhelming the system, a squandering of capital—and then . . . total bankruptcy.

PART IV

First, Do No Harm

The biomedical model, like an X ray, is ultimately a representation, one so powerful and persuasive that we often mistake it for fact. No matter how factual we consider it, the biomedical model also generates a flow of related narrative images—the body as a machine, for example, and disease as a mechanical defect—that profoundly influences how we think about our illnesses.

—David B. Morris, *Illness and Culture in the Postmodern Age*

The ideal of every science is that of a closed and completed system of truth. . . . Phenomena unclassifiable within the system are therefore paradoxical absurdities, and must be held untrue. . . . Only the born geniuses let themselves be worried and fascinated by these outstanding exceptions, and get no peace till they are brought within the fold. Your Galileos . . . and Darwins are always getting confounded and troubled by insignificant things. *Anyone* will renovate his science who will steadily look after the irregular phenomena. And when the science is renewed, its new formulas often have more of the voice of the exceptions in them than of what were supposed to be the rules.

—William James, "The Hidden Self"

There are more things in heaven and earth, Horatio,
Than are dreamt of in your philosophy.

—William Shakespeare, *Hamlet* (Act 1, Scene 5),
Hamlet to Horatio

CHAPTER 12

Asylum

I learned that a leading-edge health center I'd long admired had begun taking on affiliate practitioners. True North was an integrative healthcare practice founded on the idea that healing happens through relationship, and that patient narratives are critical to effective treatment.

The Western view of the body as machine has led contemporary medicine to extract—with near-surgical precision—what has always been a critical component of the healing process: the patient-doctor relationship. Certainly, Alice remarked on the problem, even in her time: "[A]ll great doctors are chiefly interested in the diagnosis & don't care for anything else apparently," she opined, adding, with a tinge of her trademark irony, "They ought to have a lot of lesser men, like tenders, to do their dirty-work for them, curing their patients, etc."

Things have only gotten worse. Largely because of fee-for-service rather than time-based insurance payment structures, hospitals and practices push doctors to see as many patients as possible in the shortest amount of time, and the healing potential of the patient-doctor relationship has been badly compromised. Even doctors are dissatisfied with our current system, experiencing themselves as "technicians on an assembly line," according to the writer and cardiologist Sandeep Jauhar. Under the strain of this system, one study found that doctors interrupt their patients, on average, eighteen seconds after they start speaking. This despite the fact that the best predictor of improvement in patients seeking care for a wide range of common symptoms is not, according to two separate studies, whether the doctor ordered lab tests or which medications were prescribed, but whether the patient felt truly heard in the first visit.

True North was an effort to model a healthier kind of healthcare.

———

The seed for True North was planted one day when a book landed on Kathryn Landon-Malone's foot. A pediatric nurse practitioner, Kathryn was studying for her certificate in holistic nursing when it happened. Browsing the Women's Studies section at Barnes & Noble, she reached for a book, and as she pulled it off the shelf, another one fell on her foot: Christina Baldwin's *Calling the Circle: The First and Future Culture.*

Kathryn opened the book to its preface and began to read.

When people sit in Circle, wrote Baldwin—when everybody's voice is of equal value, and people speak and listen from the heart—monumental changes can happen. Baldwin called it *circle process.* The idea—derived from Indigenous practices—was simple, but profound.

Kathryn bought the book, took it home, and read it cover to cover. Later, in another of Baldwin's books, she read that every successful change movement begins with the same phrase: "Some friends and I started talking . . ." When Kathryn and some of her friends started talking, what they envisioned turned into True North.

Using circle process, decisions were discussed collaboratively and made by consensus. In monthly CircleCare presentations, practitioners from a broad range of disciplines shared the wisdom of their modalities as they reviewed specific cases, enhancing patient care by treating the whole person.

In the early days, says Kathryn, much of the work was about learning to be in relationship with one another. She found that it grounded her before seeing patients. "Everybody felt their practice gaining in depth, and their ability to be in relationship with their patients. . . . We called it reverent participatory relationship."

––––––

True North practitioners focused on patient health and the well-being of the circle. But on a macro level, how does one measure the health of a *nation*?

The most commonly used indicator is gross domestic product. By this measure, the United States really is number one. In 2019, the U.S. GDP was $21,410,230, far ahead of the second largest economy in the world, China, which had a GDP of $15,543,710. But the GDP is a really lopsided tool for measuring a country's prosperity because it focuses on just one thing: the dollar value of the goods and services produced. It does not measure whether a transaction benefited or harmed the environment, or how it affected communities or the quality of people's health.

Here are two hypothetical scenarios that illustrate this point:

- In Scenario 1, I drive to the local grocery store weekly and stock my kitchen with processed foods like corn dogs, potato chips, and Lucky Charms.
- In Scenario 2, I choose a healthier lifestyle. I grow my own organic vegetables, using compost made from food scraps and manure from my chickens. In exchange for eggs from my hens, my neighbor, a baker, trades me bread baked with local organic grains.

Which scenario is better for the country's gross domestic product?

In the first lifestyle, I'm spending money for gas, and because the mileage on my car keeps ticking upward, it needs more service and more parts. My food is first produced by industrial farmers who spend 48 percent of their crop revenue on fertilizer, genetically modified seeds, and herbicides. (So when I buy my box of cereal, I'm also paying for the trace pesticides that come in the box.) Those crops—soy, corn, wheat, sugarcane, etc.—are processed and sent to factories where preservatives, color enhancers, and other chemicals are added, transforming these products into tasty, fattening foods that are low in nutrition. So although I develop diabetes at fifty-five and heart disease at sixty, I have added to the economy's GDP. Then I bump up the GDP even further because of the medical care and pharmaceuticals I now need to try to keep from getting sicker.

But in the second scenario, to produce my vegetables I spend money on only a few items like seeds, a hoe, and organic feed for my hens. I don't need to drive as often, so I don't purchase as much gas and my car lasts longer and needs fewer repairs. I develop a relationship with my neighbor, who stops to chat sometimes when I am out on the porch, which gives a little boost to my mood and my immune system. I'm eating healthier food and getting a good workout in the garden—which also helps me be more connected to nature—and because of all this, as well as a fair measure of genetics and good fortune, I stay healthy, so I don't need meds or frequent doctor visits.

Environmentally, in the second scenario, honeybees pollinate my broccoli and melons, which in turn provide the bees with nectar for their hives. But in the first, herbicides wipe out the bees' food sources and mess with their microbiomes, leaving them more prone to disease. Colonies collapse. And the diesel-fueled tractors, combines, and long-haul trucks release carbon into the air, speeding up climate change, negatively impacting environmental and human health.

My junk-food-eating ways were bad for me and bad for the environment, but they were so much better for the GDP.

On the day of my first True North circle, I sat down in a sleek gray chair and looked around at all the faces in the room. I was sitting in a room full of strangers, but I knew that these healers were about to become my intimate colleagues, and I hoped that some of them might also become *my* healers.

True North's medical director, Dr. Bethany Hays, for instance, had come highly recommended by some of the people in my MCS support group, and I felt fortunate when she agreed to see me on a sliding scale.

When I arrived for my appointment, one of my colleagues there, a medical assistant named Jake, did the intake and checked my blood pressure. Bethany fetched me in the waiting area and I followed her through the curving periwinkle hall to her office. We sat down across from each other at a round table. At my left, the table was piled with papers, as was her desk across the room, as if her prodigious mind was overflowing.

The truth is, as a colleague, I found Bethany a little intimidating. Strong and smart, and not one to make small talk in the hallways, she cut an imposing figure. But sitting in her office as a patient felt wholly different from crossing paths with her in the hallway. She was still strong and smart, but also compassionate, curious, and fully present. I felt that she was on my team, that she really wanted to get to the bottom of what was ailing me and help me get better.

Bethany was one of the country's foremost experts in functional medicine, which I'd heard a lot about when we discussed cases in circle. To me it sounded like the medicine of the future.

The foundations of functional medicine can be traced to systems biology, which takes a holistic approach to the complexity and interconnectedness of biological systems, synthesizing an array of scientific disciplines—including biology, physics, computer science, engineering, and more—to, in the words of the Institute for Systems Biology, "develop solutions to the world's most pressing health and environmental issues," recognizing that "the networks that form the whole of living organisms are more than the sum of their parts."

While the Cartesian approach to medicine is responsible for extraordinary advances in treating infectious disease and trauma to bones and organs, it has been less effective at preventing and treating chronic illness, which is responsible for 90 percent of healthcare expenditures in the United States. Scientists once believed in the utopic idea that the puzzle of human disease could someday be entirely solved. Most recently, many imagined that deconstructing the human genome would finally put the pieces in place. But we learned instead that human biology is more complex than that, and that genes can be switched on and off depending on a person's environment and lifestyle.

Functional medicine uses an individualized, systems-oriented approach to address the myriad interactions between lifestyle (diet, exercise, psychosocial-spiritual factors, stress, and so on) and environment (phthalates in perfume, bisphenol A in cans, mercury in fish, and arsenic in wells—or wallpaper, for that matter) that can switch certain genetic predispositions on or off.

While conventional (allopathic) medicine focuses on suppression and management of symptoms, functional medicine shifts the focus to the "upstream" biochemical pathways to treat the underlying causes. For example, an allopathic doctor with a patient who complains of heartburn generally prescribes Prilosec or some other proton pump inhibitor (PPI) to reduce stomach acid. But a widely reported 2009 study found that PPIs can actually make the problem worse in the long run. A functional medicine doctor, on the other hand, would work to identify and treat the source of the problem by starting with a detailed biopsychosocial intake with the patient, respecting the patient's knowledge of their own body. The doctor would run tests to identify digestion, absorption, and inflammation issues and nutritional and metabolic imbalances that might explain why the patient is producing too much stomach acid, or more commonly, not enough or at the wrong time. A functional medicine practitioner would also consider downstream effects. For instance, inappropriate stomach acid production can put a person at risk for a disrupted bowel microbiome and/or faulty absorption of nutrients, which can cause further problems.

Doctor and patient would work collaboratively to design an achievable action plan that may include dietary changes (like cutting out fried foods and caffeinated beverages, interventions conventional doctors might also suggest), targeted nutraceuticals (vitamins, minerals, and essential fatty acids), and lifestyle changes (slowing down over meals and chewing more, incorporating stress management techniques, increasing physical activity, and improving sleep quality and quantity). Functional medicine doctors are trained to assess a patient's readiness for change, and recognize that providing the necessary guidance and support are as important as ordering the right tests and prescribing the right treatments. Their collaborative approach to care ensures that the patient is heard, enhances the therapeutic encounter, and increases patient motivation for change.

Unlike the fragmented, organ-system-based approach of allopathic doctors, functional medicine providers view the body as a complex network of systems with weblike interconnections. These practitioners work with the physiological processes that transcend anatomical boundaries, including absorption of nutrients, cellular defense and repair, cellular communication and transport mechanisms, energy production, and more.

Given the complexity of my illness and the failure of allopathic medicine to provide any useful treatments, functional medicine sounded like exactly what I needed. So I sat in that chair across from Bethany, ready to tell her the long and winding story of my illness.

———

Alice James, of course, had her own long and winding story. In September 1881, she moved back in with her parents when she and Katharine returned from their European travels. Four months later, just a few days after an asthma diagnosis, her mother suddenly died. Alice took over the care of her bereft father. Like others in the family, she was surprised to find herself equal to the task. But when her father—lost without his stalwart wife—quit eating that November, Alice collapsed.

She sought help from a new doctor, Henry Beach, who suspected, as her aunt Kate wrote to Henry, "something lying back of her nervousness" and ultimately diagnosed rheumatic gout, a form of arthritis caused by an excess of uric acid. Her health briefly improved under her new doctor's care, but the strain of her father's impending death was too much. She collapsed again in early December.

———

After her father's funeral, Alice went to stay with Katharine, who tended to her until sometime in January. Alice then returned to Boston's Beacon Hill to live with Henry in their father's house.

But her brother's company was not enough. In May of that year, deeply depressed and still ill, Alice checked herself into the Adams-Nervine Asylum, a private establishment in Boston that had opened just three years earlier to treat, as stipulated in the will of its founder, "nervous people who are not insane." The spacious, homelike facility, which at that time treated only women, provided extended care (on average, about four months) free of charge to those who could not afford to pay, and also accepted patients from the moneyed classes, whose fees were determined on a case-by-case basis. (Today we might call that a sliding scale.) Katharine Loring's father was the treasurer.

The resident physician, Dr. Frank Page, found that neurasthenia, hysteria, and melancholia struck all classes, and according to Strouse, he and his colleagues there "did not see nervous women as overeducated malingerers shirking their proper feminine functions or as histrionic victims of imaginary ills. Instead, they saw causes of nervous distress in the strain and fatigue of quintessential feminine functions—domestic overwork and excessive caring for others."

Alice's doctor prescribed a version of the Rest Cure that included vapor baths, massage, hot air, and mild galvanic electrical currents using something called the Holtz Electrical Machine to treat her nerves and muscles. The atmosphere at Adams-Nervine was designed to feel homelike, stressing the importance of patient dignity, individuality, freedom of movement, and a sense of community. (Interestingly, the interior walls were originally painted white, but when their "glaring whiteness" was found to be "trying to the vision of nervous invalids," wallpaper was installed. I wonder how many of these newly papered walls were tainted with arsenic?)

Alice convalesced there for just over three months, returning to stay with Katharine in Beverly, Massachusetts, in early August 1882. Her health was notably improved, but not miraculously so, according to Henry. In other words, there'd been no cure.

———

By November, Alice had moved back into her father's home and was again doing poorly. She established a daily routine that included rest, massage, and galvanic treatments, and Katharine came to visit whenever she could, but she was busy caring for her consumptive sister, Louisa. Then, in February 1884, Katharine and Louisa set sail for Europe in search of a better climate for Louisa's weak lungs, leaving a desolate Alice alone in Boston. Shortly thereafter, she moved to New York City to undergo treatments with a renowned neurologist named William B. Neftel, a Russian émigré who had cared for a number of the Jameses family friends.

Like her doctors at Adams-Nervine, Dr. Neftel treated his patients with galvanic electricity, which he believed stimulated dormant electrical currents and redirected those that had gone awry. But he advised the opposite of the Rest Cure: exercise.

At first, as it was with every new treatment, Alice was infused with hope. (It was the same for me.) She told her friend Fannie Morse that she felt a "wonderfull [*sic*] change quite as if I had been transformed." Her enthusiasm had tempered by the time she returned home, when she wrote more equivocally to her friend Sara Darwin that the treatment did her "a great deal of good in many ways." She was still sick.

So many times, Alice and I got our hopes up, only to be dashed. Not even the placebo effect could cure us.

———

Of course, in Alice's time there was no health insurance. Many people paid their medical bills on an informal sliding scale based on their income. The earliest health insurance was catastrophic coverage to cover a long hospital stay—protecting both patients and hospitals by ensuring patients' bills were paid.

One of the first insurers, Blue Cross Blue Shield (now Anthem Blue Cross Blue Shield, or Emblem, depending on location), was originally a nonprofit that welcomed all comers and charged the same rate to everyone, no matter how old or how sick. Between 1940 and 1955, the number of Americans with health insurance shot up from 10 percent to more than 60 percent, and enterprising capitalists soon figured out how they could profit from this demand. For-profit insurance companies accepted only younger, healthier members and charged rates that varied depending on a person's age and other factors. By the 1970s and '80s, for-profit plans like Aetna and Cigna dominated the market. The nonprofit Blue Cross Blue Shield couldn't compete, having been left to cover the oldest and sickest Americans. In 1994, the board of directors voted to allow Blue Cross Blue Shield insurers to become for-profit corporations.

The year before going for-profit, Blue Cross Blue Shield spent 95 cents out of every dollar of premiums on medical care. This is called an insurance company's *medical loss ratio*. Now, says Elisabeth Rosenthal—a physician who is also the author of *An American Sickness: How Healthcare Became Big Business and How You Can Take It Back*— the average medical loss ratio is closer to 80 percent, and sometimes even lower, with insurers using money saved on patient care to pay for marketing, lobbying, administration, high dividends to shareholders, and exorbitant salaries for executives.

In 2017, CEOs at the nation's insurance companies earned, in most cases, more than 300 times what their average employee earned. The annual salaries for the heads of Anthem, Aetna, and Cigna averaged over $18 million, not including stock options.

Rosenthal points out that the optimistic framers of the Affordable Care Act of 2010 (ACA) attempted to curtail spending unrelated to patient care by requiring insurance companies to sustain a medical loss ratio of at least 80 to 85 percent. (Medicare spends 98 percent of its budget on treatment and just 2 percent on administration.) The counterintuitive result of this restriction is that insurance companies now have greater motivation to make big payouts in order to be sure that their 15 percent is enough to cover lobbying and marketing expenses, investor dividends, and bloated executive salaries. (As Rosenthal puts it, "15 percent of a big sum is more than 15 percent of a smaller one.") Then, to cover shortfalls, premiums are raised the following year, passing costs down to the consumer.

This helps explain why rates keep going up. In 2017, those who had individual or family coverage through their employer paid an average of $7,240 a year in employee premium contributions and prospective out-of-pocket payments to meet deductibles. This potential spending totaled 11.7 percent of the nation's median income, up from 7.8 percent a decade earlier.

―――――

Of the over fifty wealthy industrialized countries, the United States is the only one without universal healthcare, and we spend twice as much on healthcare per person, on average, than any other country—almost one-fifth of our gross domestic product. Remarkably, we nonetheless manage to rank dead last on overall performance compared to other high-income countries, including Canada, Australia, New Zealand, France, Germany, Norway, the Netherlands, Sweden, Switzerland, and the United Kingdom. More than half of all U.S. bankruptcies are due in part to healthcare expenses. In 2018, 250,000 GoFundMe campaigns requested help paying for medical treatment.

We spend more than $3 trillion a year on healthcare, yet have poorer health and shorter life expectancies than these other wealthy countries, ranking dead last in healthcare outcomes, equity, access, and administrative efficiency (and ninth on the subdomain of timeliness, contrary to some people's beliefs about how we compare to countries with universal healthcare). Many of these subpar outcomes can be attributed to our lack of universal healthcare. But even many insured Americans have incomplete and fragmented coverage and face far higher deductibles and out-of-pocket expenses than citizens of other countries. And our for-profit system is overreliant on drugs and technologies.

Lost productivity due to illness costs U.S. employers $530 billion a year.

―――――

So that they could schedule medical consultations that would allow time to integrate relationship, collaboration, and patient narratives into treatment, the on-site practitioners at True North were not enrolled with insurances. But that choice risked putting this relational form of care out of reach to many, particularly those unable to work due to their disabling health conditions. In an effort to increase accessibility, practitioners who signed on with True North, whether as on-site providers or as affiliates like me, contracted to provide 10 percent of their care for free or on a generous sliding scale for patients who would not otherwise be able to afford it.

Patients with high-deductible coverage sometimes had health savings plans that could be used to pay for their True North appointments. Others with better plans were able to send their receipts to their insurance company and get at least a partial reimbursement. Still others with good plans were financially comfortable enough to afford out-of-pocket treatment. Some were uninsured and chose to invest in the kind of healthcare that True North provided. In many cases this was because mainstream medical treatments had failed them.

———

Through the window of Bethany's office, I could see the edge of a small green forest; on the wall, a black-and-white photo of a mother lovingly breastfeeding her baby. Bethany, who had previously practiced as an ob-gyn, took a detailed history, much like Dr. Py had years before. When she asked me to describe my fatigue, I said, "Sometimes when it gets really bad, I feel like I am holding myself up, almost like I'm wearing a suit of armor."

Bethany nodded knowingly. "That's adrenaline," she said.

At the end of our hour and a half together, she prescribed a medication and several supplements to help address a suspected leaky gut issue, explaining that intestinal permeability can trigger inflammation and food sensitivities and has been linked to ME/CFS. She ordered a

NutrEval test that would assess oxidative stress, nutritional deficiencies, amino acid levels, and gastrointestinal dysfunctions that may have been contributing to my poor health. She also recommended a DetoxiGenomic profile, which would reveal my genetic risk for impaired detoxification capacity, specific chemical sensitivities, and medications that my body would find difficult to process. Both tests were designed by Genova Diagnostics, a federally licensed lab that applies a systems-based approach to its test design, guiding targeted treatment based on the web of relationships within the body. But neither of these tests was covered by my Medicare, and I couldn't afford both of them. Despite having to skip the DetoxiGenomic profile for the time being, I nonetheless left her office full of hope.

True North practitioners were encouraged to schedule introductory appointments with other True North providers so that we could get a sense of what everybody had to offer and send each other referrals. I'd scheduled a massage for immediately after my appointment, so I headed straight down the hall to Melissa's office. I'd been at odds with my body for so long, it seemed to me that a soothing massage would help put me back in it. And so it did—for a little while at least.

———

In 2009, a study in the *American Journal of Public Health* found that as many as 44,789 Americans died every year due to lack of health insurance—which among causes of death put it above kidney disease. At that time, 46 million Americans were completely uninsured. Thanks to the ACA, the number of uninsured Americans has now shrunk to 28.9 million. But that's still a heck of a lot of people with no healthcare coverage. A quick calculation, prorating deaths based on our smaller percentage of uninsured Americans, suggests that even under the ACA, up to 28,139 may die each year simply because they can't afford insurance.

It's not hard to imagine how insurance helps people stay alive. Uninsured people are more likely to postpone or forgo necessary care. They are less likely to receive preventive care and services for major health conditions and chronic diseases. A third of uninsured Americans can't afford to take their meds as prescribed. (Even 8 percent of those with private insurance cut back on their meds to try to save money.) And because people without health coverage are less likely to receive regular outpatient care, they're more likely to land in the hospital, where they receive fewer diagnostic and therapeutic services and also have higher mortality rates than those covered by insurance.

———

The Affordable Care Act has enabled almost 20 million Americans—including those with preexisting conditions—to purchase health insurance, but regardless of whether their insurance comes through their employer or the ACA marketplace, more than 25 percent of insured adults between the ages of nineteen and sixty-four are not adequately covered.

In 2009, although I had Medicare coverage, I was nonetheless spending $442 per month on out-of-pocket healthcare expenses. So, despite being insured, I was spending 20 percent of my income on healthcare. No wonder I was so stressed. A fifth of my working hours were spent earning enough to pay for the healthcare I needed in order to be able to continue to work—and maybe even recover.

Unsurprisingly, half of underinsured adults said they had problems with medical bills or debt, and two out of five reported not getting needed care due to cost.

Given these numbers, it's hard to fathom why universal coverage is even up for debate.

———

The federal government is the single largest healthcare payer in the United States, covering more than a quarter of all healthcare expenditures, and in its dual role as regulator and payer, it performs a powerful function in guiding healthcare policy. But problematically, as Elisabeth Rosenthal remarks in *An American Sickness*, "Medicare put the American Medical Association in charge of determining fair value and payment." Allowing the AMA to decide how much doctors get paid is, she says, "akin to letting the American Petroleum Institute decide what BP and Shell and ExxonMobil can charge us" for gas.

Reimbursement is based on relative value units (RVUs), which are determined by calculating the average time doctors spend on each category of visit or intervention, the average overhead incurred in delivering the service, and the cost for training and malpractice insurance. But the time assigned to procedures "is often wildly inaccurate," says Rosenthal. "The RVU panel determines the time it takes to perform a service by polling several dozen specialists who actually do the procedure, which is essentially asking them whether or not they want to be paid more." One study revealed that the 2014 estimates were longer than actual times for twenty out of twenty-four procedures, including hysterectomy, cataract removal, and upper GI endoscopy—sometimes by as much as double.

Perhaps because specialists dominate the panel that determines payment rates, the system sets rates for surgeries, scans, and other procedures that are much higher than those for checkups and management of existing conditions. For example, as primary care physician Colin West, codirector of the Mayo Clinic's Program on Physician Well-Being, explained to *Time* magazine, "If I put in an hour with a patient, I will be reimbursed for one exam—the same payment I would get for seeing that patient for 11 minutes. Meanwhile, an ophthalmologist might perform three cataract surgeries in that same hour, and each surgery might be reimbursed at twice the rate of my exam. So that doctor is making six times as much money." This fee-for-service system, which reimburses providers a certain amount for each test, diagnosis, and procedure, sets the stage for overtreatment.

As Katy Butler put it in *The New York Times*, "Medicare rewards doctors far better for doing procedures than for assessing whether they should be done at all."

———

Primary care is critical for providing consistent preventive services. People with access to regular primary care tend to build trust with providers they see regularly, and are thus more likely to follow through on the things they need to do to support their treatment, such as taking their meds as prescribed. Access to primary care is not only associated with lower mortality rates, but also, particularly for the economically disadvantaged, with more complete immunization, better blood pressure control, and improved outcomes and quality of life.

Primary care physicians order fewer tests, spend less money, and are less likely than specialists to recommend unnecessary treatments. Countries with strong primary care infrastructures have healthier populations, fewer health-related disparities, and lower overall healthcare costs. "We say primary care is critical to a healthier future," Colin West told *Time*, "but in every way we show value, it is at the lowest level." Because reimbursement rates for primary care are so much lower than for specialists, medical students saddled with debt often opt for more lucrative fields, and this means we're facing a shortage of primary care doctors.

———

In 2012, the Institute of Medicine released a report estimating that a stunning 30 percent of all healthcare spending in the United States goes toward unnecessary tests and treatment ($210 billion), excess administration costs ($190 billion), fraud ($75 billion), missed prevention opportunities ($55 billion), and other waste. In 2019, *JAMA* published an updated analysis that found that unnecessary spending now adds up to as much as $935 billion a year.

In a separate study, over 70 percent of the physician respondents believed that doctors are more likely to perform unnecessary procedures when they will profit from them. Most believed that de-emphasizing fee-for-service compensation would lower spending by reducing overtreatment. In a 2014 piece for *Harper's*, "Diagnose This! How to Be Your Own Best Doctor," the author Heidi Julavits points to research substantiating the problem. Interventions for "preference-sensitive conditions" such as hip arthritis, lower back pain, and early-stage breast cancers vary widely between hospitals. In other words, says Julavits, "the data indicate that doctors, not patients, are making the decisions, and they are doing so on the basis of financial incentives."

A study published in *JAMA* analyzed 2,552 patient-doctor discussions that took place in over a thousand office visits and found that overall only 9 percent met the criteria for fully informed decision-making. In a 2011 review of eighty-six studies, the esteemed Cochrane Collaborative found that patients given decision-making aids such as pamphlets, videos, or web-based tools describing possible benefits and harms of the options felt better informed, which reduced their internal conflict about decisions and increased the likelihood of receiving care that aligned with their values. They also had more accurate risk perceptions.

An ethic of shared decision-making is not only good for the patient but significantly reduces unnecessary medical spending.

———

In 2012, the Choosing Wisely campaign was launched by the American Board of Internal Medicine to address the problem of overtreatment. Partnering with over eighty medical specialty societies and more than seventy consumer groups, including the AARP and the National Business Coalition on Health, the campaign identifies overused tests, procedures, and treatments that sometimes don't provide meaningful benefit for patients. *Consumer Reports* translates this information into patient-friendly language and helps to get the word out. Within two years, more than 160 journal articles had been published as a result of this campaign.

———

I wish some shared decision-making had been part of the process the time I went to see my podiatrist for a mysterious pain in my foot. Worried that I might have a stress fracture, I was relieved when the med tech took me first to the X-ray room. I wanted to get to the bottom of the problem.

My podiatrist worked in a giant practice on one of the higher floors of a tall downtown building. He was a nice enough man, but brevity was one of the demands of this system. It always felt like he kept one hand on the doorknob. When he stepped into the room, he told me that stress fractures don't show up on an X-ray until four or so weeks after the initial insult, so it was impossible to know at this juncture whether I'd fractured my metatarsal. It might just be inflamed, he said. I told him I was going to be traveling to Canada in a few days and was worried about it getting worse. He said he could offer me an "air boot," one of those giant contraptions people with foot injuries wear, but he didn't seem to think it warranted, and I declined.

In the rush of the appointment, I didn't think to ask why they had bothered to radiate my foot if the X-ray wouldn't identify a fracture anyway. But I thought about it a lot afterward, and given what I have come to understand about the American medical system, I came up with two likely reasons.

First, it's more efficient. If the doctor saw me first, then determined I needed an X-ray, he would have to come back to the exam room and see me a second time after the X-ray. Second, since doctors in the United States make more money for doing procedures than they do for talking to people, it's more profitable.

So when you live in a country with a profit-driven medical system, it's radiate first, ask questions later.

I had to do a fair amount of walking in Canada, where I was visiting my father, who was dying of cancer, and the pain in my foot did indeed get worse. On a particularly bad day, I happened to mention it while the visiting nurse was at my father's house. "Oh, there's nothing they can do for that," she said. "Just tape it."

My podiatrist had never mentioned anything about tape. I drove to the nearest drugstore and bought some KT Tape and watched a YouTube video to figure out how best to apply it. The relief was instant.

Consider this. The nurse who visited my dad was paid by the provincial government, which has a system of universal healthcare rather than a bunch of private insurance companies vying for profits. My father's cancer required extraordinary amounts of care over the several months of its course, and all of it was covered by his insurance. The coverage that every single Canadian citizen has. There was no deductible, no copay. While he and my stepmother faced this terrible ordeal, one thing they didn't have to worry about was losing their house or choosing between buying groceries or paying for medicine.

So it's unsurprising, really, that the home care nurse visiting my sick father in Canada was the one who gave me the simple, inexpensive solution.

―――――

But cutting down utilization won't by itself solve the problems of excess healthcare spending in the United States. Since a system with multiple insurers is intrinsically more complex and costly than a single-payer system, administrative costs of our private insurance quagmire are higher than in any other country. In addition, healthcare providers are having to spend more time chasing patients to collect deductibles and copayments, which are on the rise and unaffordable for some. This is another administrative expense that is small to nonexistent in Canada and other countries with universal healthcare.

In my practice, I quickly learned that each insurance company had different rules; copayments and deductibles varied for every client, even those with the same brand of insurance; and reimbursement snafus were inevitable. Soon, whenever I even thought about calling an insurance company, I could feel my stress hormones shooting up. First there were the confusing automated directories, then the inevitable holds for five, ten, twenty minutes, with a recorded voice punctuating the hold music every few minutes to say something like "Your call is important to us. Please wait on the line for the next available attendant." Sometimes, by the time I finally got through to a human, I had to hang up before getting my issue resolved because my next client was sitting in the waiting room. Sometimes one customer service provider gave me a completely different answer from the one I'd talked to the week before, because they found the system as labyrinthine as I did, or maybe they just didn't care.

A majority of American doctors say that time spent on insurance billing and claims is a major problem. A study published in 2009 found that for every ten doctors providing care, almost seven additional people are needed to cover billing-related activities. A 2011 study found that American practices spend almost four times more money dealing with insurance claims, coverage, and billing than Canadian practices in my home province of Ontario. Shaving off even half the bureaucracy would be enough to cover every single uninsured American.

———

Decades before the UK had its National Health Service, in 1884 Alice decided to move to England, where she could be closer to Henry, Katharine, and some other friends. Katharine sailed across the Atlantic to meet Alice and ferry her back to the country that would become her new home. When they arrived in Liverpool on November 11 after a ten-day voyage, Henry met them at the ship. Alice was, he reported, "in a *very* knocked up condition," and had to be carried off the ship by two stewards. It took her nine weeks to recover enough strength to leave her room.

On the recommendation of Dr. Beach, in December Alice called a Dr. Garrod to her house. In a letter to her sister-in-law, William's Alice, she described that initial appointment as "the most affable hour of my life." Her new doctor had "listened with apparent interest and attention to my oft-repeated tale," which, she quipped, "by the way to save breath and general exhaustion I am going to have printed into a small pamphlet." After a thorough examination, Dr. Garrod assured her there was no organic source for her symptoms and that the weakness in her legs would not lead to paralysis.

But by the end of the month her legs would not move at all. In January 1885 the disillusioned Alice wrote to her aunt Kate,

My doctor turned out as usual a *fiasco.* . . . The gout he looks upon as a small part of my trouble, "it being complicated with an excessive nervous sensibility," but I could get no suggestions of any sort as to climate, baths or diet from him. The truth was he was entirely puzzled about me & had not the manliness to say so. . . . My legs have been entirely useless for anything more than hobbling about the room for three months & a half & and most of the time excessively painfull [sic]. I asked the doctor whether it was not unusual for a person to be so ill & have no organic trouble & he said, "yes, very unusual indeed."—I should have thought he would therefore have liked to do something for me—but it was only my folly in going to a great man their *only* interest being diagnosis, & having absolutely no conscience in their way of dealing with one.

In June 1885, after other family members came to care for Louisa, Katharine left her sister's bedside to move in with Alice. On sunny days, Katharine took Alice out into the world in her Bath chair, an early three-wheeled wheelchair. By the fall, although Alice's overall health was still poor, her energy was the best it had been since arriving in London and she was able to enjoy a rich social life. She even began to host a London salon.

———

And a hundred and twenty-some years later, I in my little downtown office and my colleagues at True North—and many other healthcare providers around the country—did our best to push against the shortcomings of the U.S. healthcare system and provide the empathic and substantive healing work of the "tenders" a frustrated Alice once envisioned so long ago.

CHAPTER 13

Bedlam

In 2018 the pharmaceutical industry employed over 1,400 lobbyists to represent its interests in Washington—more than two for every member of Congress—and spent more money to influence lawmakers than any other industry. Its $285 million expenditure was almost twice that of the next industry on the list: insurance. Lobbyists and campaign donations have long influenced congressional decision-making. In the 2019–2020 election cycle, the pharmaceutical industry endeavored to secure its influence by making more than $50 million in donations to congressional candidates of both parties.

In a culture where the pharmaceutical industry holds so much sway, it's unsurprising that in 2003 lawmakers passed legislation that forbade Medicare from negotiating drug prices, making the United States one of the only industrialized countries in the world to allow drug companies to set their own prices. As a result, Americans pay almost twice as much as other wealthy countries for the very same drugs. The Inflation Reduction Act of 2022 aims to address that problem by allowing the government to begin negotiating the costs of a limited number of drugs. It's a start, but its actual impact remains to be seen.

As of 2020, prescription drugs account for almost 11 percent of healthcare spending in the United States, up from 8.2 percent in 1999. Excessive drug prices are the biggest source of healthcare overspending in the United States, even greater than our exorbitant administrative costs or overuse of CT scans and MRIs. Name-brand drugs account for almost three-quarters of the total amount spent on pharmaceuticals in the U.S. Between 2011 and 2016, their prices doubled, with the consequence that Americans spent $333 billion on prescription drugs in 2017, almost three times what they spent in 2000. The pharmaceutical industry is thus one of the economy's most lucrative sectors, with profit margins twice those of the automobile or the petroleum industries.

Without question, when prescription drugs work, and when their side effects are manageable, they reduce suffering and save lives. But in the face of this degree of corporate control, the U.S. government's system to ensure the safety and efficacy—not to mention the affordability—of pharmaceuticals could bear some scrutiny.

Pharmaceutical executives defend high prices by citing the cost of research and development, but the numbers don't bear this out. An analysis in the *BMJ* found that for every dollar that big pharma spends on basic research, it invests $19 in marketing. And more than 80 percent of all funds for research to discover new drugs and vaccines comes from public sources, not corporations. Furthermore, wrote the authors, "the pharmaceutical industry devotes most research funds to developing scores of minor variations that produce a steady stream of profits." They added that 85 to 90 percent of new pharmaceuticals over the past fifty years "have provided few benefits and considerable harms."

In the late nineteenth century Charlotte Perkins Gilman was prescribed Elixir Coca (cocaine and alcohol) by a doctor, and her husband was able to purchase Essence of Oats (morphine and alcohol) for her over the counter. While we may now look askance at the use of these addictive concoctions, we would do well to remember that doctors today prescribe benzodiazepines for anxiety and of course OxyContin and other opioids for pain. While these drugs can be addictive, sometimes they play a critical role in patient well-being.

Cannabis was used interchangeably as a painkiller or a stimulant. Shortly after Alice's disastrous overseas trip to Europe, her new physician, Dr. Garrod, prescribed pills made with cannabis, but in December Alice suffered a mysterious attack that caused "great distress of the heart." She thought she was dying, and afterward was unable to move her legs. Dr. Garrod suggested that in the process of applying galvanism (electrical currents) to the back of her neck to relieve a headache, she must have hit the pneumogastric nerve (now known as the vagus nerve), possibly causing some kind of paralytic stroke. But Alice believed it was a reaction to the cannabis and stopped taking the pills. Alice's experience notwithstanding, contemporary researchers are beginning to understand the therapeutic applications of cannabis.

Other nineteenth-century medicines are, to the contemporary eye, more concerning. Doctors prescribed nux vomica or its derivative strychnine to stimulate the central nervous system. Tonics and fortifiers could include ingredients like arsenic or phosphorus, both poisons that accumulate in the body. The drug calomel, made from mercury chloride, was a popular panacea not only for some of the symptoms of neurasthenia, but also for problems as wide-ranging as teething and syphilis. Belladonna and ergot were thought to relieve neurasthenic headaches, but could provoke side effects like nausea, vomiting, or convulsions.

If, as F. G. Gosling points out in *Before Freud*, "it is impossible to estimate the damage" of the prolonged use of some of the treatments prescribed by nineteenth-century physicians, the same could be said of contemporary killers like Vioxx, fen-phen, Darvocet, and Meridia, all of which were eventually pulled from the market.

Cynthia Atkinson, a gentle-hearted True North energy medicine practitioner, started each treatment session with a brief conversation about the issue I wanted to work on. The fatigue was a given, but I brought up other difficulties as well, including my low threshold for stress and my permeability—the chemical sensitivities, of course, but also my emotional permeability; my general sense of not feeling safe in the world; and childhood experiences that I believed continued to influence my life in unproductive ways.

I then lay fully clothed on her table focusing on the issue I'd brought to the session as Cynthia held her hands over me, assessing each part of my energy system, she said, to determine which areas were most out of balance. While I lay quietly or talked in more depth about an issue, she repositioned her hands intermittently on or above my body, allowing energy to flow through her and into me as she reminded my entire energy system—physical, emotional, mental, and spiritual—how to return to its inherent wholeness.

Cynthia was also trained in a therapeutic approach called Internal Family Systems (IFS), which recognizes that people have many different internal parts, and these parts all have helpful qualities, but sometimes due to life circumstances they get out of balance and cause distress. For instance, I had a part of me that felt guilty for being sick. Maybe that part even thought the illness was my fault. And there was another part that got defensive and angry at the prospect that my illness was imaginary or that I was in some way to blame. These parts needed acknowledgment, acceptance, and love from *me*.

By following the IFS process, I could get to know these parts better, honor them for the hard work they'd been doing on my behalf, and help them to trust that they were now safe and could relax. So while Cynthia helped my energy systems to come into balance, we also used the IFS process to bring my conflicted parts some much-needed respite.

At the beginning of our seventh session, I told her that I'd felt an internal shift: after a full day of seeing clients, I now still had some energy left over. "That's unheard of," I said. "Usually I'm tapped right out."

———

We have few studies on the efficacy of energy treatments. Of those available, none indicate that these treatments cause physical harm, and plenty of anecdotal testimony like my own indicates they can be helpful.

On the other hand, we're inundated with studies about pharmaceuticals. Which seems like a good thing, except those studies aren't always trustworthy. In a 2005 essay for *PLoS Medicine*, damningly entitled "Medical Journals Are an Extension of the Marketing Arm of Pharmaceutical Companies," Richard Smith, the former editor of the *BMJ*, revealed that "between two-thirds and three-quarters of the trials published in the major journals—*Annals of Internal Medicine*, *JAMA*, *Lancet*, and *New England Journal of Medicine*—are funded by the [pharmaceutical] industry." He cited a systematic review published in the *BMJ* that found that studies bankrolled by a company were four times more likely to have results favorable to the company than those funded by other sources. As Richard Horton, the editor of another esteemed British medical journal, *The Lancet*, put it, "Journals have devolved into information laundering operations for the pharmaceutical industry."

Smith lists several ways that researchers can manipulate data to get the results their funders are seeking. These include conducting a trial using too low a dose of a competitor drug (to make it appear the new drug is more effective) or too high a dose of a competitor drug (to give the illusion that the new drug causes fewer side effects), or conducting a trial against a treatment known to be inferior, or conducting a trial too small to reveal differences from a competitor drug. Another way researchers and pharmaceutical companies manipulate data is by suppressing unfavorable results. Most of the time, negative, neutral, or inconclusive results are not reported. Basically what this means is that we're getting only the good news. The studies that show a drug doesn't work rarely see the light of day.

The Food and Drug Administration Amendments Act of 2007 (FDAAA) was meant to curtail the problem of publication bias, but when the *BMJ* looked into the issue in 2012, it found that four out of five trials covered by the legislation had ignored the requirements.

———

In June 2009, I returned to Bethany's office for the results of my NutrEval test.

She had already looked over the printout. "Well, we have some pretty interesting data here that answer some of our questions and give me some ideas for a course of treatment," she said as we sat down. She handed me a copy so that we could review it together. Twenty-seven pages long, it included colorful charts and diagrams, with a detailed narrative at the end.

"So," she said, pointing to a section entitled Gastrointestinal Dysfunctions, "you have some markers characteristic of intestinal malabsorption and/or dysbiosis, just like we suspected. And a number of your amino acids were low." She explained that amino acids are the structural elements of proteins and have many important functions in the body, including synthesizing hormones and neurotransmitters, regulating immune function, and boosting energy. "If you're deficient in any particular amino acid, or any assortment of them, a whole function of your body can get blocked."

She flipped through a few pages and then stopped. "You can see here on page 12 that most of your essential and metabolic fatty acids are in the reference range, but one of your omega-6 fatty acids—called dihomo-gamma-linolenic—was low, and one of your saturated fatty acids—tricosanoic acid—was high. Evening primrose oil contains gamma-linolenic acid, and a vitamin B complex supplement with biotin can help lower your tricosanoic acid. And there are some other imbalances shown here that can be righted with the help of fish oil. Do you have any questions so far?" Bethany looked up to check in with me.

"Not yet," I said. "But this is pretty cool. I'm excited. Keep going."

"Okay," she said, and flipped a couple more pages. "See here? Your oxidative stress markers look pretty good, but some of your inflammation markers show a tendency toward inflammation, which is not good for your overall health if it's chronic."

When we'd gone through the whole document, Bethany sat back in her chair. "So where do we go from here? A hydrochloric acid supplement will help you break down proteins better so that your body can absorb them. A probiotic will help your overall gut health. And this test provides a personalized amino acid supplement protocol that can be compounded for you at a specialized pharmacy not far from here. That should help your energy and strengthen your immune system. Let's give it a go and check in again in a month."

Finally, a test showed an imbalance that we could target and treat.

————

Sometime during his tenure as dean of Harvard Medical School in the 1930s and '40s, Charles Sidney Burwell famously quipped to an incoming class, "Half of what we are going to teach you is wrong, and half of it is right. Our problem is that we don't know which half is which." In 2010, when I read David H. Freedman's "Lies, Damned Lies, and Medical Science" in *The Atlantic*, I learned that Dr. Burwell's joke still holds true.

Freedman described the work of the meta-researcher John

Ioannidis, one of the world's leading experts on the credibility of medical research, who, with his team, has demonstrated in widely cited studies in the field's top journals,

> again and again, and in many different ways, that much of what biomedical researchers conclude in published studies—conclusions that doctors keep in mind when they prescribe antibiotics or blood-pressure medication, or when they advise us to consume more fiber or less meat, or when they recommend surgery for heart disease or back pain—is misleading, exaggerated, and often flat-out wrong.

In one of his papers for *PLoS Medicine*, entitled "Why Most Published Research Findings Are False," Ioannidis and his team reported findings that 80 percent of non-randomized studies (by far the most commonly published) are erroneous, and even randomized trials, which are considered the gold standard for reliability, are wrong 25 percent of the time. Freedman's *Atlantic* article described Ioannidis's belief "that researchers were frequently manipulating data analyses, chasing career-advancing findings rather than good science, and even using the peer-review process—in which journals ask researchers to help decide which studies to publish—to suppress opposing views."

In a separate 2005 study published in *JAMA*, Ioannidis scrutinized forty-nine of the most widely cited papers published between 1990 and 2003 in the most cited journals, and found that 41 percent were wrong or significantly exaggerated.

Ioannidis has found that even when research errors are identified, they generally persist for years, and sometimes even decades. As he told Freedman, "Even when the evidence shows that a particular research idea is wrong, if you have thousands of scientists who have invested their careers in it, they'll continue to publish papers on it. . . . It's like an epidemic, in the sense that they're infected with these wrong ideas, and they're spreading it to other researchers through journals."

———

Additionally, the FDA's ties to the pharmaceutical industry appear to be clouding the judgment of those who are charged with protecting Americans from dangerous or ineffective medications. Vioxx, for instance—an anti-inflammatory pain reliever touted as safer than aspirin for extended use due to lower risk of ulcers—was approved by the FDA in 1999 despite one reviewer's concerns about data suggesting that the drug might increase the risk of heart attack. It was a lifesaver for its maker, Merck, as it arrived on the scene just as patents on several of the company's popular drugs were about to expire, allowing competing generics to enter the market. The drug became a blockbuster, with $2.3 billion in sales in 2003.

Several studies supported the FDA reviewer's concerns, and Merck went on the offensive, arranging ghostwriters for industry-backed studies in more than a dozen medical journals, including *The New England Journal of Medicine* and *JAMA*.

By September 2004, when Merck withdrew Vioxx from the market, the drug had caused an estimated 88,000 heart attacks, almost half of them fatal. In 2011, the company pled guilty to criminal charges for its misleading marketing and sales tactics and paid a fine of $950 million to the U.S. Department of Justice. It also agreed to pay out $4.85 billion to settle 27,000 lawsuits.

In a 2010 piece for the *Boston Review*, Marcia Angell, former editor in chief of *The New England Journal of Medicine* and author of *The Truth About the Drug Companies: How They Deceive Us and What to Do About It*, reported that five years earlier the FDA had convened a panel to discuss whether painkillers in the same class as Vioxx—called COX-2 inhibitors—should also be pulled from the market. After three days of hearings, the panel determined that although the drugs did increase the risk of heart attack, the benefits outweighed the risks and all three drugs—including Vioxx—should remain available to patients. "A week after the panel's decision, however," wrote Angell, "*The New York Times* revealed that of the 32 panel members, ten had financial ties to the manufacturers, and that if their votes had been excluded, only one of the drugs would have been permitted to stay on the market." The negative exposure prompted the FDA to reverse its decision and allow only one of the drugs, Celebrex, to remain on the market, now with a clear warning on the label.

Other popular drugs eventually pulled from the market since the 1970s due to health risks include Accutane, an acne medicine (birth defects, miscarriages, inflammatory bowel disease); diethylstilbestrol (DES), a miscarriage preventative (cancer to both the patient and her offspring); Zantac, a heartburn treatment (probable carcinogen); and over thirty more.

———

When I saw Bethany again in July, I told her that shortly after I initiated the supplement protocol, I felt much better. I started the amino acids two weeks after that, but reacted to the maltitol, a sweetener that the compounding pharmacist had added to the formula, and started feeling less good. So Bethany called in a new order, telling the pharmacist to cease and desist with the maltitol, and my energy continued its upward trajectory.

———

In 2003, when he was worldwide vice president of genetics at GlaxoSmithKline, Dr. Allen Roses admitted, "The vast majority of drugs—more than 90 percent—only work in 30 or 50 percent of the people." This, he said, is largely due to genetic variants that in some way interfere with the medication.

This is what makes functional medicine so exciting: the patient's genetics are incorporated into the treatment plan.

In early October 2009, I swabbed my cheek and sent it off to the lab for the DetoxiGenomic profile. The results arrived by the end of the month, and I returned to Bethany's office hopeful and curious. On the first page of the profile, Bethany wrote, "Not a good detoxifier." To address this problem, she recommended some supplements to enhance my detoxification pathways.

The test also gave us some information about how I metabolize specific drugs and even anesthesias, based on my genetic polymorphisms. With this crucial information, I would be able to collaborate with any of my doctors to find the best drugs for me, when necessary.

When I returned to her office in November, I was ebullient. "It's been a long time since I felt this good," I told her. "My energy and mood are great, my MCS is radically better."

During the AIDS crisis in the late 1980s, under pressure from ACT UP and other advocacy groups, the FDA sped up its approval process to get treatment to patients sooner, allowing the antiretroviral drug azidothymidine (AZT) on the market after just one clinical trial instead of the standard three. This was a critical move in the face of a deadly pandemic, but it took just a decade before drugmakers began abusing the resulting accelerated approval (AA) protocol for financial advantage. In *An American Sickness*, Elisabeth Rosenthal quotes Thomas R. Fleming, a professor of biostatistics at the University of Washington, who said, "Not only does the AA process allow sponsors to get marketing approval much sooner and with much less research expenditure, but also, quite frankly, it allows them to market products that likely are biologically active but less likely to provide truly important effects."

And there's no mechanism to revoke FDA approval or pull drugs off the market if later studies prove them to be without benefit, says Rosenthal, adding that a 2014 in-depth data investigation found that a shocking "74 percent of cancer drugs approved by the FDA during the previous decade ultimately did not extend life by even a single day."

In addition to undermining drug efficacy, the FDA's expedited approval process compromises drug safety. In a piece for *Harper's*, Alicia Mundy reported that of the thirteen drugs pulled from the market between 1997 and 2004 due to health risks, "at least seven are now known to have been approved over the objections of FDA safety reviewers, who either had warned of serious potential dangers or had refused to sign official approval letters." More recently, in 2021 two members of an FDA advisory panel resigned when the agency approved the drug Aduhelm for treatment of Alzheimer's despite unconvincing evidence of efficacy and known risks of brain swelling and hemorrhage.

In 2019, Dr. Raeford Brown, a pediatric anesthesia specialist and chair of the FDA Committee on Analgesics and Anesthetics, expressed concern about the amount of money the pharmaceutical industry invests in influencing legislators. "Congress is supposed to have oversight of the FDA. If the FDA isn't going to hold pharma accountable, and Congress is getting paid to not hold pharma accountable," then this is a big problem.

A 2018 *Science* investigation found significant evidence of conflict of interest in members of FDA advisory boards, some of whom had previously received payments for consulting, lectures, or research from the companies whose drugs they were now tasked with reviewing, and others who received similar types of payments within four years after approving such drugs. As Vinay Prasad, an associate professor of epidemiology and biostatistics at the University of California, San Francisco, who studies such financial conflicts, explained, "The people who are asked to weigh this evidence impartially often stand to gain tremendously in their further professional careers from a positive relationship with the company. . . . It's in their best interest to play nice with these companies."

In 2010, despite discovering what it called "egregious" and "pervasive" violations at a major pharmaceutical testing lab, the FDA nonetheless allowed almost a hundred drugs to stay on the market regardless of the fact that their safety and effectiveness were now uncertain, even approving one additional drug after the fraudulent activities had come to light.

When agencies like the FDA and the CDC (not to mention the EPA) betray the public's trust, they contribute to government mistrust, paving the road for conspiracy theorists. Trustworthy government agencies are critical to public health and a robust democracy.

———

About two-thirds of the pharmaceutical industry's $30-billion-per-year marketing budget is spent on "educating" doctors, and a good portion of this is invested in influencing med students via gifts, free lunches, and industry-sponsored educational sessions. A 2011 review of several studies found that up to 90 percent of students in clinical rotation received educational materials like textbooks and journal reprints from pharmaceutical companies. And 93 percent of third-year students were asked or required by a superior to attend industry-sponsored lunches. A year before that review's release, Marcia Angell wrote that "drug companies support educational programs even within our best medical schools and teaching hospitals, and are given virtually unfettered access to young doctors to ply them with gifts and meals and promote their wares." And it works. This became clear when researchers found that graduates of residency programs that limit engagement with pharmaceutical sales reps were able to think more critically about the pharmaceutical industry.

Studies show that residents tend to believe they're entitled to gifts due to their long work hours and financial hardship, even when they think that gifts are inappropriate. Some wrongly believe that, unlike their peers, they're immune to improper influence.

Even seasoned doctors are unduly influenced by visits from pharmaceutical reps, prescribing newer, more expensive (and less tested) drugs, even when they've not been proven to be more effective, or even prescribing meds when otherwise they wouldn't have. A 2016 study published in *JAMA Internal Medicine* found that for the price of a $20 meal, doctors upped their prescriptions for branded drugs. And if the meal was more expensive or a doctor was treated to additional meals, prescription rates were likely to rise even higher. Of course, all these prescriptions lead to inflated healthcare spending, which would explain in part why this category is such a significant proportion of our GDP.

Have you seen your doctor using a pen or a clipboard with the name of a new drug on it? That was a gift from a visiting pharmaceutical rep, designed to influence your physician's prescribing behaviors.

———

Forty-three percent of Americans believe that only "completely safe" drugs are allowed to be advertised, but in reality the *Journal of Internal Medicine* found that 57 percent of claims are misleading and another 10 percent entirely false. In 2015, the industry spent a record-breaking $5.4 billion on direct-to-consumer (DTC) marketing; that same year, Americans dropped an unprecedented $457 billion on prescription drugs.

In an article called "Can You Trust Drug Ads on TV?" *Consumer Reports* declared, "Drug ads should be banned. . . . For one, they encourage patients and doctors to turn to medication when nondrug options might work. And when drugs are needed, ads often promote more expensive options, not the best or the safest." The American Medical Association (AMA) and the American Society of Health-System Pharmacists (ASHP) have voted to ban DTC marketing for just these reasons. One study of oncology nurse practitioners found that 74 percent of them had been asked by patients for inappropriate drugs due to DTC marketing. Sometimes medical practitioners succumb to the pressure to prescribe the drugs against their better judgment to avoid friction in the relationship.

———

In 1999, three years into a study of an AIDS vaccine, it became clear the vaccine wasn't working and the trial was stopped. Executives at the Immune Response Corporation, the biotech company sponsoring the study, at first suggested and then insisted that the university researchers tweak the data to show that the vaccine had some effect on viral loads on a subset of participants. When the researchers refused and submitted their findings to *JAMA*, the Immune Response Corporation sued. The company's president gave *The Baltimore Sun* a telling sound bite when he complained, "I spent over $30 million. I would think I have certain rights."

CHAPTER 14

Pulse

We tell stories about our health, about patients, about doctors, about diseases. Of all the narratives running through contemporary medicine, one of the most consequential and little told is that of the culture in which doctors in the United States are educated and trained, and the downstream impacts of that culture on patient care.

Elisabeth Rosenthal, who worked as an ER physician before becoming a journalist and then the author of *An American Sickness*, describes medical residents as "the worker bees that keep hospitals going," and argues that "there is much to suggest that hospitals have turned residencies into another profitable business."

Residents work grueling hours treating emergency room patients, assisting in operating rooms, teaching the medical students assigned to their wards, drawing blood, and taking care of a host of other tasks. In exchange, they gain valuable training and experience on their path toward licensing and board certification. Hospitals receive federal and state subsidies to support graduate education: in 2018 this averaged about $171,000 annually per resident.

Before 2003, residents routinely worked 100 and even 120 hours per week, with single shifts sometimes as long as 48 hours or longer. Then, in a successful bid to stave off federal regulations, the

Accreditation Council for Graduate Medical Education (ACGME) implemented new rules, capping the number of hospital hours residents can work at an average of 80 per week (which means that they can feasibly work 100 hours one week and 60 the next), and limiting the maximum shift length to 16 hours for first-year residents and up to 28 for more seasoned ones. To me, this still sounds like an awful lot of hours on the floor.

And perhaps unsurprisingly, surveys have found that the ACGME rule hasn't precipitated significant change. As one writer pointed out in *The Atlantic*, "the reforms simply require residents to do the same amount of work in less time." Often this is physically impossible, and a survey in *JAMA* revealed that 83 percent of residents work more hours than permitted. Other research reveals that the vast majority submit false reports of their hours to their programs and the ACGME. Since hourly restrictions pertain only to time spent in hospitals and clinics, residents also take substantial amounts of work—such as writing patient notes, filing reports, and reading up on research to aid diagnosis and treatment—home with them. Twenty percent of residents report sleeping an average of five hours or fewer per night. This is bad for more than the residents: a 2004 study found that those in that 20 percent were more likely to report making significant medical errors.

In the European Union, residents are limited to a workweek of no more than forty-eight hours, a little more than half what American residents are supposed to be limited to per the ACGME restrictions.

Furthermore, the modest salary paid to residents in the United States, when divided by the number of hours they work, amounts to the approximate hourly wage of the hospital janitors. The annual value of each resident's work adds up to $232,726, which means, according to Rosenthal, that even without a subsidy "having residents is a better than break-even deal."

Mistreatment and bullying are systemic in medical training. A large national survey of residents and fellows in 2016 found that a full 48 percent of respondents reported having been bullied at work in the previous year. Over a third of respondents indicated more than one source of bullying. An earlier survey found that "most of the negative behaviors were perpetrated by other doctors, in a pecking order of seniority."

Abuse took several forms, including belittling and undermining, unjustified criticism and attempts to humiliate, intimidating use of discipline, destructive innuendo and sarcasm, ignoring and excluding ("freezing out"), setting impossible deadlines, and more. Three percent of respondents even reported experiencing physical violence. BIPOC and female trainees were significantly more likely to be targeted.

Almost one in four medical students in one study disclosed clinically significant symptoms of depression, and 7 percent said that they had considered suicide sometime in the previous two weeks. Elsewhere, one doctor recalled, "I definitely graduated med school with PTSD. . . . We had two suicides and . . . another serving life in prison for murdering a classmate after a delusional episode after not sleeping for a month. . . . It takes a lot for me to cry, but I cried all the time, along with everyone else, but we hid it from each other, of course." Med students are compelled to conceal their emotions, as Judith Graham explained in *Stat*, because they face "withering criticism from faculty who have little tolerance for ignorance, signs of weakness, or emotional displays."

This problem only gets worse in residency, where 29 percent of residents suffer from depression. As Graham notes, the fact that their symptoms escalate within a year of starting their residency indicates that the programs themselves are contributing to the issue. In this atmosphere of overwork and intimidation, it's not at all surprising that so many residents suffer depression at some point during their internship. Nor is it surprising that they would emerge on the other side with a certain amount of entitlement. As one doctor put it, "We develop a bond because we go through some tough experiences together that the rest of the world doesn't have. Since you put in that kind of effort and pay those kinds of dues, you come out thinking you're pretty special and are owed something for your suffering."

When their training culture teaches them to suppress their feelings and attempts to abuse their human frailties out of them, doctors learn to cope with the pressure by objectifying their patients. This creates a psychological shield that prevents them from connecting authentically with their patients and blocks their ability to pick up cues that would help them monitor how they wield their power. And this leads to problems. Because a therapeutic relationship is critical to healing. This is why in 2002 physician Rita Charon developed the field of narrative medicine: to nurture, as she describes it, "clinical practice fortified by narrative competence—the capacity to recognize, absorb, metabolize, interpret, and be moved by stories of illness. Simply, it is medicine practised by someone who knows what to do with stories."

———

Alice despaired of finding a doctor who could both hear her and cure her. As she wrote to William,

> It may seem supine to you that I don't descend into the medical arena, but I must confess my spirit quails before any more gladiatorial encounters. It requires the strength of a horse to survive the fatigue of waiting hour after hour for the great man and then the fierce struggle to recover one's self-respect. . . . I think the difficulty is my inability to assume the receptive attitude, that cardinal virtue in woman, the absence of which has always made me so uncharming to and uncharmed by the male sex.

But she did try again. In September 1886, she told William that she had consulted with another English physician, Dr. Townsend, who was in agreement with Dr. Garrod and a Dr. Torry that an "abnormally sensitive nervous organization" predisposed her to gout, and the problem in her legs was caused by "anxiety & strain." She liked Dr. Townsend, but all he could offer her were some "very strong tonics," and Alice gave him up.

But through it all she never gave up her self-respect. When William wrote her a pitying letter that included his perception of her "stifling slowly in a quagmire of disgust and pain and impotence," she parried by informing him that she and Katharine had "roared" over his letter . . . "for I consider myself one of the most *potent* creations of my time." She threw in a dig at her professor brother: "Though I may not have a group of Harvard students sitting at my feet drinking in psychic truth, I shall not tremble, I assure you, at the last trump."

Nor did she.

———

In a 2015 TEDMED talk, physician Pamela Wible declared that despite her predisposition for optimism, "after a decade of seven-minute visits at assembly-line clinics," unable to adequately care for her patients' needs or even her own, "even I felt suicidal." The profession is facing an escalating crisis of depression, burnout, and suicide, with about three hundred to four hundred suicide deaths annually.

Every year the Physicians Foundation takes the pulse of the medical profession by surveying thousands of doctors. In 2018, the survey found that almost a quarter of respondents described themselves as "overextended and overworked" . . . and this was *before* the pandemic.

Research shows that "empathy burnout" can set in after seeing ten patients in a day, but doctors average twice that many, working an average of fifty-one hours a week, and sometimes much more. Even before COVID-19 turned hospitals into war zones, 40 percent of doctors said they suffered from professional burnout often or all the time. A separate 2018 survey of over 15,000 physicians found that 15 percent reported feeling depressed. The greatest contributor, they said, was the job.

So America's healthcare industry isn't just bad for patients; it's bad for doctors too. In 2018 a startling 27 percent said that if they had it to do over again, they would not choose the medical profession.

A big part of the problem, says Wible, is that insurance and pharmaceutical companies, government regulators, and new technologies have all "inserted themselves into the sacred patient-physician relationship." Indeed, while the Physicians Foundation survey found that the patient/physician relationship is the thing that doctors say is most satisfying about medical practice, respondents listed the "least satisfying" elements of their jobs as regulatory/insurance requirements, electronic health records, and the loss of clinical autonomy.

In "Doctors Tell All—and It's Bad," Meghan O'Rourke quotes Sandeep Jauhar, the cardiologist author of *Doctored: The Disillusionment of an American Physician*, who says that doctors no longer see themselves as "pillars of any community," but as "pawn[s] in a moneymaking game for hospital administrators." The mechanization of their professional selves dehumanizes them *and* their patients. In this context, Jauhar admits, "I realize that in many ways I have become the kind of doctor I never thought I'd be: impatient, occasionally indifferent, at times dismissive or paternalistic."

The authors of a 2019 *Medscape* opinion piece suggested that the term *burnout* is the wrong name to give what doctors are experiencing. This isn't burnout, they said; this is "moral injury."

"Healthcare systems have looked for easy fixes for physician distress," they added, "focusing on wellness (yoga, retreats, and self-care lessons), but this is misguided. Finding solutions requires that we address the problem for what it really is: a challenge inherent in the structure of the healthcare industry."

When healthcare spending soared in the 1980s, managed care was touted as a way to control costs. Under this new system, doctors and other healthcare providers were required to keep detailed records to justify their treatment choices. Insurance companies then performed "utilization reviews" to determine whether they would reimburse for the visit.

The resulting administrative burdens now add up to hundreds of billions of dollars in additional costs every year. Between 1980 and 2019, the number of healthcare administrators skyrocketed by 3,000 percent. Spending has continued to rise, but now a good percentage of that income is going into the pockets of CEOs, corporate shareholders, and the people whose job it is to deny treatment.

Burnout, depression, stress, and lack of sleep have been shown to increase the risk of medical error, as can the breakdown in communication that happens in hierarchical environments where disrespect and bullying are a systemic part of the culture. But since there are no federal laws requiring hospitals to report patient deaths and injuries caused by error, it's hard to know exactly how often it happens. A 1999 report from the Institute of Medicine found the number of unnecessary deaths to be somewhere between 44,000 and 98,000 per year, making medical error the eighth leading cause of death. A 2016 study published in the *BMJ* put that number even higher, estimating more than 250,000 U.S. deaths annually—the third leading cause of death. And these figures account only for hospital deaths, not those happening as a result of error in doctors' offices, walk-in clinics, or nursing homes. In *When We Do Harm: A Doctor Confronts Medical Error*, Danielle Ofri points out that in academic circles the methodologies of these papers have been criticized by some, but "researchers are in agreement that the number of errors is not small at all."

And of course medical errors can cause undue suffering even when death isn't the outcome. Catherine Guthrie, the author of *Flat: Reclaiming My Body from Breast Cancer*, writes that although her surgeon did a double mastectomy, he somehow missed the tumor, so she had to go under the knife a second time. Tressie McMillan Cottom, the author of *Thick: And Other Essays*, lost her baby when dismissive healthcare providers failed to identify signs of early labor, something she attributes to her being a Black woman. Katherine Standefer, the author of *Lightning Flowers*, took three 850-volt shocks to the heart when the implantable cardioverter-defibrillator (ICD) that she may not have needed was programmed at inappropriate settings. Susannah Cahalan, the author of *Brain on Fire: My Month of Madness*, went suddenly psychotic and catatonic and was diagnosed with "stress" and then bipolar disorder until an astute neurologist properly diagnosed and treated her for a rare autoimmune disorder. Surgeons have been known to amputate the wrong leg or, like Freud's colleague, leave surgical materials in the body.

Doctors are human and humans make mistakes. Shouldn't we be doing what we can to create a culture that would keep mistakes to a bare minimum?

———

In addition to the overwork, the bullying, the expense, and the big pharm influence, there are other ways that the U.S. medical education system fails its students . . . and their future patients. A 2004 survey found that two-thirds of doctors felt inadequately trained to treat the chronically ill. More than two-thirds of med schools fail to include anything about ME/CFS in their curricula, and the disease receives scant mention in just 40 percent of textbooks, and none in the rest. Nearly a quarter of all med students are taught nothing about diagnosis and treatment of illnesses caused by toxic chemicals. In 2013, a survey of med school graduates by the Association of American Medical Colleges (AAMC) found that a third of respondents believed that they received "inadequate" instruction in environmental health, this despite the fact that two years earlier the AAMC released a report asserting that "health is the product of the interactions among biology, genetics, behavior, relationships, cultures, and environments." Doctors are also given little training in nutrition.

One thing they *are* taught, as one cardiologist told author Maya Dusenbery, is "to be on the lookout for hysterical females who come to the emergency room."

─────

In July 1887, on the advice of Dr. Garrod, the thirty-nine-year-old Alice moved into a boardinghouse in a spa town known as Royal Leamington Spa in the county of Warwickshire. There she could "take the waters," drinking and bathing in the mineral springs that were believed to be the remedy for a wide swath of ills, including some of those that plagued Alice: gout, rheumatism, and digestive issues. She had found her rich social life in London "altogether too stimulating for jangled nerves," as she told her friend Sara Darwin, and was consigned, as a result, to total rest. "I shall be densely dull and lonely of course, but the sands of my little hour-glass will run out as swiftly here as anywhere." She led a much quieter existence in Warwickshire, spending mornings in bed and afternoons on the couch in the drawing room, reading, writing, and gazing out the window.

Just a few months earlier, in December 1886, Alice had begun jotting down favorite quotes in the pages of a leather-bound commonplace book. Strouse notes that her entries "show her absorption in the idea of triumph over worldly adversity, of private peace in the face of pain and death."

A month after Alice had settled in, Katharine was called back to the United States to care for her ailing father and sister. Now, with Katharine gone, a Leamington man named Bowles took Alice out in her Bath chair. Perhaps on her outings with Bowles, she looked up at the sky and recalled from her commonplace book the words of *War and Peace*'s Prince Andrei as he lay wounded in battle: "How was it I did not see that lofty sky before? And how happy I am to have found it at last. Yes! all is vanquished, all is a cheat except that infinite sky. There is nothing, nothing but that."

But even as she was trying to accept her fate, she was also longing to break out of it. This is the confounding dialectic of illness.

Alice added quotes to her commonplace book all through 1887 and 1888. Then, writes Strouse, in the spring of 1889, the forty-year-old Alice "relinquished this form of ventriloquism. At the end of May, she turned to a fresh page in the leather-bound volume and began to keep a diary":

> I think that if I get into the habit of writing a bit about what happens, or rather doesn't happen, I may lose a little of the sense of loneliness and desolation which abides with me. . . . and it may bring relief as an outlet to that geyser of emotions, sensations, speculations and reflections which ferments perpetually within my poor old carcass for its sins; so here goes, my first Journal!

In December of that year, in the midst of a three-month visit from Katharine, two entries in a row reflect Alice's frustration with the constraints put upon her. "How sick one gets of being 'good,'" she wrote on December 11, 1889. "How much I should respect myself if I could burst out and make every one wretched for 24 hours; embody selfishness. . . . It might enrich the soul a bit."

And then she added this sharp addendum: "And then the dolts praise one for being 'amiable!'"

The next day, she wrote of a time

when my shawls were falling off to the left, my cushions falling
out to the right and the duvet off my knees, one of those crises of
misery in short, which are all in the day's work for an invalid, Kath.
exclaimed, "What an awful pity it is that you can't say *damn*!" I
agreed with her from my heart. It is an immense loss to have all
robust and sustaining expletives refined away from one! At such
moments of trial refinement is a feeble reed to lean upon.

The writing became a familiar comfort. In May 1890 she wrote,
"If I can get on my sofa and occupy myself for four hours, at intervals,
thro' the day, scribbling my notes and able to read the books that
belong to me, in that they clarify the density and shape the formless
mass within, Life seems inconceivably rich."

What she could not have known is that just two years from making
her first entry, Alice would be chronicling her final year of life.

———

From the doctors we consulted, Alice and I sought both effective
treatment *and* empathy. But 56 percent of contemporary doctors feel
they lack the time to be empathic, which is unfortunate because empathy
appears to be the antidote to burnout.

Studies show that empathy declines during medical training.
This isn't surprising given the culture of stress that med students
and residents endure and how little empathy they're shown. They
are also trained to avoid getting too close to their patients in the belief
that keeping distant is a way to avoid pain and burnout. But the
absence of empathy causes harm to patients *and* their doctors, and
trickles down to others . . . even patients' therapists, like me. And
here's what the research reveals: connecting with patients makes
doctors happier and more fulfilled, and *that* is a buffer against burnout.
Connection builds resilience for doctor *and* patient. That can
trickle down, too.

Empathic communication skills are critical to good care—not only because they increase patient satisfaction and improve adherence to recommended treatments, but also because they're associated with a decrease in medical errors and an increase in positive outcomes, including reduced pain, lowered blood pressure, alleviation of depression and anxiety, and enhanced healing. Patients also make fewer malpractice claims against empathic doctors, which is why a number of malpractice insurance companies provide online Empathetics® education courses for their insureds.

Luckily, empathy can be learned (or relearned, as the case may be). A 2012 study found that residents randomly chosen to participate in an empathy course were judged by patients to be significantly more empathic than a control group who did not receive the training.

But ultimately, physicians are up against a system that doesn't support a critical aspect of healthcare: the therapeutic relationship. As Pamela Wible points out, once third-party payers started running the show, both doctors and patients were the casualties. "Some administrator on the fourth floor turned up the speed on the assembly line, and before we knew it, we were churning patients through and skipping bathroom breaks."

In this environment, ordering tests and prescribing drugs are the logical shortcuts. Pharmaceuticals "make it possible for doctors to move fast," says Wible. They also make it possible for doctors to earn more. A medical appointment that results in a prescription is considered more complex and thus eligible for higher reimbursement.

"It's much easier for doctors on the assembly line to write a prescription and escape," says Wible, "than spend an hour with a patient." One of the problems with that approach, she says, is that "the idea of a magic pill teaches people that the answer is somewhere outside of them: 'if I just get the right medicine, I'll be fine.' This disconnects patients from their natural healing capacities."

———

Pamela Wible was so distressed by her rushed, dehumanizing career choice that in 2004, she walked off the line and took to her bed, too depressed to work. For six weeks, she was dogged by thoughts of suicide. But then one day she was "jolted out of bed" with a radical idea. She decided to host a series of healthcare forums to ask patients what they desired in healthcare . . . and then create their ideal clinic. "I did eight community forums in all and got about a hundred pages of written testimony, which became my business plan."

She opened her clinic just a few months later, in April 2005. She accepts insurances, gives a 40 percent discount to uninsured patients who pay at time of service, and offers a sliding scale and even barters with patients to make sure that every person who needs care gets it. Rather than rushing through seven-minute appointments, her appointments are thirty to sixty minutes long, and she works from a whole-person orientation in partnership with her patients. Her overhead is very low, as she does all her own billing and doesn't have a receptionist. She practices part time, walking or bicycling to the office, and rewards patients who walk or cycle to their appointments with small gifts like locally made handcrafted soaps. Remarkably, when she published an article about it in the *Journal of Family Practice* six months after opening, she predicted that her earnings would probably exceed her previous full-time salary. "I've reduced my costs," she says, "by humanizing the experience."

Wible now helps other doctors launch their own community-designed practices. "All it takes to run a community-designed ideal practice," she says, "is self-confidence and basic arithmetic."

———

Even in Royal Leamington Spa, Alice's health continued to deteriorate. Then on August 2, 1890, she "went under," as she later put it, with an excruciating bout of what she inimitably described as "squalid indigestions." Other than the company of her nurse and Bowles, and the three-month visit from Katharine in the fall of 1889, Alice had spent her three years at Leamington alone. Now Henry, who'd been in Italy, rushed to her bedside, and Katharine set sail from America. When she arrived, Katharine wrote to their friend Fanny, "I never have seen any one so thin as she was, so full of pain and altogether wretched."

Alice thought she might be dying—wished for it, in fact. "There seems a faint hope that I may fizzle out," she wrote in her diary, "but the Monster *Rebound*, which holds me in its remorseless clutch, I am sure will gather itself up for many another spurt." When Henry and Katharine asked a doctor if Alice might die, he gave what Alice later described as a "consoling answer": "They sometimes do."

In September, Katharine moved Alice back to London, where they took rooms at a hotel not far from Henry's apartment. Henry wrote to William that Alice was "really, too ill to be left," and Katharine had thus determined that she must stay in London to nurse her.

By the end of the month, Alice had begun to gain weight. In her journal she lamented "the dreary snail-like climb up a little way so as to be able to run down again" that was also so familiar to me, especially from the early days of my illness, when my energy waxed and waned so unpredictably. "And then these doctors tell you that you will die or *recover*! But you *don't* recover. I have been at these alternations since I was nineteen and I am neither dead nor recovered—as I am now forty-two there has surely been time for either process."

Alice and Katharine had hoped to move to a town forty miles outside of London, but by November Alice had once again "gone into pie," and they were forced to change their plans. Frustrated, she complained of "the ignorant asininity of the medical profession in its treatment of nervous disorders."

———

A course called "The Healer's Art," developed for healthcare providers in 1991 by Rachel Naomi Remen, MD, at the UCSF School of Medicine, is now an elective taught to first- and second-year med students in over ninety schools in the United States and around the world. Its mission is to "explore the human dimensions of medicine rarely discussed in medical training" and facilitate the growth of a new paradigm for medical education. The fifteen-hour experiential course incorporates principles from contemplative studies, humanistic and transpersonal psychology, storytelling, and the creative arts to cover topics including presence, acceptance, deep listening, loss, grief, healing, relationship, encounters with awe and mystery, and self-care practices. To counter the shaming culture of traditional medical education, students and faculty work closely to a build a safe and supportive learning atmosphere that is nonjudgmental and non-competitive. Every year, more med schools have added this course to their curriculum. In this small way, schools and students are working to rewrite the narrative of what makes a doctor.

———

Thanks to David B. Morris's *Illness and Culture in the Postmodern Age* and Arthur W. Frank's *The Wounded Storyteller: Body, Illness, and Ethics*, I was able to form a perspective on my illness that was a radical departure from the one imposed upon me by the U.S. medical system. I wasn't a malingerer, a hypochondriac, or a hysteric: I was in the *vanguard*.

That day that I dragged myself home from the clinic back in 1989, wondering if my fatigue was in my mind or my body, I'd fallen prey to the dichotomized thinking of modernist medicine—attempting to impose logic and certainty on a bodily experience that was by its very nature complex, illogical, uncertain, and interconnected.

In *Illness and Culture in the Postmodern Age*, Morris writes that each era can be defined by certain emblematic diseases. Those that dominated the narrative in the modern era before the introduction of penicillin in 1944 were infectious diseases like polio, typhoid fever, and tuberculosis. But the postmodern era is characterized by chronic, gradually debilitating illnesses (the kind so few doctors are trained to treat).

"Postmodern illness," says Morris, "often involves a crucial element of ambiguity about whether the disorder really exists." He lists several examples, including ME/CFS and MCS, arguing that one of the postmodern perspectives most disorienting to traditional thinkers is the understanding that illness is not "a purely biological state . . . but rather something in part created or interpenetrated by culture."

Morris's view is supported by an influential 1977 piece for *Science* by internist and psychiatrist George L. Engel, "The Need for a New Medical Model: A Challenge for Biomedicine," which introduced the biopsychosocial perspective—a groundbreaking approach to medicine recognizing the overlapping influences of biology, psychology, and social context. This is the model that informed my education as a social worker. Postmodern illnesses, which confound the modernist belief that a biological understanding of a disease is enough to cure it, are most effectively viewed through a biopsychosocial lens.

I learned of Arthur W. Frank's *The Wounded Storyteller* when Morris cited the book in *Illness and Culture in the Postmodern Age*. The two books appear to be in conversation with each other. Frank writes that "modernist medicine claimed the body of its patient as its territory, at least for the duration of treatment." It did this in part by claiming the narrative. In modernist medicine, says Frank, "The story told by the physician becomes the one against which others are ultimately judged true or false." For those facing the diseases that could be described as modernist, "the colonization was judged worth the cure, or the attempted cure." But for those who suffer from postmodern ailments, this medical colonization doesn't work; the territory is too uncertain, too protean.

Morris argues that postmodern illness calls for us to reevaluate our sources of medical knowledge.

Laboratory tests and scientific studies cannot reveal everything that doctors need to know. The social, cultural, and personal dimensions of illness must be understood through other means, and one neglected but useful resource is narrative. Narrative, we might say, constitutes a mode of understanding appropriate for situations too variable and too untidy for laboratory analysis.

While the modern era privileged the voice of the doctor, the postmodern era is skeptical of singular, totalizing perspectives and instead acknowledges the complexity of the body and the diversity of stories that might be told about it. In the postmodern age, people tend to be suspicious, says Frank, of "medicine's reduction of their suffering to its general unifying view." As Morris writes, "The modernist narrative of biomedicine, with its heroic doctors and researchers struggling to find a cure . . . has begun to give way to a far more complicated and confusing narrative that contains painful moments of breakdown and failure." It is, he says, "a fragmentary narrative."

Frank also says that the postmodern experience of illness begins "when ill people recognize that more is involved in their experience than the medical story can tell."

This is a robust refutation of Talcott Parsons's theory of the sick role, a modernist perspective that includes the expectation that the ill cede authority over their bodies, positioning the physician as an agent of social control whose sympathy, says Frank, "is to be limited by the overriding message that the sick person's task is to get well and return to normal obligations of work and family."

When the ill body becomes, as Frank says, "an 'it' to be cured," the self becomes dissociated from the body. The reprobate Frank drew upon his own encounters with cancer and cardiovascular disease in another book, *At the Will of the Body: Reflections on Illness*, where he declared, "The body is not to be managed, even by myself. The body is the means and medium of my life; I live not only in my body but also through it. No one should be asked to detach his mind from his body and then talk about this body as a thing, out there."

Postmodernism recognizes the importance of the patient's story, the power vested in the patient's voice, and the inherent wisdom of the body. The physician and sociologist Howard Waitzkin interprets the frequency with which doctors interrupt patients as "basically attempts to curtail storytelling by patients." As Morris points out, "This is not dialogue but medical monologue punctuated by the patient's desperate efforts to be heard."

More recent research shows that patients are now fighting to claim their own narratives, initiating at least half of the interruptions, two-thirds of which introduce important new information. Postmodern patients refuse what Arthur Frank calls "narrative surrender."

"Modernism," says Frank, "made the physician . . . into the hero of illness" and defined heroism by *doing* rather than, say, persevering. Postmodern medicine requires a different approach, he says: ill people must be viewed as heroes of their own stories—and in a postmodern era, many kinds of heroism may be recognized.

I spent years—decades, really—feeling like a failure because I was sick and couldn't get better. I couldn't *do* enough. But these words of Frank's changed my relationship to my illness.

———

One way doctors can prepare for the complexity of patient stories and increase empathic connection is by studying narrative medicine. Learning how to do close readings of literature, says physician Rita Charon, helps providers build their skills of clinical attention so that they can absorb all that their patients have to tell—in their body language, tone, facial expression, *and* words.

By discussing literature in small groups and writing and sharing their own narratives about their work, healthcare providers increase the ability to recognize other people's perspectives and tap into their own built-in empathy. "The writing renders the doctor audible, the patient visible, and the treatment a healing conversation between them," writes Charon, who is the founder and director of the Program in Narrative Medicine at Columbia University. "Until the writing, there are two isolated beings—the doctor and the patient—both of whom suffer, and both of whom suffer alone. By virtue of the writing, there is hope for connection, for recognition, for communion. . . . The movements of attention and representation spiral together toward the ultimate goal of narrative medicine: affiliation."

Illness is a profoundly isolating experience. The sick person often feels cast off by society—disconnected not only from loved ones but from a formerly harmonious relationship with their healthy body and from the person they always knew themselves to be. The practice of medicine involves a co-creation of story, says Charon, calling upon the provider's creativity in "*inhabiting* without colonizing the lived experience of the one who suffers." Connection in this way reduces the isolation and thus increases the resilience of both patient and doctor.

Narrative medicine curricula and projects are proliferating throughout the United States, Canada, Great Britain, Latin America, the Middle East, and Australia, a sign that this approach to healthcare is both needed and effective.

———

Working with patients as whole people—through their stories—is critical to healing. As Ken said in that support group so long ago, even when a cure is unlikely, *healing*—an internal transformation—is nonetheless possible.

Arthur Frank delineates three different illness narratives: the chaos story, the restitution story, and the quest story. In the United States, we are partial to the restitution story. This is not surprising, given our amped-up version of capitalism and the way it expresses itself in our medical system. In the restitution narrative, says Frank, "the active player is the remedy: either the drug itself . . . or the physician. Restitution stories are about the triumph of medicine." In the U.S., the restitution imperative can become just another form of commodification. As Frank puts it, at the core of the American restitution story is the belief: "So long as there is more to buy, whatever needs fixing will be fixed, and I will continue to be." The restitution story is the fulfillment of Parsons's sick role, with its goal to return the ill person to the status quo, "because getting well," says Frank, "is the only outcome Parsons considers as acceptable."

But not everybody gets to have a restitution story. For those who live with chronic illness, there will not likely be a restitution.

In the early days of my illness, I was ensconced in a chaos narrative, what Frank describes as "the pit of narrative wreckage." Shattered, I felt infinitely broken. None of it had any meaning and it seemed there was no way out.

It's so tempting for friends, loved ones, and healthcare providers to try to haul the person out of the wreckage, but this "only denies what is being experienced and compounds the chaos," says Frank. I learned this again and again in my work many years later as a therapist. My clients who were in the very pit of a chaos story resisted my efforts to pull them out of it. What they needed first was to be fully heard. They wanted me to *join* them in their chaos narrative. Only when I was willing to do that could we eventually begin to look together for a path to a different story.

In the quest story, says Frank, the illness motivates its host to undertake a journey, using the experience for self-actualization. By this means, she gains a voice. Rather than being colonized by the dominant medical narrative, the sufferer becomes a storyteller, reclaiming her own experience of suffering and transforming that suffering into testimony. The ill who choose to undertake the quest return from their journey with new wisdom and perspectives to share. As Frank points out, people tell stories "not just to work out their own changing identities, but also to guide others who will follow them."

––––

Some of Arthur Frank's work was informed by Joseph Campbell's influential treatise *The Hero with a Thousand Faces*. Campbell was an anthropologist who studied the myths of cultures around the world and concluded that the archetypal hero goes through a series of predictable challenges across cultures. He called this the hero's journey, and it has influenced screenwriters and therapists alike. George Lucas relied heavily on the book when he wrote the *Star Wars* scripts, and was the first Hollywood filmmaker to credit Joseph Campbell as his influence.

I studied up on Campbell's work, and it helped to think of what I was going through as a hero's journey with a Departure, an Initiation, and (hopefully) a Return. I began to think of my illness as a Call to Adventure.

But not all of the hero's journey mono-myth seemed like it applied to me.

"Woman as Temptress," for instance. "The mystical marriage with the queen goddess of the world represents the hero's total mastery of life, for the woman is life," writes Campbell, "the hero its knower and master." And a little later, "No longer can the hero rest in innocence with the goddess of the flesh; for she is become the queen of sin." I was not capable of the mind-twisting required to make sense of these statements in the context of *my* life, *my* quest.

––––

With the help of Morris, Frank, and Campbell, I was rewriting my narrative. In the early years I'd tried to *refuse the call*, but it dogged me unrelentingly. Eventually I had no choice but to step across the *threshold*. I could remain a victim of my illness or I could embrace what it might teach me. I endured a *road of trials* that lasted a quarter of a century. I met many *teachers*.

Over the years, I'd aligned with a mission: I would do my best to reconnect my body, my mind, and my emotions, and to understand the impacts of the culture that enfolds them. I practiced listening to my body, honoring it, slowing down when it asked me to slow down. I didn't always do this perfectly, but I was determined to *cross the return threshold*. I sought the *freedom to live*.

The truth is, I wanted full recovery and couldn't imagine accepting anything else. But Campbell's framework does not require restitution. The hero who crosses the return threshold simply returns from the adventure with the wisdom gained from the quest and finds a way to share it. The freedom to live comes from learning how to live in the moment without fear of (bodily *or* metaphorical) death.

————

The stories we tell depend on the frameworks that guide our perceptions. Social workers like me are trained to look at things from a biopsychosocial perspective, which means that we see a fluid interplay between biology, psychology, and social context. In the world of ME/CFS, however, the term has been a thin disguise for a calamitous *psycho*social perspective of the illness. In a letter about ME/CFS published in the *BMJ* in 1996, the NIH's Stephen Straus betrayed his bias when he erroneously defined the biopsychosocial approach as "one which stresses the complex interplay of social, behavioural, and emotional factors in the presentation and perpetuation of symptoms."

Do you see what he did there? He forgot to mention the biological part of the equation. Genetics, for instance. And he seems to misunderstand the "social" part of the biopsychosocial perspective, implying that it has to do with enabling the "perpetuation of symptoms" rather than contributing to disease. The stress of being underpaid, uninsured, and unable to afford treatment, for instance, is a social context Straus appears not to consider.

Imagine how the country could change if we truly practiced bio-psychosocial medicine. We could still benefit from lasers, MRI scanners, and pharmaceuticals, when necessary, but we could also help patients better access their own inner healers through their stories.

Patients whose narratives matter become patients whose self-efficacy matters, and these patients are empowered to engage in their own well-being—to choose to exercise, to make healthy eating choices, to listen to their bodies, to rest, to ask for nurturance from loved ones, to offer nurturance to others in need. On a larger scale, as a culture viewing health through a biopsychosocial lens, we would be empowered to implement a gross domestic well-being program to complement our measures of gross domestic product. As Morris puts it, "At its most revolutionary" biopsychosocial medicine "can spark a major reallocation of financial resources toward prevention, as we seriously begin to address the cultural causes and contexts of illness."

CHAPTER 15

Treasure House

When I first looked up *neurasthenia* in my Merriam-Webster's dictionary, it defined the illness as "an emotional and psychic disorder that is characterized esp. by easy fatigability and often by lack of motivation, feelings of inadequacy, and psychosomatic symptoms." But in 1881, George Beard thought differently. Contradicting the beliefs of many of the doctors of his day, including some of those that Alice had consulted in the early years of her illness, he declared in *American Nervousness: Its Causes and Consequences* that neurasthenia "is a physical not a mental state, and its phenomena do not come from emotional excess or excitability." Beard and S. Weir Mitchell both saw the mind and body as intrinsically interconnected and believed that one day science would find somatic causes for all mental illness.

Alice's brother William explored the flip side of this perspective in his 1890 essay "The Hidden Self," one of the earliest American documents exploring the role of the unconscious in illness. William suggested that even some illnesses considered organic might be triggered by "some perverse buried fragment of consciousness . . . inhibiting the normal flow of life." Later, he dedicated an entire chapter of *The Varieties of Religious Experience* to the growing mind-cure movement, which embraced the idea that all disease was rooted in mental dis-ease. In some cases, he observed, the mind-cure worked remarkably well. These results, he wrote, "plainly show the universe to be a more many-sided affair than any sect, even the scientific sect, allows for."

Why not make room for that?

"Science succeeds in preventing and curing a certain amount of disease," he continued, while "mind-cure gives to some of us serenity, moral poise, and happiness," thus also helping to prevent disease. Both, he suggested, can be "genuine keys for unlocking the world's treasure-house." And at the same time, neither needs to be "exclusive of the other's simultaneous use."

———

Almost a century later, psychoneuroimmunology was born.

In the 1970s, while studying memory and taste aversion in lab rats, psychologist Robert Ader made a serendipitous discovery. First, he gave the rats a saccharin solution accompanied by an injection of cyclophosphamide, a drug that induces nausea and gastrointestinal upset. The rats soon learned to avoid the saccharin solution. But that wasn't as remarkable as what happened next. Cyclophosphamide also happens to be an immunosuppressant, and even when Ader halted the drug and administered the saccharin solution by itself, some of the rats were dying of bacterial and viral infections. What was happening here? "A hypothesis that seemed reasonable to me," Ader said in a 2010 interview, "was that, in addition to conditioning the avoidance response, we were conditioning the immunosuppressive effects [of cyclophosphamide]." In other words, the taste of the saccharin alone was triggering neural signals in the rats' brains that suppressed their immune systems.

Further studies confirmed Ader's groundbreaking theory, contradicting the long-held belief among scientists that the immune system was autonomous and that emotions did not have an effect on health. This discovery led Ader to develop the field he called psychoneuroimmunology.

In 1981, John M. Williams and David L. Felten discovered one of the first indications of neuroimmune interaction when they found a network of nerves leading to the thymus and spleen and terminating near clusters of lymphocytes, macrophages, and mast cells—all of which help control immune function. A decade later, Felten coedited the second edition of Ader's groundbreaking book *Psychoneuroimmunology*, which laid out the abundant evidence indicating that the brain and immune system represented a single integrated system of defense.

————

Candace Pert was just a grad student at Johns Hopkins University Medical School when she located the elusive opiate receptor, the first receptor ever discovered that admitted drugs originating from outside the body—in this case, opium, morphine and heroin. She published her groundbreaking findings in the March 1973 issue of *Science*.

"Unofficially," she wrote in her memoir,

> it was the beginning of my apprenticeship in neuroscience, a discipline that did not yet exist, and would not for almost a year. I didn't know it then, but I had walked right into the center of a revolution that was brewing, one in which the boundaries of distinct disciplines such as biochemistry, pharmacology, neuroanatomy, and psychology would dissolve to make way for the new interdisciplinary field of neuroscience.

The opiate receptor was the first of what she came to call the *molecules of emotion.*

Receptors, each comprising a single molecule, are found on the surface of cells in the brain as well as in the rest of the body. In her memoir, Pert explained that receptors are usually compared to keyholes. The "keys," which are also just one molecule, are called ligands. But she said that this metaphor, while apt for the mechanistic paradigm, doesn't adequately convey the reality, which is more fluid and poetic—perhaps even spiritual. "Receptor molecules respond to energy and chemical cues by vibrating. They wiggle, shimmy, and even hum as they bend and change from one shape to another." To Pert, it is more a dance than a lock and key. "The word *ligand*," she explained, "comes from the Latin *ligare,* 'that which binds,' sharing the origin with the word re*lig*ion." Receptors transmit messages from ligands to the cell interior, triggering a chain reaction of biological responses depending on the message received.

Pert's discovery set off a mad rush to find the natural ligand *within* the body that fit into the opiate receptor. Three years later, a triumphant team of Scottish researchers published a paper identifying the body's own feel-good ligand, now known as endorphin, which stands for "endogenous morphine," or the morphine made by the body itself. Endorphins are the neurochemicals that reduce pain and boost pleasure.

These discoveries spurred a new wave of research that would permeate every field of medicine, "uniting endocrinology, neurophysiology and immunology," wrote Pert, "and fueling a synthesis of behavior, psychology, and biology." Pert and her team went on to find the norepinephrine receptor, the GABA receptor, and the dopamine receptor.

Overall, there are three different types of ligands: neurotransmitters like norepinephrine, GABA, dopamine, serotonin, acetylcholine, glycine, and histamine; steroids, which consist of the sex hormones testosterone, progesterone, and estrogen; and peptides, such as endorphin, oxytocin, and insulin, which constitute about 95 percent of all ligands and play a broad role in regulating virtually all life processes. Peptides are produced in many parts of the body, including the brain. Pert calls them "information molecules" because they act as messengers, distributing information throughout the body.

With her team at the National Institutes of Health, Pert located peptide receptors in all parts of the brain. She and her team also made the astounding discovery that there are immunopeptides in the nervous system and neuropeptides in the immune system. In other words, the brain and the immune system communicate back and forth through their peptide messengers.

William James believed we experience sensations first and then interpret those sensations as emotions. His student, Walter Cannon—a physiologist who later coined the term *fight-or-flight response* and wrote the 1932 classic *The Wisdom of the Body*—said the emotions come first and the physiological changes in the body occur in response. But Pert's research convinced her that the communication goes both ways, and that our emotions can affect our immune system and vice versa. "Peptides serve to weave the body's organs and systems into a single web that reacts to both internal and external environmental changes with complex, subtly orchestrated responses. Peptides are the sheet music containing the notes, phrases, and rhythms that allow the orchestra—your body—to play as an integrated entity."

In 1985, Pert and three colleagues published their paradigm-smashing theory of the molecules of emotion in *The Journal of Immunology*: "Neuropeptides and their receptors . . . join the brain, glands, and immune system in a network of communication between brain and body, probably representing the biochemical substrate of emotion."

She expanded on these ideas in her memoir:

> The mind as we experience it is immaterial, yet it has a physical substrate, which is both the body and the brain. . . . The mind, then, is that which holds the network together, often acting below our consciousness, linking and coordinating the major systems and their organs and cells in an intelligently orchestrated symphony of life.

This perspective, she says, runs counter to the "mechanical universe, peopled by clocklike organisms, as conceived by Cartesian and Newtonian models."

———

It took Sarah Ramey twelve years to complete her delightfully titled memoir *The Lady's Handbook for Her Mysterious Illness*. Unbeknownst to each other, we toiled in different parts of the country to write books about what our illnesses were teaching us about the shortcomings of America's medical culture and the health risks of capitalism.

Ramey's ordeal started with a urinary tract infection she picked up while swimming in Walden Pond, fifteen miles north of where the James family had lived in Cambridge, Massachusetts. She went to the ER for treatment the very next day, but when the pain failed to resolve after six long months, Ramey sought the help of a leading urologist. He convinced her to submit to what he described as a "gentle" surgical procedure that would interrupt the muscle spasm he believed was causing the pain. But the local anesthetic he applied was no match for the searing pain Ramey experienced that day in his office, and by the time she got home, something felt profoundly wrong. The next day she was rushed to the hospital with a case of sepsis that almost killed her. Even after the infection had cleared, the broken-glass sensation in her pelvis persisted, only now it radiated out to the surrounding muscles in the vagina, rectum, and bladder as well. The doctors couldn't find anything wrong and eventually sent her home with a bottle of painkillers and portable IV antibiotics.

But Ramey did not recover. Instead, she toppled into an incapacitating mystery condition with multiple symptoms—debilitating fatigue, stopped bowels, and excruciating daily pain—and embarked on a long, harrowing quest to regain her health.

Like me, Ramey tried to explore her struggles through the lens of the hero's journey, but she could never quite make it fit. She wondered about the *heroine's* journey, and discovered that psychotherapist Maureen Murdock had written a book exploring Joseph Campbell's mono-myth through the unique experience of women, and it offered an entirely new lens through which Ramey could view her illness.

————

In 1981, Murdock asked Campbell for his thoughts on how the heroine's journey might be different from the hero's, and to her surprise he told her that women don't need to *make* the journey. "In the whole mythological tradition the woman is *there*," he said. "All she has to do is to realize that she's the place that people are trying to get to. When a woman realizes what her wonderful character is, she's not going to get messed up with the notion of being pseudo-male." Murdock found this answer deeply unsatisfying and set out, well, on a *journey* to find her own answers. And then so did Ramey.

Across numerous cultures and across centuries, the Goddess has frequently been represented as the great transformer/destroyer. In order to meet her, travelers had to find their way into the Underworld. As Ramey puts it, "While these stories on the surface look like they are about death," they're in fact "an exercise in exploring the shadow, the interior, the unconscious, the heart." The descent story to find the Goddess was about "the destruction of the ego, the reassembly of the true self, and regeneration." In other words, says Ramey, "the heroine's journey is a journey *in*."

It turned out, as Ramey discovered, that "a *lot* of women had already written about the female underworld initiation . . . but somehow their work had ended up relegated to the dusty, unread shelves of the Women's Issues sections tucked in the farthest, most untraveled corners of used-book stores."

After reading several such books, she came to see that the heroine's journey isn't about slaying the dragon; it's about connecting to the darkness, "learning how to grow strong roots, and to thrive in connection, cyclically, with everything else." In other words, she says, it is an "*ecological* initiation."

With an acknowledgment that people can fall anywhere on the spectrum of masculinity and femininity regardless of sex or gender identity, historically "connection over domination, empathy over trying to immediately fix a problem," and sensitivity instead of stoicism in response to poor environments have been viewed as more feminine ways of being in the world.

Ramey says that the mythic heroine is the protector of the interior, the root system, the soil, the psyche, the body, the cycles of life and death, and "the vast and often invisible systems that nourish, nurture, and support everything." The heroine is also the protector, she says, of the cultural body, the cultural psyche. We need the feminine to balance the masculine, the yin to the yang.

This journey inward gives the heroine "a fluency with darkness," an ability

> to deal with pain, or illness, or emotional upset—without pathologizing it, without othering it, and without shutting it down. . . . Indeed, nonempathetic responses, like trying to fix something that can't be fixed . . . or closing down in the face of someone else's suffering—these are all ways of denying the dark, and staying safe up in the light. Empathy is not sweet or sugary or nice—it's about the strength it takes to go down and be with the dark.

For all the progress made by women, says Ramey, we still live in a hierarchical culture where traits seen as masculine rank higher than those viewed as feminine. She urges women to reclaim their feminine traits with pride. "What has been used against us—our sensitivity—in its strongest form is the ability to respond to something negative before it snowballs into an uncontrollable problem." The feminine capacity for going down into the darkness, for plumbing the depths of our emotions and for connecting with empathy to the emotions of loved ones supports our ability to evolve, to transform, and to be a healing presence for others. "What is considered soft and weak . . . is some of the strongest medicine there is on Earth."

Ramey's words were a revelation to me. I always believed the way to be a good feminist was to be strong, competent, rational, and independent. When I was first struck down by a mysterious fatigue, one of my initial responses—in an argument conducted inside my head—was to deny my weakness and defend my strength. I exiled the delicate-flower part of myself. Which likely took a certain amount of energy to do—energy I really needed for other things, like healing.

While Ramey directly refers to women when she speaks of the feminine, I think that she and I would agree that what we are calling the feminine can be found in all of us. "If a person has no understanding that she has the absolute right to be feminine," says Ramey, "to be sensitive to her underworld's signals," well, then, "instead of going down and in, she will brush her shoulders off and soldier on. And she will be applauded for this."

> But if the environment is unsafe, the endocrine system, the nervous system, and the immune system *do not want the body to fight, toughen up, paper over, or ignore them.* These systems want the person to slow down, drop in, listen, and respond wisely—sooner, not later. Something is wrong in the root system and it needs to be attended to. . . .
>
> Thus the sensitive body requires that it be strong in this other, important way—the way that is not valued almost at all—the strength it takes to make time, to be willing to change behavior, to change the environment, and to tell other people that something subtle is wrong and needs tending before it snowballs out of control.
>
> This is wisdom, not weakness.
>
> Yet it is perceived and treated as the exact opposite.

In America's culture of unfettered capitalism, we exalt the "solar aspect of our lives," says Ramey, always striving for more. But bodies aren't built for infinite ascent. All of us (and some of us more than others) need time to connect to the root system.

And of course the same is true of physicians, no matter their sex or gender. The doctor who was so cold with me when I was at my most delicate, my most vulnerable, and my least capable, was trained by a system designed by—and *for*—men. She'd had to subvert her feminine side to survive the patriarchal world of medicine.

Doctors are trained "to slay dragons," says Ramey, "shoot at symptoms, kill disease, and surgically remove or fix problems." America's medical system "quite simply, is missing its other half."

The darker half.

The slower half.

The more compassionate half.

The half that is willing to descend, to search and figure out what is truly going on, no matter how inconvenient it is—so the patient can finally, genuinely ascend. . . .

This imbalance is a big part of the reason we excel at acute (heroic, eliminate the bad guy) illness and can't for the life of us solve chronic (heroinic, root system) illness.

In order to survive and thrive, all cultures need to respect the darkness and the shadow. And for this reason, the feminine initiation story is as essential as the masculine one. "Nothing grows without a relationship with the fertile void."

But when a country, or a medical system, is in "a deeply unbalanced state—where only the logical mind is valued, where only striving and achievement are valued, when the lights never turn off . . . when symptoms are repressed instead of understood, when empathy is uncommon, and when the algorithm trumps the story—this is when the need for the feminine corrective balloons."

Ramey asserts, "The Feminine . . . is the missing medicine in Medicine."

She suggests that functional medicine provides the balanced approach we need. It's science-based and logical while also being collaborative and empathic, and it treats the root causes of what ails the patient, viewing the human body as an ecosystem rather than a machine. Of course we don't want to throw out the machinery and medicine that work so well for acute illness, but functional medicine needs to be embraced as a coequal partner.

To make a fourteen-year story short, Ramey finally convinced a doctor to do a transvaginal sonogram to investigate a suspicion she'd confided to skeptical doctors throughout her ordeal. And sure enough, the scan revealed a large mass of scarring and fibrous tissue that was ensnaring all the nerves on one side of her vagina—almost certainly caused by the urologist's botched job fourteen years earlier—which had triggered a parallel inflammatory syndrome of the central nervous system. With the surgical removal of four of those nerves, Ramey experienced immediate partial relief from the pain, inflammation, and bowel dysfunction. She is still working to recover her health. Which has meant in part recovering her voice. "My case went unsolved for fourteen years because no one would listen to me," she writes. "And the reason they would not listen to me is because I am a woman."

———

Much was gained when Descartes devised the scientific method, with its emphasis on objective observation. We have Descartes to thank for iPads, global positioning systems, and the ability to diagnose and treat illnesses like pneumonia, cancer, and heart disease.

But Descartes's legacy glorifies the mind and repudiates the body. It privileges thinking over feeling, the objective over the subjective, the extraction of emotion from the acquisition of knowledge. We have become disconnected from our feelings and our intuition. We've lost our ability to perceive the whole.

————

Emotions aren't just the realm of women and they aren't frivolous or inconsequential. In fact, they've played a key role in our survival as a species. As neurologist Antonio Damasio points out in *Descartes' Error*, emotions are a critical element in rational decision-making. Without them, each of us would need to spend inordinate amounts of time carefully analyzing all the possible outcomes of every decision we make. We might even have to pull out a pad of paper or sit down at a computer and begin making complex mathematical calculations. Often, especially when various outcomes are more uncertain, we would get so lost in our calculations and analysis we'd *never* come to a decision. I get the image of someone sitting at a desk, scribbling, scribbling, scribbling for all eternity, never getting frustrated or lonely or even happy.

While we all vary in the ways we experience and process emotion, Damasio suggests that we're biologically predisposed to make decisions with the help of the sensations in our bodies—good and bad feelings we experience as a result of prior outcomes of similar situations. Much of this learning happens in childhood as part of the socialization process, but it continues throughout life. Damasio calls these feelings *somatic markers* and explains that the bad feelings we get—both in our gut and in other parts of our body—help us pay attention to possible negative outcomes. Similarly, the good feelings help us weigh the possibility of positive ones. This ability helps us narrow down the options and increases the efficiency of the decision-making process. It also helps us project into the future, expanding our willingness to endure short-term suffering for long-term gain.

Doctors, too, can't just be "rational" and "evidence-based" when diagnosing and treating illness. Their bodies also help them make decisions, both consciously and unconsciously. And this is why it's so important for them to have the time and training to attune to their patients and to be mindful of their own biases.

————

In the 1990s, Dr. Jay Goldstein, a psychiatrist and psychopharmacologist, developed a theory that ME/CFS was triggered by an insult to the limbic system, which is the part of the brain involved in memory, emotion, and the regulation of the autonomic nervous system. The illness was thus not psychosomatic but "neurosomatic," a disorder of central nervous system processing caused by a complex interaction between genetic, developmental, and environmental factors. In his book *Betrayal by the Brain*, he chided the major journals concerned with psychosomatic medicine for rarely discussing neurobiology. The belief that the illness was psychosomatic, Goldstein wrote, led social anthropologists to consider ME/CFS a "'culture bound syndrome' that displaces the repressed conflicts of patients unable to feel or express their emotions," leading to fruitless treatments. He wrote that cognitive rehabilitation didn't work well for this patient group, "since the problems are caused by a biochemical neural network of dysfunction, rather than by maladaptive or deficient learning strategies." Goldstein's limbic hypothesis stated that no matter what originally triggered the ME/CFS, the reason for its chronicity was a limbic system injury that caused widespread neuroimmune dysfunction.

————

In 1992, Iris Bell, Claudia Miller, and Gary Schwartz published the first paper suggesting that multiple chemical sensitivity might be the result of kindling, a sensitization of the brain's limbic system caused by repeated low-level exposure to chemicals. Their work was influenced by Graham V. Goddard's 1967 discovery that electrical stimulation to the brains of rats, administered over a period of several weeks at a low intensity, below the threshold for triggering seizures, eventually nonetheless provoked convulsions. Goddard and others found it was also possible to induce kindling through chemical stimulation.

Bell and her colleagues noted that a large body of animal research suggests that both acute and long-term exposure to a variety of chemicals impacts neurophysiological function and triggers limbic kindling. They added that "people often trace the onset of the MCS to an initial high-dose exposure such as a chemical spill or repeated, lower level exposures" such as home pesticide treatments or office building toxicants, and the intermittent nature of low-level chemical exposures in daily life facilitates kindling. Listing a range of MCS symptoms that includes headaches, fatigue, concentration and/or memory difficulties, insomnia, heart palpitations, irritability, depression, hives, and for some people seizure disorders, they added,

> Central nervous system symptoms are prominent and perhaps the most common feature of the illness in the otherwise diverse clinical symptomatology. . . . Once the syndrome has been initiated, a "spreading phenomenon" reportedly occurs, in which sensitivity generalizes from the original agent to low doses of multiple, chemically unrelated substances, such as perfume, tobacco smoke, auto exhaust, and newsprint.

Psychologist Leonard Jason and his team applied this theory to myalgic encephalomyelitis/chronic fatigue syndrome in 2009. Their article in the *Journal of Behavioral and Neuroscience Research* was the first peer-reviewed paper to suggest that limbic kindling may play a role in ME/CFS. Noting that chronic stress sensitizes neural processes and the resulting overactivation might lead to fatigue, they theorized that kindling among patients with ME/CFS might appear after prolonged stimulation of the limbic hypothalamic-pituitary-adrenal

(HPA) axis, either due to high-intensity stressors or to chronically repeated low-intensity stressors. Once this system is "charged," they explained, it becomes reactive to even very small stimuli. They cited Ashok Gupta's 2002 paper in *Medical Hypotheses*, which suggested that a pathogen or a chemical or physiological stressor may alter the brain in a way that leads to impaired immune response. Gupta proposed that in such periods of stress, the amygdala—which is a part of the limbic system—may become chronically sensitized to negative sensations experienced in the body. This triggers a vicious cycle in which unconscious negative reactions to symptoms provoke chronic stimulation of the sympathetic nervous system, which can cause immune reactivation and dysfunction, physical and mental exhaustion, and a host of secondary symptoms.

In 2009, a Norwegian research team synthesized a persuasive integrative biopsychosocial theory expanding on Gupta's concept that persistent autonomic nervous system arousal is the primary mechanism in ME/CFS and noting, among other things, that polymorphisms in genes related to the autonomic nervous system have been associated with ME/CFS. They called their hypothesis the CFS sustained arousal model, and concluded that this model "holds the capacity to explain *all* main findings concerning CFS disease mechanisms within a unifying theoretical framework."

———

In one of the more poetically expressed scientific insights that changed the way we view the world, meteorologist Edward Lorenz made a discovery he came to call "the butterfly effect." It was the science behind the possibility that something so seemingly innocuous as the flap of a butterfly's wings in Brazil could create changes in the atmosphere leading to something as momentous as a tornado in Texas. Lorenz had found that even minute discrepancies between two starting points could produce vastly disparate outcomes. The scientific expression for this was "sensitive dependence on initial conditions."

Lorenz's butterfly effect is just one of several principles of chaos theory, an interdisciplinary system for understanding nonlinear phenomena that otherwise appear infinitely random and complex.

I wondered whether chaos theory might be applied to the human body, and found a 1997 paper called "Chaos and the Limits of Modern Medicine," written by James Goodwin, MD, and published in *JAMA*. Before Lorenz made his discovery, wrote Goodwin,

> the traditional scientific outlook was that everything was predictable, given enough information. Lorenz was in essence stating that to predict weather long range would require individual data on every molecule in the earth's atmosphere, and, of course, measuring the molecules would alter them. [*Author's note*: This we know from quantum physics.] In other words, some systems are unpredictable and always will be unpredictable.

Bodies, too—like weather, like the environment—are complex systems. Goodwin points out that medical researchers in the past century or so have studied, taught, and valued only what they could measure, with little interest in what he calls "the true core of medical practice"—subjective experience and individual differences. But chaos theory "gives us the concepts and vocabulary to articulate the fact that much of the practice of medicine is outside the realm of the modernist reductionist model of science."

> The physician labors in a sea of uncertainty, but our vocabulary— the product of scientific medicine—communicates a degree of determinism that does not exist. Chaos theory will provide us with a new vocabulary, equally "scientific" and respectable as that of scientific medicine, with which to do battle with our reductionist

colleagues. . . . When complete understanding is abandoned as a goal, the traditional tasks of the physician—listening, witnessing, relieving suffering—will no longer be relegated to a small corner of medicine, the so-called art of medicine, but will be returned to the core of medical practice and medical education.

If the traditional healthcare system actively incorporated chaos theory, our care might be dramatically different.

Cartesian medicine sections our bodies into parts (and our healthcare system into specialties), but chaos theory shows us that all these "parts" are connected, and what happens in one part of the body, even something small, can have a cascade effect on overall health, sometimes in surprising and unpredictable and larger-than-expected ways.

Ten years before Goodwin's paper came out, James Gleick published the first popular book about this revolutionary theory, *Chaos: Making a New Science*. In the early pages, he explored science's resistance to radical new ideas, quoting from Thomas Kuhn's 1962 bestseller, *The Structure of Scientific Revolutions*: "Under normal conditions the research scientist is not an innovator but a solver of puzzles, and the puzzles upon which he concentrates are just those which he believes can be both stated and solved within the existing scientific tradition." In other words, most research scientists are limited by the existing understanding of science.

Of course, there's great value in medical research in the Cartesian tradition. It has saved countless lives and improved the quality of life for even more people. I'm really grateful for my cataract surgery: so linear, so logical, so elegantly completed. My vision got cloudy and my ophthalmologist did an exam, found the problem, and solved it surgically.

But when the existing scientific tradition is no longer large enough to contain all our questions, the people who take the discipline to cutting-edge places tend to be the ones who do not fit well into the recognized categories. As Gleick puts it,

A new science arises out of one that has reached a dead end. Often a revolution has an interdisciplinary character—its central discoveries often come from people straying outside the normal bounds of their specialties. The problems that obsess these theorists are not recognized as legitimate lines of inquiry. Thesis proposals are turned down or articles are refused publication.

Chaos theory helped to connect scientific (and other) disciplines that were previously considered distinct entities, influencing physics and physiology, of course, but also chemistry, seismology, and probability theory, among others. Medical research and treatment can join this revolution by respecting the overlaps and interconnections that will help us treat the body as a whole system, one that interacts with its environment through its senses, its memories, and the chemicals of emotions.

Decades before he won the Nobel Prize in 1918 for his contributions to quantum theory, Max Planck had firsthand experience with the intransigence that Gleick describes when he submitted his doctoral dissertation, which worked out some novel ideas on the second law of thermodynamics. His disinterested professors—one of whom Planck suspected never bothered to read it and another who was openly disapproving—gave the paper an unenthusiastic pass. In his 1949 autobiography, he famously wrote, perhaps a little bitterly, "A new scientific truth does not triumph by convincing its opponents and making them see the light, but rather because its opponents eventually die, and a new generation grows up that is familiar with it."

In 2001 a study by the Institute of Medicine found that there is in fact a long lag between when health scientists learn something significant and when doctors incorporate that new research into their patient care: it's seventeen years.

———

Like Planck, polymath Benoit Mandelbrot saw his ideas ignored or ridiculed by his colleagues. Trained as a mathematician, over the course of his life he performed groundbreaking work in economics, engineering, geometry, and physics. Because of his cross-disciplinary proclivities, he referred to himself—using the language of mathematics, of course—as an outlier.

He saw patterns where others saw chaos. One day, he stepped into a colleague's office and noticed that the professor's blackboard diagram of cotton prices looked *just* like his own diagram of income distribution. The data for neither fit within the traditional bell curve, so the numbers *looked* disorderly, but when he ran the data through the computer and viewed it in terms of *scaling*, he could discern a pattern that no one else had seen. He was onto something, but for decades he didn't know quite what. He described his process in his memoir:

> I started looking in the trash cans of science for such phenomena, because I suspected that what I was observing was not an exception but perhaps very widespread. I attended lectures and looked in unfashionable periodicals, most of them of little or no yield, but once in a while finding some interesting things. In a way it was a naturalist's approach, not a theoretician's approach. But my gamble paid off.

Mandelbrot found patterns in the clusters of interference on phone lines, and then in certain aspects of nature, such as ferns, Romanesco broccoli, the scattering of galaxies, and even rainfall patterns. It took thirty years, but eventually he realized that his intuitive curiosity, which at first had seemed so random, so *chaotic*, was neither of these things. He was on the trail of a dynamic that no one else had identified.

He came up with the name *fractals* for these "self-similar" systems that looked alike at all scales, and devised a way to measure irregular, or what he called "rough," forms, from stock market graphs to coastlines.

Before Mandelbrot made his discoveries, only smooth geometric Euclidian forms like squares, circles, and trapezoids could be measured. But, as Mandelbrot famously put it, "Clouds are not spheres, mountains are not cones." In a 2010 TED Talk shortly before his death, he explained that he had created a geometry for "branching systems for which there was no geometry." The mathematics of fractals is one element of chaos theory.

By the end of his life, Mandelbrot had won many awards and taken prestigious positions at Harvard and Yale. But for most of his career he was swimming against the tide. When he couldn't get peer-reviewed journals to publish his papers, he wrote books instead, his most influential being *The Fractal Geometry of Nature*. First published in the U.S. in 1982, it brought fractals into mainstream consciousness.

Rivers and trees have fractal-like structures, and so do cardiovascular systems and lungs. Think about rivers flowing into streams that trickle into creeks. Envision tree trunks and their branches, and the smaller branches that bifurcate from the larger ones. In the cardiovascular system, the large arteries branch into smaller arteries called arterioles, which branch into capillaries, which branch into small veins called venules, which branch into larger veins and back to the heart. In the lungs, the bronchi branch into bronchioles, which branch into tiny air sacs called alveoli, where an exchange occurs so that oxygen can be absorbed into the blood and carbon dioxide can be exhaled. Theoretical biologists have discovered that many other systems in the body also bear fractal elements, including the urinary collecting system, the biliary duct in the liver, and the lymphatic system.

The fractal design of the lungs makes for a tremendously efficient packing system. Remarkably, a pair of human lungs, spread out, would cover an area the size of a tennis court. This is important because any animal's ability to absorb oxygen is more or less proportional to the surface area packed into its lungs. Even our breathing patterns are fractal.

With the help of Mandelbrot's formulae, scientists are exploring the ways that chaos is health. For instance, researchers discovered that heartbeats, like economic phenomena, follow fractal laws. The tension between the sympathetic nervous system (which prepares the body for action) and the parasympathetic nervous system (which helps the body relax) keeps the heart at a "critical point," ready to slow down or speed up as needed. The associated small, fractal variances help the heart last longer. Just as any of our muscles tire if we repeat the same movement over and over, the heart, too, would wear out more quickly if it beat in exactly the same rhythm every time.

Interestingly, the heartbeats of people with heart disease don't follow fractal patterns. As Mark Ward suggests in *Beyond Chaos: The Underlying Theory Behind Life, the Universe, and Everything*, "Older bodies tend to be less adaptable than younger ones and have a more limited fractal repertoire. As a result the responses of their bodies to illness or trauma are not as creative." In other words, the nonlinearity of chaos is vital to our survival.

Crystal Ives Tallman, a physician and assistant professor at UCFS Fresno's School of Medicine, explained it succinctly in a paper she wrote several years ago as a student:

> A linear process, given a slight nudge, tends to remain off track. A nonlinear process, given the same nudge, returns to its starting point. For this reason, nonlinear systems can withstand small jolts and operate over a broad range of environmental conditions. Systems disordered in the right way are highly adaptable and poised at a critical point, ready to react swiftly to any change.

Chaos theory is now being applied to research in Parkinson's, atrial arrhythmias, epilepsy, and other health conditions. In 2020, researchers were able to predict the early course of the COVID-19 pandemic in several countries despite limited reliable data using an approach based on chaos theory.

There's an elegant beauty to fractals. Gleick quotes the German physicist Gert Eilenberger, who eloquently articulated what chaos theory reveals to us about aesthetics. "Our feeling for beauty is inspired by the harmonious arrangement of order and disorder as it occurs in natural objects—in clouds, trees, mountain ranges, or snow crystals. The shapes of all these are dynamical processes jelled into physical forms, and particular combinations of order and disorder are typical for them." Our bodies are also natural wonders, nonlinear systems that are ordered and disorderly at the same time, a web of networks in a continuous state of flux.

Gleick comments that a fractal understanding of the world prepares us for a shift in how we view our relationship to "untamed, uncivilized, undomesticated" nature.

> At one time rain forests, deserts, bush, and badlands represented all that society was striving to subdue. If people wanted aesthetic satisfaction from vegetation, they looked at gardens. As John Fowles put it, writing of eighteenth-century England: "The period had no sympathy with unregulated or primordial nature. It was aggressive wilderness, an ugly and all-invasive reminder of the Fall, of man's eternal exile from the Garden of Eden. . . . Even its natural sciences . . . remained essentially hostile to wild nature, seeing it only as something to be tamed, classified, utilized, exploited."

Rather than try to master nature in the way this country's colonizing and capitalist European forebears did and still do, we would serve our planet and our bodies better if instead we engaged with them in awe and wonder.

———

Awe—the sensation of being in the presence of something vast, something greater than ourselves—is related to the ancient conception of mystery. Awe inspires humility. It reminds us that our rational understanding of the world is finite. That there are things beyond our knowing. Awe can open us up to our nonlinear ways of experiencing the world. It can connect us to our curiosity, our creativity, our higher selves. It can seed patience, wisdom, compassion. The American allegiance to the march of forward progress and the pragmatics of hard currency has caused us to turn our backs on this way of experiencing the world.

While chaos theory can answer some of the questions that previously were unanswerable, what I like about the theory is that it also leaves room for mystery. It tells us that although we can understand some phenomena better, we'll never be able to predict *everything*. In other words, the whole is greater than its parts. This is what we've learned from Candace Pert's revelations about the way the molecules of emotion move through the body until they reach the ligand that fits them just right. And this is what we know about our ecosystems, too.

A paper influenced by chaos theory—and cowritten by three family members: a biologist, an ecologist, and an environmental scientist—suggests that "pulsing" may be critical to sustainability in ecosystems.

> In all the scales of nature from tiny fast systems of biochemistry to the largest galaxies of the cosmos, we observe systems that pulse. Host-parasite and predator-prey cycles are examples. . . . Growth of one part of nature consumes and pulls down another part of nature temporarily. Then a cycle is completed with retrogression and regrowth.

The earth's ecosystem, like a beating heart, balances at the critical point between order and chaos.

PART V

Recovery

We live in capitalism. Its power seems inescapable. So did the divine right of kings. Any human power can be resisted and changed by human beings.

—Ursula Le Guin

The protest is part of the American way of life.

—Thurgood Marshall

Yes, we can change the world because we have many times before.

—Rebecca Solnit, *Hope in the Dark*

We are all musicians in a great human orchestra, and *it is now time to play the Save the World Symphony*. You are not required to play a solo, but you are required to know what instrument you hold and play it as well as you can. What we love we must protect. That's what love means. From the right to know and the duty to inquire flows the obligation to act.

—Sandra Steingraber, as quoted in Robert
Shetterly's *Americans Who Tell the Truth*

CHAPTER 16

Rewiring

Functional medicine and other treatments had helped to improve my energy and endurance, but I was still plagued by food and chemical sensitivities and I was running out of treatments to try, running out of foods I could eat. I couldn't walk down the laundry aisle or pump gas or fly in a plane without wearing my carbon filter mask. It felt like the world kept getting smaller and smaller, and I had to be prepared, be prepared, be always prepared for the next assault. It could strike out of anywhere, and then came the eye pain and headache and brain fog to ruin my whole day and maybe the next one, too.

I was doing so much better, but full recovery felt just beyond my reach.

One morning in 2009, sitting at my desk in the house with the red door, I opened an email from an MCS blogger and learned of an entirely new treatment, unlike anything I'd seen before. Its website was touting some miraculous recoveries. Too good to be true, it seemed.

But then . . . what if it wasn't? What if *this* was the answer?

———

Annie Hopper, the developer of the Dynamic Neural Retraining System (DNRS), was a therapist, a newspaper columnist, and a regular talk radio guest expert in emotional wellness when she started to feel inexplicably unwell. She had just moved to a new office in Kelowna, British Columbia, painted it, and bought all new furniture, but it wasn't until months later, when she returned from a two-week vacation, that she realized it was the *office* that was responsible for her headaches, muscle pain, and insomnia. Further investigation revealed that her building was moldy and her office—which abutted the janitor's supply room—poorly ventilated. Not one of all the healthcare providers she consulted during that time had asked her about the air quality in her home or office.

A few months after this revelation, she walked past a scented candle display at a bookstore, and as she later wrote in her book *Wired for Healing*, "within five minutes I could barely speak or focus. Light was painful, sound was painful and it felt like I had knives piercing through my head. . . . The pain continued to get worse until it felt as if I was having some kind of brain hemorrhage." Since doctors had been no help to her, she went home to bed, hoping to feel better in the morning, rather than risk any further exposures at the hospital. But when she awoke, "the entire world had changed. I woke up feeling like a different person in a different body, and I was now the star of my own personal horror film. I literally felt like I was being poisoned by everything around me." She reacted with headaches, nausea, rapid heart rate, difficulty breathing, cognitive impairment, and loss of voice upon any initial exposure, followed by days of muscle pain and twitching, and total exhaustion.

When she developed an additional sensitivity to electromagnetic fields, she was forced to move into a broken-down houseboat with the electricity switched off. She stayed there for five months, with only her dog for company. Although she underwent the detoxification treatments generally advised by environmental doctors and alternative healthcare providers, her years of professional study in brain-based research led her to suspect that her symptoms might be due to a brain impairment. In a desperate bid to find a route to recovery, she did a deep dive into the literature.

———

In the November 1890 diary entry in which Alice castigated the entire medical profession for its "ignorant asininity," she revealed perhaps an equal frustration with her body—one deeply familiar to me, and to Hopper, too, I'm sure. She described herself as "a collection . . . of fantastic *un*productive emotions enclosed within tissue paper. . . . Animated by a never-ceasing belief in and longing for *action*, relentlessly denied." Elsewhere, Strouse notes, Alice referred repeatedly to her "restricted career" and described her body as a "little rubbish-heap."

"Behind this barrage of self-mockery hid a strong, frustrated will," writes Strouse. "Again and again, Alice connected her incapacity to her ambition—just as she noted on feeling within herself the 'potency of a Bismarck' that her 'sense of vitality' was 'simply proportionate to the excess of weakness.'"

To William, Alice wrote gamely: "There is little change in my state, the only variety in the day being the varying degrees of discomfort, and I find much entertainment therein."

In February 1891, Katharine found a four-story Italianate townhouse to rent in London, spacious enough to house Alice's nurse and maid, as well as the live-in cook whose services were included in the lease. The house, an elegant white building with arched bay windows, had a flower garden out back. When summer came, the garden bloomed with poppies, cornflowers, daisies, pansies, and nasturtiums. In this peaceful setting with Katharine, Alice described herself as "absurdly happy."

———

Thirty-five years later, Walter Cannon, the American physiologist who'd once been William James's student, introduced the concept of homeostasis. Suggesting that our bodily systems have set points, Cannon proposed that when the body is confronted with external conditions that disturb normal functioning, homeostasis is the mechanism that helps it return to internal stability. So, for instance, if the body is getting dehydrated, the kidneys, in an effort to preserve the water in the body, produce less urine. Under this paradigm, "normal" biology is based on statistical modeling, including population averages, and health is defined as an absence of disease.

In 1988, neuroscientist Peter Sterling and biologist Joseph Eyer expanded on the reductionist modernist idea of homeostasis when they introduced a postmodern paradigm: allostasis. "The major thrust in physiological research for the last century has been to study isolated organs and tissues," they wrote. "It turns out that most organs function remarkably well when they are disconnected from the rest of the body and brain and placed in a petri dish. . . . But when measurements of the internal milieu are made in an intact, unanesthetized organism, the results fit the homeostatic model very poorly."

And in fact, because of the way the body's systems are interrelated, they wrote, clamping down on one parameter with, say, a blood pressure medicine, tends to cause compensatory changes in other parameters that then also require medication. For example, long-term treatment for mild to moderate hypertension did indeed reduce the risk of dying from stroke, they wrote, citing several 1986 studies, but it *increased* the risk of dying from heart disease.

They argued that the latest evidence supported a new conceptual model. The *brain* is the wizard behind the curtain, assessing the external environment, predicting what's going to happen based on past experience, and orchestrating the rest of the body's systems to make anticipatory changes. Unlike the linearity of homeostasis, allostasis recognizes the body as a complex ecosystem that is constantly adjusting in response to changing variables of the external environment. In order to be able to do that successfully, any given set point is likely to be regulated cooperatively by a variety of internal systems.

———

A 2019 paper about allostasis by Sung W. Lee, who is an MD with a master's degree in philosophy, echoes perspectives connecting chaos theory and heart rate. Lee describes what he calls "optimal anticipatory oscillation," which may be demonstrated, for instance, "as patterns of variability in heart rate, indicating a capacity for rapid recalibrations of cardiac output in context-sensitive ways," thus decreasing the risk of morbidity or mortality. In other words, the heart is able to adjust swiftly to complex and changing environments by balancing at a critical point "on the border between order and disorder, also described as 'the edge of chaos.'"

From an allostatic perspective, says Lee, optimal health then might be described as a "dynamic capacity for recalibration." Allostatic health also fulfills the definition of health offered by the World Health Organization: a "state of complete physical, mental, and social well-being, and not merely the absence of disease."

———

The book that became prerequisite reading for Annie Hopper's Dynamic Neural Retraining System, the one that most influenced her design of the program that ultimately cured her, was *The Brain That Changes Itself*, by the Canadian psychiatrist and psychoanalyst Norman Doidge. The book introduced Hopper to the concept of neuroplasticity. As Doidge explains it, for four hundred years, scientists believed that after childhood, brain anatomy was unchangeable. One reason for this conviction, he writes, is that the brain was believed to be "like a glorious machine. And while machines do many extraordinary things, they don't change and grow."

But in the 1960s and '70s, some iconoclastic scientists began to discover that the brain is in fact surprisingly malleable. Doidge tells the stories of several of these researchers and the patients whose lives were changed as a result of their work. Hopper used that research to build her own program of targeted brain retraining based on the idea that her limbic system had gone into overdrive in its effort to protect her from further harm, wreaking havoc on her entire body. As she explained in *Wired for Healing*, "This cascading stress response can trigger the hypothalamus to release specific neurotransmitters that may keep the brain and body in a chronic state of stress, which, in turn, can negatively affect multiple systems."

She came to believe that MCS, ME/CFS, fibromyalgia, chronic Lyme, and similar poorly understood illnesses were triggered by trauma, whether it be chemical (like the various pesticides I used over the years), viral (like the Epstein-Barr virus that caused my mononucleosis), bacterial (like Lyme disease), fungal (toxic mold), or extraordinary physical stress (head trauma or overtraining syndrome) or emotional strain (abuse, for instance). Emphasizing that "the root of the condition is located *physically* in the brain and is a form of an *acquired brain injury* that affects many systems of the body," Hopper explained that when the body is in a state of chronic fight or flight, "energy is taken away from other mechanisms associated with growth and regeneration, like communication between cells, absorption of nutrients, production of energy, excretion of waste products, or rest. Research has shown that chronic or excessive stress inhibits synaptic function and neuronal growth." Limbic system dysfunction can also impair detoxification processes.

Hopper learned from *The Brain That Changes Itself* that "neurons that fire together wire together." In other words, when neurons fire repeatedly at the same time, the connection between them gets stronger and stronger. A benign example: many of us associate movie theaters with popcorn.

Hopper hypothesized that her chemical and mold exposures had caused what she called a "cross-wiring" in her brain that triggered her symptoms, and that limbic kindling was making the problem worse and worse. One analogy that helped Hopper understand neural pathways is that they are like the ruts made by a sled on a snowy hillside. The more the sled shoots down one path, the smoother and speedier the groove gets, making it harder and harder to carve a new trail.

Hopper was going to have to figure out a way to calm down her limbic system and rewire her brain. But how?

———

Chronic stress or trauma may lead to "allostatic impairment," says Sung W. Lee, remarking that such persistent assaults on the brain can impact all of the systems of the body, "even if these influences originate from mental, social, cultural, or other 'non-physical' sources." He adds that Peter Sterling has suggested "that since social disruption is the ultimate cause for the brain to predict a need for elevated arousal, then it is repair of the social fabric that is ultimately necessary for the brain to revise its prediction and thereby re-orchestrate its downstream regulation."

Lee writes that social change accompanied by individual commitments to disciplines that can help the brain change its predictions, such as "mental training," exercise, yoga, and similar strategies, can help adjust set points so that the stress response system does not get so easily activated.

The allostatic paradigm could enhance many fields, he says, including medicine, mathematics, physics, architecture, urban planning, anthropology, epidemiology, nutrition, pharmacology, and education. Alluding to the precepts of chaos theory, and the butterfly effect in particular, Lee writes that such allostatic approaches "may show that even subtle forms of well-placed intervention can have compounded consequences."

———

From Doidge's book, Hopper also learned about constraint-induced movement therapy (known as CIMT), introduced in 1981 as a groundbreaking new way to help survivors of stroke and brain injury to rewire their brains and recover hand mobility.

Wearing a mitt to constrain the functional hand, patients perform small repetitive tasks that get incrementally more difficult. Gradually, the patient regains dexterity in the paralyzed hand. Research confirms that CIMT restores reduced neuronal brain maps. In one study, scientists measured before-and-after brain maps of six stroke survivors, each with a hand and arm that had been paralyzed for an average of six years—long after any spontaneous recovery could be expected. After just two weeks of CIMT, not only had the patients' motor functions substantially improved, but the size of the brain map determining hand movement had doubled. Another study revealed that neuroplastic changes can reach across brain hemispheres.

Hopper began thinking about how she could adapt CIMT to limbic system dysfunction.

———

Despite the joy of moving with Katharine into their heavenly home, three months later Alice found herself "going downhill at a steady trot" and sought the care of prominent London physician Sir Andrew Clark.

Finally, and to her great relief, she was lifted "out of the formless void" and set down "within the very heart of the sustaining concrete." A diagnosis: breast cancer. As she exulted in her diary, "To him who waits, all things come!"

Sir Andrew, "the blessed being," had also "endowed" her with "not only cardiac complications," but also a "most distressing case of nervous hyperaesthesia" (hypersensitivity of one or more of the senses of sight, sound, touch, and/or smell). These, she wrote triumphantly, added to a spinal neurosis that has taken me off my legs for seven years; with attacks of rheumatic gout in my stomach for the last twenty, ought to satisfy the most inflated pathologic vanity. It is decidedly indecent to catalogue oneself in this way, but I put it down in a scientific spirit, to show that though I have no productive worth, I have a certain value as an indestructible quantity.

To William, she described it as

the most supremely interesting moment in life . . . and I count it as the greatest good fortune to have these few months so full of interest & instruction in the knowledge of my approaching death. It is as simple in one's own person as any fact of nature, the fall of a leaf or the blooming of a rose, & I have a delicious consciousness, ever present, of wide spaces close at hand, & whisperings of release in the air.

In this same letter, just as Strouse had quoted it in the introduction to her biography, Alice beseeched William, "so when I am gone, pray don't think of me simply as a creature who might have been something else had neurotic science been born." And then: "notwithstanding the poverty of my outside experience I have always had a significance for myself."

Within four months, the pain from the cancer had become unbearable and the morphine that had worked for a time seemed now to be the cause of intolerable anxiety and insomnia. In December, after Alice, Katharine, and Henry read an article by a nearby doctor about hypnosis, Katharine immediately hired him. Alice enthused later that the session helped her float "for the first time into the deep sea of divine *cessation*." While it didn't stop the pain, she found it profoundly calming. The specialist taught the technique to Katharine, who began regularly hypnotizing her.

Alice wrote in her diary that she believed hypnosis could open up a "vast field of therapeutic possibilities," and had come to the conclusion that she was "simply born a few years too soon." Finally she'd found a way to get a break from "the individual watch dog, worn out with his ceaseless vigil to maintain the sanity of the modern complicated mechanism." But she would never be able to explore the full benefits of this treatment: she was dying.

———

Well over a century after Alice, Hopper, too, felt herself on the cusp of a vast field of therapeutic possibilities. She became her own case study, designing a program for herself that involved an hour of concerted brain retraining every day. She started by just *imagining* herself being exposed to an everyday chemical such as perfume or air freshener. Then she simply *noticed* the fear that was arising in her body, and as though putting a mitten on the part of her brain that was afraid, she interrupted her old pattern of thinking and feeling and reminded herself of her *new* understanding that her problems were actually caused by cross-wiring in her limbic system.

From her reading, she knew that in order to calm her limbic system and rewire her brain, she had to flood her system with calming biochemicals when she encountered toxicants, mold, or electromagnetic fields. Given how constricted and stressful her life had become, this seemed impossible to do safely. But in *The Brain That Changes Itself,* she'd learned of neuroscientist Alvaro Pascual-Leone, whose work helped Hopper realize that neurologically, the brain doesn't wholly distinguish between imagining an act and actually doing it. Pascual-Leone directed a piano-based study that compared before-and-after motor function skills and brain maps of two groups of people, none of whom had ever studied the instrument. His subjects were taught to play a simple series of notes. The "physical practice" group was directed to play the sequence two hours a day for five days. The "mental practice" group was instructed to sit in front of an electric keyboard for the same amount of time each day and *imagine* both playing the sequence and hearing it played. On the third day, the mental practice group played as accurately as the group that had actually played the notes. By the end of the fifth day, both groups showed similar brain map changes. This research helped Hopper conceive that by visualizing happy memories in vivid detail during her daily brain retraining practice and whenever exposed to triggering stimuli, she could successfully rewire her brain.

Then she took her brain retraining one step further, *also* devoting time to visualizing as specifically as possible the free and joyful future she wanted for herself. If her brain didn't distinguish between her reality and her imaginings, then she could manifest the full recovery she sought with the help of her imagination. She was changing her prediction so she could alter her body's allostatic response.

As she grew healthier, Hopper incrementally exposed herself to challenging stimuli, both in her structured daily practice and in the unstructured encounters she faced when she ventured back into the world she'd been forced to leave. She thought of this process as neuroplasticity boot camp.

Over time, writes Hopper, her limbic system calmed.

The cingulate cortex stopped focusing so intensely on the perceived threat. This reduced the fear messages sent to the amygdala, which decreased the production of stress hormones in the pituitary and adrenal glands and calmed my entire system. Eventually, my sensory perception normalized, and my body resumed . . . functions like growth and repair. My hippocampus had a chance to relearn the association to a particular stimulus, which helped to alleviate the anticipated fear. This prevented the cycle from reinitiating itself. My threat mechanism began to regulate itself. I had successfully changed the structure and function of my brain!

After six months of rigorous brain retraining, Hopper had achieved something few others with MCS had done: she recovered.

————

For so long I'd wondered if recovery was even possible. I'm sure Hopper did, too.

The titanic power of industrial capitalism can feel equally insurmountable. How easy it would be to sink into helpless resignation.

But we can't afford to do that. Now more than ever, we need to *act*. The Trump administration and its aftermath have shown us that our democracy is in peril. When the chasm between rich and poor gets too wide, a country becomes vulnerable to fascism.

During those bleak Trump years, I was seduced by the title of Rebecca Solnit's 2004 *Hope in the Dark*. Revised and reprinted in 2016, this book gave me a new reference point for viewing this country's trajectory and potential for change. Solnit writes that many activists have "a mechanistic view of change . . . They expect finality, definitiveness, straightforward cause-and-effect relationships, instant returns." But this isn't how change happens, and the resulting disappointment triggers "bitterness, cynicism, defeatism, knowingness." Who among us has not slipped into despair and cynicism these past several years?

Our world and its social systems are infinitely complex, however, and sudden groundswells can take us by surprise. Solnit describes social change in terms of chaos theory: small acts can give rise to monumental shifts. "Histories usually pick up when the action begins," says Solnit, but social change starts in the imagination. "This means, of course, that the most foundational change of all, the one from which all else issues, is hardest to track. It means that politics arises out of the spread of ideas and the shaping of imaginations. It means that symbolic and cultural acts have real political power."

With all that's wrong in America, it's sometimes hard to remember all that is good. This country has never lived up to its fullest potential, but what that means is that there's room to fight for better. And we have a long history of doing just that . . . and *succeeding*.

For several demoralizing decades, for instance, the queer community fought for the right to marry, and then suddenly several states legalized gay marriage, and then President Obama signed it into federal law. Women campaigned for the right to vote for almost three-quarters of a century before a young Tennessee legislator chose to do his mother's bidding and cast the deciding vote to ratify the 19th Amendment in 1920. Abolitionists agitated for the end of slavery for thirty-five years until the Civil War finally put it to a stop. The people who worked on these projects in the early decades did not fail; they laid the groundwork. Many discouraged people believe Occupy Wall Street achieved nothing, but it changed how we talk about capitalism, and how often.

———

In 2008, just two years after her life was turned upside down by a bookstore's scented candle display, Hopper began traveling North America giving five-day trainings to teach others with limbic system disorders how they could recover, too. But she wasn't booking near our area and I couldn't afford the training combined with the travel and lodging.

Then, in September 2011, *The New York Times* published a photo essay by Thilde Jensen, who was known among us in the online MCS community. Jensen's career as a documentary photographer had been cut short by MCS in 2003. She'd been forced to move out of her Brooklyn apartment and live outdoors for two years, in tents or trailers or under the stars. During that time, she photographed others like her who were living on the outskirts of society due to extreme chemical sensitivities, documenting the toll the illness took on some of the most very ill, who were mostly invisible to society.

Thanks to the DNRS course, Jensen significantly recovered—enough to devote more energy to her project, called "Canaries," and get it out into the world. When I emailed Annie Hopper to see what it would take to get her to the Portland area (more, it turned out, than our little MCS group could manage), she told me that an instructional DVD series would be available soon.

———

Around the time of Jensen's *New York Times* photo essay, another member of our MCS support group told us about a similar program designed by a man in England with ME/CFS, Ashok Gupta, who, like Hopper, had fully recovered. The woman was in a Gupta Program peer group on a website called Planet Thrive and said that many in the group were reporting improvement. Gupta, the author of the paper I wrote about in chapter 15, called ME/CFS, MCS, and similar illnesses *neuroimmune conditions*.

The theory underlying both programs resonated with me. After all, I had tried just about everything else. It made sense to me that the trauma of the illness and its aftermath had carved a trail in my neural pathways.

———

Unfortunately, even Hopper's five-DVD set was unaffordable to many of us in our MCS group. Of course Hopper deserves to make a good living for sharing her life-changing discovery, but I couldn't help but feel that once again the system was stacked against people with disabilities, many of whom live close to the bone because they can't work full time, or in some cases, at all. And like just about every other MCS and ME/CFS treatment, DNRS was considered experimental, so it wasn't covered by insurance.

A group of us figured out a work-around; we pitched in together to make the purchase and took turns borrowing it. Finally, one gusty January day, it was my turn. I picked up the set at a group member's house and began watching the recommended one DVD per day. The production was pretty low-tech, with Hopper standing in the front of a conference room at one of her live trainings sharing her illness and recovery story and then explaining the ideas behind limbic system dysfunction and its relation to MCS, ME/CFS, and other illnesses. The DVDs included testimonials from people who had seen significant improvements even within the five days of the training and others who had fully recovered from severe illness after previous trainings and daily practice.

Like me, Hopper had been motivated by her illness to learn about the many health risks of toxicants. In her DVDs, at the same time that she enjoined her viewers with MCS to remember that small exposures are not typically harmful, she also emphasized that it's better for everyone's bodies and for the environment to use natural products when possible. And then she trained her students in what she called "the steps." She offered helpful advice and cheerleading, and told viewers there were DNRS coaches available if needed for further support. The DVD training made it clear that brain retraining is a dedicated, laborious, structured, incremental process of rewiring the brain. It would require my full commitment.

Using Hopper's steps as the template, I immediately began designing my own program. I asked a perfume-loving friend to spray samples of three of her perfumes onto scraps of fabric and seal them up in separate jars. I also squirted a sample of the hand soap from my office restroom into a baby food jar. The soap was relatively mild, but it gave me headaches nonetheless, which meant I was left to simply rinse my hands when I was at work.

On the first day, I opened the lid of the baby food jar and took a tiny whiff. Then I closed it again and began doing my steps, starting with interrupting my brain's old pattern with a loving "Stop! Stop! Stop! My brain is stuck in a rut and it's sending me false messages."

Hopper recommended an hour a day of brain retraining, which included thanking the limbic system for its valiant protective efforts and letting it know it could now relax, visualizing happy past memories and vividly imagining the details of a healthy future.

Due to my busy work schedule, I was already getting just seven hours of sleep a night—one or two hours fewer than I actually needed—but in order to fit in time for brain retraining, I began setting my alarm a half-hour earlier. It was the most I could fit in. Hopper urged viewers not to miss a single day in her six-month program, because the limbic system could so easily slip back into the more familiar neural pathway, and so no matter how much I wanted to skip it, I didn't. I thought of it as short-term suffering for long-term gain.

When I could, I did my braining retraining standing up, as she recommended, but if my energy was low, I did it lying down. I said everything aloud, because that's what she advised, and there were movements to go along with the verbal steps of the program, preferably with great enthusiasm, all to help the limbic system forge and integrate this new, healthier pathway.

I've never liked meditating and I didn't enjoy brain retraining, but that didn't matter because I'd tried everything else and Hopper's theory felt right, at least for me. I was going to try this thing.

I envisioned the monarch caterpillars I raised as a girl—the magic moment when the newly hatched butterflies took flight from my open hand. I envisioned the tree fort I built with my best friend, how we talked to the tree and believed it talked back to us through the wind in its leaves. I envisioned the river where I now swam, the curious little fish that gathered around my legs when I stood hip-deep on the other side, the silvery glint of their scales.

I envisioned my future self pushing my cart down the laundry aisle without donning my mask, checking in at a hotel without having to call first to ask them to clean my room with nontoxic products, and—the pièce de résistance—sitting on a plane en route to a visit with my brother and his family in their small town on the coast of Tasmania.

———

It's natural to feel discouraged sometimes, even most of the time; but we can't just acquiesce. "Your opponents would love you to believe that it's hopeless, that you have no power, that there's no reason to act, that you can't win," says Rebecca Solnit. "Hope is an embrace of the unknown and the unknowable, an alternative to the certainty of both optimists and pessimists. Optimists think it will all be fine without our involvement, pessimists take the opposite position; both excuse themselves from acting."

And so we must step up and do this work and tell our stories. Our stories of injustice *and* our stories of hope. When we join together, our voices and actions can change the world.

Right this very moment, all over the country, little fires are kindling, and nobody knows when any of them will ignite or what the outcomes might be. Two months into the COVID-19 pandemic, when George Floyd was murdered by White police officer Derek Chauvin, suddenly people were marching in the streets in unprecedented numbers. Confederate statues fell, racist executives were forced out of their jobs, and cities began to reallocate police funding to invest in community services instead. Later, in a history-making triumph, a jury pronounced Chauvin guilty and he was sentenced to twenty-two and a half years in prison—almost as many years as I had been ill.

———

Reasons for hope are all around us if we care to look. In Maine, by partnering with the state chapter of the Nature Conservancy (which is a member of an informal umbrella group of land trusts, timber companies, philanthropies, and conservation groups dedicated to returning land to Maine tribes), the Passamaquoddy Nation recently reacquired almost the entirety of a 150-acre island that was stolen by the state in the mid-nineteenth century.

And in 2014, after years of pressure from environmental groups like the Campaign for Safe Cosmetics, healthcare groups like the American Nurses Association, and concerned parents, Johnson & Johnson began removing known and probable carcinogens and other hazardous chemicals from their baby products.

In 2002, the people of Porter Township, Pennsylvania, were the first of hundreds of American communities to adopt an ordinance nullifying corporate personhood. Then four years later, the Pennsylvania borough of Tamaqua became the first community on earth to enact an ordinance recognizing the rights of nature. Now, roughly forty U.S. communities have formally decreed the rights of nature, and Ecuador has written these rights into its constitution.

"We need litanies or recitations or monuments to [our] victories," writes Solnit, "so that they are landmarks in everyone's mind."

———

On top of the structured daily practice, Hopper also said it was critical to do as many of the steps as feasibly possible when out in public and exposed to real-world toxicants like bus exhaust or cleaning products or fresh paint.

If you had asked me before taking the DNRS program if I had a lot of fearful thoughts about chemicals, I would have denied it. But the program turned me into an observer of my own fears, and I realized how common they were and how much they ruled my life. So every time I had a fearful thought, even if I was out in the world, I did whatever steps I could, in my head and sometimes with the subtlest of hand motions.

Hopper developed her program based on her research, deductions, and intuitions about what might work. What fortitude it must have taken to stay motivated, to allow her whole life to be taken over by this experimental practice. As far as she knew, what she was trying to do had never been done before.

I know that *I* had lots of doubts. What if it didn't work? What if this was all a waste of time?

But what else did I have left? If what it took to recover was an act of sheer will, then nothing would stop me. My will had kept me alive when I was filled with such despair I wanted to die. It had helped me stay faithful to an increasingly restrictive diet. It kept me striving—reaching for health and for the fullest life possible. I'd always had the will, but I didn't have the tools. My will needed a focus. And now it had one.

I had to give *everything* to this. It could be the answer I'd been seeking for twenty-four years.

Some DNRS trainees experience improvements on the very first or second day. For others, it can take months before seeing any benefits. In my case, it took two weeks. I was getting up every morning and moving through the steps on faith tempered by a fair amount of skepticism, given my many years of dashed hopes.

But one morning, I opened the lid to the hand soap and inhaled, and something felt different. I didn't get the signal pain behind my eyes. My body didn't clench up. The soap smelled . . . innocuous. At the office later that day, I squirted some into my hands and took a whiff. I smiled (because even a forced smile produces feel-good chemicals in the brain and would help to rewire my experience of the soap as positive rather than negative), took a deep breath (to help activate my parasympathetic nervous system), and ran through a few of the steps in my mind, reminding myself that my past experiences were due to a cross-wiring in my limbic system and that I was successfully retraining my brain. Then I lathered up.

———

The things that once seemed impossible here in America eventually became so much a part of the status quo as to be taken for granted. Women with careers, for instance. Black people and Whites swimming in the same pools and drinking out of the same water fountains. A Social Security safety net so that the elderly and disabled could pay their bills and keep a roof over their heads.

Environmentally, we can be grateful for the recovery of the bald eagle due to the banning of DDT. Gasoline that doesn't have lead in it. Cleveland's Cuyahoga River not being on fire. As Solnit points out, "Most environmental victories look like nothing happened; the land wasn't annexed by the army, the mine didn't open, the road didn't cut through, the factory didn't spew effluents that didn't give asthma to the children who didn't wheeze and panic and stay indoors on beautiful days. They are triumphs invisible except through storytelling."

———

I rinsed the soap off my hands, dried them, then strode down the hall and back to my office. And I was fine. Fine. After collapse and incapacity, after twenty-four years of suffering, I must say that the thrill of being fine—just fine—was exhilarating. I sat with my next client, and the next, wrote my notes, used the toilet again and washed my hands with soap just like anybody else, and all day long I was *fine*.

And with this little soupçon of evidence, I knew that finally, after all these years, I was truly on the road to recovery.

My faith was often tested. There were challenges and setbacks, but I kept on.

One Sunday afternoon, as I moved through the steps, I yawned. This, I knew, was cause for celebration. Although I'd triggered my sympathetic nervous system with a whiff of my friend's perfume, the yawn signaled that the DNRS was engaging my parasympathetic nervous system. My limbic system really was calming in response to the brain retraining!

From that point on, the brain retraining yawns came frequently. Eventually my system became inured to my friend's perfume. And when a new client showed up to my office wearing a scent, I could just do a few quick steps in my mind to reassure my limbic system that everything was okay, and it was.

Gradually I found myself able to face all the toxicants that had previously made me so ill. I could walk through the laundry aisle without wearing a mask. I could fly in a plane. I could stay in a hotel, even when the room smelled of cleaning products. Sometimes it was hard to recognize the magnitude of my recovery. I'd walk into a conference room that might normally have triggered a headache and not even notice that I didn't get one, because how do you notice something that isn't there?

And my energy, which for years I'd described as being on the low end of normal, was finally just *normal*. I didn't crash anymore. I didn't have to curl up in a ball to try to recover lost energy.

Perhaps because I was practicing only half an hour each day, it took a year and a half to fully recover from the ME/CFS and MCS. All that was left was the food sensitivities. Avoiding specific foods had long been the *only* thing I could do—other than rest for the ME/CFS and avoidance for the MCS—that gave me any kind of control over my symptoms. When I avoided sweeteners, all grains, dairy, and plants from the evening nightshade family, I felt better. When I ate foods with any of those ingredients, I suffered from various combinations of fatigue, depression, joint pain, itching, and other symptoms.

Before I tackled this final frontier, I needed a break from the tedium of brain retraining. And so I took a year and a half off. But just a few months before I was to fly to my first artist residency—where all meals would be provided—I picked up where I left off and started in on my food sensitivities.

I began doing at least a few steps of DNRS immediately before eating any food that contained triggering ingredients, almost like saying grace. A key element of brain retraining is incremental challenges, so I didn't immediately head to the gelato parlor. But soon I was eating pumpkin pie sweetened with maple syrup in a gluten-free crust. And then I was eating potatoes. And raspberries with honey in yogurt. And cheese! Dairy had always clogged my ears, but after several months of delighted consumption, I asked my doctor to look in my ears and they were clear. Clear!

When I'd fully recovered, I allowed myself sugar treats twice per week. At the bakery, I could barely contain my excitement. I felt like a kid and could barely restrain myself from jumping up and down with glee.

I'd done it. It took twenty-seven years, but finally I'd gotten my life back. All of it. Every last drop.

———

New stories, new movements, tend to start on the margins and move to the center, just like some of our most groundbreaking scientific discoveries. The phrase *Me Too* was coined by Tarana Burke in 2006 to empower sexual assault survivors in underprivileged communities. How could she have imagined that just over ten years later those words would fuel a worldwide movement?

In 2017, a few days after actor Ashley Judd accused producer Harvey Weinstein of sexual harassment in *The New York Times*, actor Alyssa Milano made #MeToo a Twitter hashtag and the internet exploded with women's stories of sexual harassment and assault. Altogether over eighty women came forward with accusations against Weinstein, and in 2020 he was sentenced to twenty-three years in prison. Since 2017, a swath of executives and performers have lost their jobs because finally when women spoke out, people listened.

Of course, the fact that a number of men lost their jobs or went to prison doesn't make this—or the Derek Chauvin conviction, either, for that matter—a happily-ever-after story. As Solnit is quick to point out, there is rarely if ever such a thing as an *ending* when it comes to activism. We make beautiful strides, and still, no country will ever be a utopia.

But just because we can't create paradise on earth doesn't mean we should give up trying to solve the problems we see. As philosopher Bertrand Russell once wrote, "It is not a finished Utopia that we ought to desire, but a world where imagination and hope are alive and active."

———

Many Americans erroneously equate capitalism with freedom and democracy, and Republicans have weaponized the word *socialism* by falsely associating it with the communism of Soviet Russia. But social democratic countries, and particularly Nordic nations—which consistently rank among the happiest in the world—embrace socialist policies like universal healthcare, generous maternity leave, publicly funded day care, and government regulations that distribute resources more evenly.

Defenders of unfettered capitalism say that competition generates innovation. While this is true, it's also true that sometimes the best innovations happen thanks to government. Energy-saving lightbulbs, for instance. Improved technologies to lower smokestack emissions. Safer cars. The internet. The Human Genome Project.

Of course, the U.S. already has a number of popular socialist programs, including Social Security, Medicare, Medicaid, police and fire departments, snow removal, garbage collection, and several services that begin with the word *public*, including schools, beaches and parks, and libraries. We pay for them with our taxes for the benefit of all Americans.

But we can do better. It's entirely possible for the U.S. to change its economics and remain a democracy. We can borrow ideas from Scandinavian and European countries and from Canada, too. These and other nations offer any number of economic, environmental, and healthcare models that favor people and planet over corporations.

———

Studies are beginning to confirm that it's possible to regain health by rewiring the brain. Between 2016 and 2018, Dale Guenter, MD, an associate professor at McMaster University in Hamilton, Ontario, conducted the first ever study of Annie Hopper's DNRS outcomes, and the results were striking. For one year, his team followed 102 people with multiple chemical sensitivity, ME/CFS, and/or fibromyalgia (among other health problems) who took the five-day in-person DNRS training. Forty percent of them reported that their symptoms had begun more than twenty years previously. Participants filled out six standardized health surveys prior to the training, and then follow-up surveys at three, six, and twelve months. The study was presented in 2019 at the annual conference of the North American Primary Care Research Group.

The quality of life survey (known as SF-36) measures eight indicators: physical functioning, social functioning, emotional functioning, bodily pain, general health, mental health, vitality, and physical activities at work or home. The average healthy Canadian generally scores between 70 and 90 percent. At the three-month mark, participants' average quality of life on all measures had significantly improved. As Guenter commented, "One important thing to note is that most of the improvement is in the first three months. Another important thing is that it lasts." Most notably, after a full year the indicator with the lowest score—the ability to take on responsibilities at work and home—soared from just 13 percent to 68 percent. Overall, the average pre-DNRS score among participants was 44 percent, while their post-DNRS score a year after the training was 71 percent, on the low end of the normal range for the average healthy Canadian.

Of the 102 people studied, 39 percent qualified for the MCS diagnosis prior to learning DNRS, while just 6 percent did one year later. Almost 72 percent of the participants met the cutoff for chronic fatigue before the training, and that number dropped to 29 percent. And 77 percent scored above the diagnostic cutoff for fibromyalgia before taking the course, but just 27 percent did one year later. Anxiety and depression rates were also significantly reduced.

A year after Guenter presented his findings, in October 2020 the *Journal of Clinical Medicine* published the first randomized controlled trial of a brain retraining program. The study, which measured the effects of the Gupta Program on fibromyalgia, found that after eight weeks the group practicing the program had a 37 percent reduction in their fibromyalgia scores, while the control group—which spent an equivalent amount of time doing relaxation techniques—had none. In addition, for those who practiced the program there was a reduction in a biochemical that plays a critical role in a variety of neuroplasticity processes—including pain modulation—and that some studies have found elevated in people with fibromyalgia. There was no reduction at all for the control group.

These studies demonstrate the promise of brain retraining.

———

We're a nation born out of resistance. The Boston Tea Party. The Declaration of Independence. The American Revolution. I suspect that, like me, almost everyone concerned with issues of social justice feels they're not doing enough when it comes to resisting the runaway train of industrial capitalism. We're so inundated by all the bad news, and not one of us can fix it all. The sense of helplessness can be immobilizing, which feeds the helplessness, and so on, twisting us into Gordian knots.

Many of us think of activists as those people outside on the front lines, carrying their picket signs down city streets, chaining themselves to bulldozers, prepared to risk arrest, or worse. But activism can take many forms. It's marching in the streets, yes, but it's also writing letters to the editor; testifying at town council meetings; calling legislators; organizing rallies; making political art; feeding protesters; donating to progressive causes; collecting signatures for petitions; calling or texting or sending postcards to prospective voters to get out the vote; registering voters; driving voters to the polls; canvassing; boycotting; writing a letter to the doctor who misdiagnosed your disease as psychosomatic; educating loved ones, students, the public, prisoners, the community, and legislators about social justice issues; volunteering for campaigns of candidates who support your values; performing political street theater; strategizing with others; taking issues to court; forming business co-ops, whistleblowing, tabling in public settings to educate people about issues; organizing a union; striking for better wages, safety, and benefits; serving on a tenants' rights board; providing child care for other activists; partnering in advocacy with BIPOC, LGBTQIA+ folx, survivors of sexual assault, domestic violence survivors, and the unhoused; publishing position papers; speechifying; working with state or federal legislators to write a new bill; testifying before state or federal committees about bills; and supporting the next generation of activists of all ages. Ultimately, to co-opt a phrase used by Spencer Tracy's character in *Inherit the Wind*, the activist's work is to comfort the afflicted and afflict the comfortable.

For some more specific ideas, see the Appendix at the end of this book.

––––––

A month before her death, and with Katharine as her amanuensis, Alice wrote of her "long slow dying," musing, "One sloughs off the activities one by one, and never knows that they're gone, until one suddenly finds that the months have slipped away and the sofa will nevermore be laid upon, the morning paper read, or the loss of the new book regretted; one revolves with equal content within the narrowing circle until the vanishing point is reached, I suppose."

She was ready to go. As for her soul,

> I never felt so absolutely uninterested in the poor, shabby old thing. The fact is, I have been dead so long and it has been simply such a grim shoving of the hours behind me as I faced a ceaseless possible horror, since that hideous summer in '78 when I went down to the deep sea, its dark waters closed over me, and I knew neither hope nor peace; that now it's only the shriveling of an empty pea pod that has to be completed.

She died on a sunny afternoon, March 6, 1892.

––––––

The final entry in Alice's diary, composed by Katharine, reveals that Alice was a writer to the very end.

> All through Saturday the 5th and even in the night, Alice was making sentences. One of the last things she said to me was to make a correction in the sentence of March 4th "moral discords and nervous horrors."

This dictation of March 4th was rushing about in her brain all day, and although she was very weak and it tired her much to dictate, she could not get her head quiet until she had it written: then she was relieved.

When William received the cable from Henry that Alice had finally passed, he sat down and wrote his brother a letter. "Now that her outwardly so frustrated life is over, one sees that in a deeper sense it was a triumph. In her relations to her disease, her mind did not succumb." William believed she kept the illness "from invading the tone of her soul. . . . And if one regards the working out of that particular problem as the particular burden that was laid on her, one can only say that it was well done, and that her life was anything but a failure."

———

The era that followed on the heels of the first Gilded Age was the Progressive Era, and this is another story that brings me hope. As a result of the excess and corruption of Alice's time, people got mad, came together, and agitated for change . . . and it *worked*.

In the early 1900s, one in fourteen laborers belonged to unions— a total of 2 million people—but since almost all of them were White men and the unions included few unskilled workers, in 1905 socialists and radical trade unionists from all over the country formed the Industrial Workers of the World (IWW), which excluded no one. Although the IWW never had more than five thousand to ten thousand enrolled members at any one time, their influence was far-reaching, as they rallied strikers all over the country, delivering rousing speeches in the streets, singing political songs, distributing educational pamphlets, organizing mass meetings and parades, and holding strong when arrested and brutalized. In the 1890s, there were about one thousand strikes in the United States per year; by 1904 that number had risen to four thousand. (In 2019 there were just twenty-five work stoppages, more than any year since 2001.)

The socialist movement grew rapidly. At its peak, the Social Democratic Party had 100,000 members, and 1,200 office holders in 340 municipalities. A half million people subscribed to its most prominent party newspaper, *Appeal to Reason*.

The dramatic upswing in magazine sales established audiences for investigative journalism, which—tapping into the widespread discontent sparked by the negative effects of the Industrial Revolution—exposed corruption and provoked political pressure for reform. Writing for *McClure's Magazine*, for instance, Ida Tarbell took on John D. Rockefeller's Standard Oil Company in a series of revelatory articles. Other muckrakers revealed unscrupulous dealings between politicians and businessmen, fraud in patent medicine advertising, and unsafe working environments. Upton Sinclair's bestselling novel *The Jungle*, which portrayed unsanitary conditions and worker exploitation in the meatpacking industry, was serialized in *Appeal to Reason* before being published by Doubleday.

All this activism led to a time of labor reform, trust breaking, the broadening of rights, and the narrowing of the income gap. The Sherman Antitrust Act was passed in 1890 and then, soon after, the Meat Inspection Act and the Pure Food and Drug Act (which led to the creation of the Food and Drug Administration). The Department of Commerce and Labor (DOCL) was created in 1903 to monitor corporations, dissolve monopolies, and ensure fair business practices. (In 1913 the DOCL was split into the Department of Commerce and the Department of Labor, both of which continue to be responsible for regulating business.) And under Theodore Roosevelt's administration, five national parks were created, and 150 national forests.

The 16th Amendment, which introduced a graduated income tax, was ratified during the Progressive Era, as was the 17th, which mandated that senators be elected directly by Americans rather than appointed by state legislatures, thus limiting the power of political machine bosses. The creation of the Federal Trade Commission allowed investigation of unfair trading practices such as monopolization, bribery, and false advertising. And the Clayton Antitrust Act strengthened the Sherman Antitrust Act, exempting labor from antitrust prosecution and legalizing strikes and peaceful picketing—at least until the courts got their hands on it.

During the Progressive Era many states introduced initiatives and referendums as ways for citizens to pass laws without the involvement of legislature, primary elections to reduce corruption, and recalls to allow for the removal of underperforming or crooked legislators. Several states passed worker's compensation bills.

In New York, the parades for women's suffrage kept growing. In Washington, DC, over 5,000 women marched in a 1913 parade down Pennsylvania Avenue—the largest women's march in history up until that time, a prelude to the 470,000-person women's march on Washington protesting Trump's inauguration in 2017, which, nationwide, became the largest single-day protest in U.S. history. The 19th Amendment, conceding women's right to vote (although racists would still find a multitude of ways to prevent women of color from voting), was finally ratified in 1920.

By the end of the Progressive Era, America's cities were cleaner and healthier, governments less corrupt, workplaces safer, monopolies fewer, wages higher, work hours lower, housing upgraded, and children better educated. These advances would not have been made without the work of activists.

———

There are many lifestyle choices we can make to try to protect the health of our bodies, our populace, our democracy, and our planet . . . such as buying less stuff, shopping at local small businesses, working less (if we can afford to), driving less, flying less, avoiding personal care products made with chemicals that have known—or unknown—health effects, cleaning with environmentally friendly products, refraining from using plug-in air fresheners, and growing organic vegetable gardens or shopping at farmers markets. But for perspective, while one individual can save 2.4 tons of carbon dioxide per year by going carless, in 2020, Shell alone emitted the equivalent of 1.38 *billion* tons of carbon dioxide. As professor of atmospheric science Michael E. Mann pointed out in *Time*, "There is a long history of industry-funded 'deflection campaigns' aimed to divert attention from big polluters and place the burden on individuals."

While small, individual actions matter, ultimately the changes we need to make cannot be achieved by refraining from using plastic straws or bringing our own bags to the grocery store. David Wallace-Wells, the author of *The Uninhabitable Earth: Life After Warming*, put it this way on the podcast *Still Processing* in 2019: In the United States, "we're told that we make our mark on the world through how we consume.... That's such a diversion from actual political action.... If you're defining that as the core of your political relationship to the world, you're leaving aside so much power that you have in a country like ours to really make change." The change we need to make is at the foundational level—and that we have to do together.

———

Here's an idea: Write down all the forms of activism you have engaged in. Start with a list of all you've done in your life. Then list all you've done in, say, the past four years. Some people will find they have done a lot; some will find they have done little or perhaps even nothing.

Now check in with yourself: Do you feel like you're doing enough, given the state of things? Is there anything more you can take on right now? And also, might you be willing to stretch yourself a little beyond your comfort zone—or perhaps even a lot—and try something new? Maybe your answer is no to both of these. Perhaps you're a single parent with two full-time jobs and three children and no money or time or energy to spare. In that case, you can focus on your individual choices and on teaching your children the values of connection, authenticity, and social justice over consumerism.

But if your answer is yes, write down one or two things more you can do in the upcoming year (and forward) to move our country in the direction of social justice rather than the pursuit of infinite economic growth.

I believe that if each of us steps it up just a notch or two, we can power remarkable shifts.

———

I've also come to believe that we can make the biggest impact by acting locally. In my city, my husband (who'd never done such a thing before) led the charge to stop a hotel from building a ballroom on a public park. And just across the bay from where I live, the city of South Portland has been successfully blocking a local pipeline corporation from transporting Canadian tar sands to load onto tankers docked in our shared bay. At Standing Rock, Sioux tribes have led the fight against the Dakota Access Pipeline that would run near their reservation, putting the earth, water, and wildlife at risk. Activist and biologist Sandra Steingraber, author of *Living Downstream*, focuses her activism on fracking, because it's the issue in her backyard.

What's happening in *your* neck of the woods?

Changes in state laws often produce the frontline momentum that ultimately yields change on the federal level. Most recently, this was the path to gay marriage. And when individual states like Maine, California, and Minnesota passed laws to develop their own chemical regulatory systems, industry got nervous enough that—with additional pressure from a coalition of hundreds of organizations and businesses—it finally endorsed the Frank R. Lautenberg Chemical Safety for the 21st Century Act. (While the 2016 reform was substantially watered down due to industry influence and is not adequately protective, it's nonetheless an improvement on the 1976 Toxic Substances Control Act. Unfortunately, this law was passed three years after Senator Lautenberg, the act's longtime champion, had died.)

Where I live, we say, "As Maine goes, so goes the nation," but this is true for every state. North Dakotans overwhelmingly voted to effectively ban chain store pharmacies from their state. And across the country from Maine, in the other Portland, city councilors voted to take all the city's investments out of corporations—including those with ties to the Dakota Access Pipeline. Each state, city, or town can set an example and show the rest of us how it's done.

CHAPTER 17

Web

Why did I get sick? This is the question that dogged me from the beginning.

I mean, it started with a case of mononucleosis, but I don't even know how I got *that*. At the time, I was employed as a temp worker at an ice cream factory, so maybe the doctor was right that I picked it up from the water fountain? But that seems far-fetched. More likely it was latent in my system and erupted as a result of the stress of my move to America. I will never know.

But why did I *stay* sick?

One thing I know is that genetic testing shows that I was born with the MTHFR polymorphism, which, when activated, causes methylation difficulties, leading to problems with immunity, inflammation, and detoxification. I also have a polymorphism in my COMT gene, another methylation gene, one linked to ME/CFS in the 2009 Norwegian study. People with this polymorphism tend to feel emotions more strongly than those who don't (check), and their stress reactivity is heightened (and check). I wonder about the effects of these two polymorphisms in combination, and how they might have compromised my ability to return to a healthy state of allostasis.

So I had a genetic predisposition to fall ill in this way . . . but what stressors, in association with my genetic inheritance, may have cumulatively impacted my health and resilience?

While it's impossible to answer this question with any certainty, I faced a reasonably significant number of those. Of course, the virus that triggered the mono was its own biological stressor, requiring my body to marshal its forces to kick the invader out. I had a months-long war going on inside my body: Is it any wonder my resources were depleted?

And it seemed like the illness would never end, which provoked even more stress. Ashok Gupta's paper in *Medical Hypotheses* about the impact of fear conditioning on ME/CFS perfectly describes my experience of that time.

> The person may begin to monitor the body for the symptoms of stress and the virus in anticipatory concern, especially given the prolonged nature of the illness, and the person's urgency to return to full health in order to deal with the source of the psychological stress. Areas of the prefrontal cortex, orbital cortex, and the anterior cingulate are involved in attention to dangerous or negative stimuli. There may be associated anxieties about the prolonged length of the period of post-viral fatigue and anticipatory concern about long-term illness. These concerns contribute to fear conditioning in the amygdala. It is important to bear in mind that fear conditioning can occur whilst the person still has the viral illness (or other physical stressor) and/or even once the viral illness has passed during a period of post-viral fatigue.

It was also stressful being uninsured—having to pay out of pocket for my healthcare even though I wasn't able to work.

My doctor's dismissiveness was stressful and traumatizing.

The stigma of chronic fatigue syndrome was stressful.

And although I wasn't aware of it at the time, I now understand that it was stressful for my entire system that I was largely unable to acknowledge—even to myself—when I *was* stressed or anxious or grief-stricken. I was *strong*. I was *moving forward*. I was *getting things done*. Living in my head in order to disconnect from my body and suppress my emotions—what might properly be called the Cartesian way—generated more work for my body, predisposing me to illness.

The anxiety that was a natural response to falling so ill just as I launched into what was supposed to be my economic independence helped to keep me in a prolonged state of fight/flight/freeze. As Gupta suggested in *Medical Hypotheses*, the adrenaline pumped through the body when someone is in fight or flight "is particularly potent in maintaining muscle contraction," keeping the muscles "primed for reaction to dangerous stimuli." Ultimately, he wrote, this can cause lasting fatigue, a sort of "freeze" reaction.

Any time it seemed the fatigue was finally starting to lift, relief and happiness flushed through my body. Like many in this situation, I would then do the things I couldn't do when I was laid up—maybe wash all my laundry, or walk to the library instead of drive, or dance a bit to Little Richard . . . and then I would crash, which filled me with fear and despair and even resentment. Could I not even dance along to a few Little Richard songs?

Each time my body gave way again, it alarmed me. And that alarm jangled through my entire system. And each time this happened, my limbic system, in its effort to protect me from further harm, grew more alert to such apparent threats. This is what Gupta calls the CFS vicious circle. Limbic kindling in action. The more this happened, the more hyperalert my limbic system got. All in a misguided effort to do its job, which was to protect me.

As a True North affiliate, I'd learned of the import of the birth experience and first days of life from the pediatric nurse practitioner Kathryn Landon-Malone, and this made me consider my birth story in a new way. My mother had told me things were tightly regimented at the military hospital where I was born in San Antonio, Texas, during the Vietnam War. There were several other women also laboring in the delivery room, contributing to an environment that felt to my mother like, as she put it, "army mass production."

Born jaundiced, I'd been whisked away from her at birth, and she didn't get to hold me until she was out of the delivery room. Feeding happened on a strict schedule, and she and the other moms were led into a room with straight-backed chairs all lined up in a row and handed their babies, whom they were advised to awaken for nursing with a flick to the soles of their feet. Due to the jaundice, I was otherwise being poked with needles for blood tests or lying under blue lights, naked but for a diaper and a protective eye covering, alone. My mother and I didn't get the critical hours of connection so key to forming the wiring that helps babies produce calming biochemicals.

Norman Doidge points out in *The Brain That Changes Itself* that "trauma in infancy appears to lead to supersensitization . . . of the brain neurons that regulate glucocorticoids." As a result, survivors of early trauma may be more easily stressed for the rest of their lives. The reason for this, says Kathryn, is in part because the immature nervous/endocrine system is in a critical imprinting time. So when the amygdala alerting process is set off in response to a frightening event—such as being separated from mama, the newborn's only known life-force—the cascading endocrine stress response wires right in with the experience.

Kathryn confirms that what I describe of my birth and postnatal experience would qualify as an early trauma. She says that stressed infants initially cry more and have more trouble digesting food and being in the world, so it makes sense that I was also a colicky baby. And a mom, stressed with a new and unhappy child, gets thrown into her own state of dysregulation. "So it's a shared experience," says Kathryn. I think of it as a positive feedback loop between mother and infant, keeping them in a cycle of dysregulation.

———

But even before I was born, the chemical stressors started in utero, just a routine by-product of "better things for better living." The Pledge my mother used to polish the furniture, for instance. The Aqua Net hair spray she used to coif her hair. The neurotoxic pesticides on the golf course she walked once or twice every week with my father while she was pregnant with me, which may have had a long-term impact on my developing brain, endocrine system, and immune system.

And then, through my childhood and on through adulthood, I was exposed to many, many chemical stressors. The weed and feed pellets my father scattered onto the lawn where I played, the fabric softener in our laundry, the polish I brushed onto my nails, the pesticide I sprayed on my cat, all the mercury dental amalgams fused into my teeth from early childhood on, the exposure to DDT in Belize, the Freon at the refrigerator tubing factory, and then, when when my body was already compromised by ME/CFS, the roach treatments in two different apartments, the volatile organic compounds in fresh paint, the rotenone I powdered onto my guinea pig, the malathion on the garden, the mercury in the fish I ate, the air pollution that wafted across the country from coal-fired plants all the way to Maine, and on and on and on.

Who knows what genes were switched on as a result of these exposures, or when?

Then there's my Adverse Childhood Experiences (ACE) score, which includes my depressed mother's flight from the family when I was eleven. My total score adds up to four, putting me at greater risk for ME/CFS.

More than half of patients in a 1997 study believed stress played a role in developing CFS. Given all that I've learned, I now believe the depleting effects of the virus combined with my genetic predisposition combined with the long-term impacts of my neonatal trauma combined with the stress of taking care of myself alone in a new city combined with my isolation of affect combined with the stress of the stigma combined with the detrimental impact of pesticides and other chemicals was just more than my autonomic nervous system and immune system could handle. I got stuck in a state of fight, flight, or freeze, and I couldn't get out of the loop.

Limbic system impairment could be the unifying theoretical framework that explains ME/CFS, MCS, and similar illnesses, like fibromyalgia, electromagnetic hypersensitivity, chronic pain, food sensitivities, mold sensitivity, chronic Lyme disease, and irritable bowel syndrome. Hopper claims that DNRS has helped people recover from all these as well as PTSD, depression, anxiety, inflammatory conditions, and other chronic illnesses, including long COVID.

Although brain retraining worked for me and has helped many others, that doesn't mean it's the answer for all people suffering from ME/CFS, MCS, and similar illnesses. Just like one specific treatment will not put 100 percent of all cancers in remission, the same is true of brain retraining.

Jennifer Brea, director of the 2017 Sundance Award–winning

documentary *Unrest*, whose TED Talk on the psychologizing of ME/CFS has so far garnered more than 2 million views, first fell ill after a viral infection in 2011. She consulted a series of specialists, trying in vain to find a diagnosis and treatment. When she was a year into the illness, her neurologist diagnosed her with conversion disorder, aka conversion hysteria. Just the day before, a psychiatrist had told her it was clear she was very ill, but once again a doctor mantling himself in Freud's antiquated theory of hysteria explained to a very ill woman that her body was converting unacknowledged emotions into physical symptoms.

Eventually Brea was diagnosed with ME/CFS. With treatment, she improved somewhat, but in 2018, after some symptoms worsened, she was diagnosed with craniocervical instability and learned that this was causing her skull to push down on her spine and compress her brain stem, impairing her autonomic nervous system and triggering neurological symptoms. Brea underwent a risky craniocervical fusion surgery. When she awoke, she says, she felt fully relaxed and fully in her body for the first time in her life.

Prior to surgery, Brea was largely bedbound and walked an average of just 250 to 300 steps a day; after recovering from it (and two follow-up surgeries for tethered cord syndrome), she walked 4,000 to 7,000 steps a day. Within five months of surgery, Brea announced that she no longer met the criteria for ME/CFS. When I spoke to Brea in January 2021, she told me she was still in remission from ME/CFS. In fact, she'd recently hiked thirty-two miles in four days.

Many illnesses overlap with ME/CFS, including Ehlers-Danlos syndrome (EDS), postural orthostatic tachycardia syndrome (POTS), mast cell activation syndrome (MCAS), small intestinal bacterial overgrowth (SIBO), Lyme disease, celiac disease, and hypothyroidism, among others. Brea says that she has a total of seven diagnoses, and some of those diseases still cause problems.

When people try brain retraining and it doesn't work, they often get the message that they're not trying hard enough, instead of the consideration that there's something more going on. "People are look-ing for one answer [for ME/CFS treatment]," says Brea, "but I don't think that exists." The reason, she believes, is that most people with ME/CFS have more than one thing wrong with them, and *all* their diagnoses require treatment.

Other people with ME/CFS have experienced significant improve-ments from taking antivirals, receiving intravenous immunoglobulin therapy (IVIg), or even hyperbaric oxygen therapy (HBOT). Targeted supplement treatment can also help.

It's possible that brain retraining is most likely to be helpful after underlying issues have been addressed. As Brea put it in a January 29, 2021, tweet, "I think of brain retraining as something that might help some people turn off the alarms once the fire has been put out." She added: "The problem is, we have no way of confidently distin-guishing between a person who has an alarm that won't turn off and a person who still has (possibly several) smoldering or raging fires. It is dangerous to try to turn off the alarm when there is still an un-controlled fire."

By the time I learned of brain retraining, I felt that I'd tried everything else. My ME/CFS was significantly improved, and for the most part I could manage my MCS and food sensitivities through avoidance. But it seemed to me that without some kind of funda-mental understanding of the illness I would never fully recover. When I learned of the theory that my limbic system had slipped into an alarm loop that was causing a cascade of harm throughout the sys-tems of my body, a process that I could interrupt with dedicated daily practice, I was empowered with the knowledge to make meaningful steps toward recovery.

Unfortunately, many people—doctors and sufferers alike—misconstrue brain retraining programs as simply "thinking positively." But, as Annie Hopper emphasizes, "rewiring the limbic system is not an intellectual process, but rather an experiential one."

While there's now some preliminary research indicating that

DNRS and the Gupta Program are effective, we need more random-ized controlled studies; larger studies; studies comparing the effects of DNRS and the Gupta Program; studies that track and quantify the number of participants who drop out (and why); studies comparing the benefits of these treatments to other treatments; studies tracking whether brain retraining is more likely to work for people in early stages of illness who haven't tried other treatments or those who, like me, have tried just about everything; studies identifying which illnesses have the highest rates of recovery from brain retraining and which the lowest; studies establishing the potential harms of these treatments; studies revealing the rate of relapse after brain retraining recovery and comparing that to the rate of relapse in others who went into spontaneous remission; and so on. And could there be other treatments that would work faster and require less time and effort?

For these studies, we need funding.

Brea felt *great* on her four-day hiking trip . . . until she got home to L.A. It seemed, she said, like the polluted air had a *texture*, "and it just smacked me in the face." This got her thinking about the "health tax" all of us pay due to the chemicals in our environments.

————

At the risk of doing exactly what Alice asked William not to do, I can't help but wonder how her life might have been different had she had access to the treatment that finally restored me to robust good health, and possibly other interventions as well, like, perhaps, hor-mone therapy or surgery for endometriosis.

But even then, there would still be the matter of her death. Was her breast cancer the result of chance? Unfortunate genetics? The stressors of industrial capitalism? Pollutants in one or more of her abodes, in her clothes, in the water or the sky? Or some combination of all these things? Her body, like mine, tells a story; tells many of them, in fact, interwoven.

———

A body is an ecosystem, and the planet's ecosystem is a vast living organism that embodies all of us, and the lesson of the butterfly effect is that change isn't entirely predictable and sometimes small shifts can lead to substantial outcomes. It's impossible to know how the actions each of us take might reverberate.

Just as we can apply the related theory of allostasis to the breathtakingly complex workings of the human body, we can also use it as a framework for understanding our social systems and our relationship to the planet.

In a series of columns about this for the *Psychology Today* blog, Jessica Del Pozo interviews the founder of the nonprofit Emergent Resilience, Kevin Gallagher, who suggests that while from a homeostatic perspective "we are separate, independent entities that try to maintain our internal equilibrium in the face of external changes," the allostatic paradigm, on the other hand, "recognizes that the world around us is in constant flux and that our bodies are in an ongoing conversation with that world, anticipating our current needs and then adapting as circumstances change." He adds: "Allostasis recognizes the inherent interconnection between our own bodies and the external environment, the essential interrelationship between ourselves and the world around us."

Here in America's culture of runaway capitalism, we've been inculcated with two problematic and interrelated ideologies. One is the belief that our economic standing is a reflection of our value; the other is the Social Darwinist notion that the only way to rise to the top is to climb over each other, and that the ones at the top are the best of us and the ones who fail to thrive in this culture are the worst, the weakest, and the most deserving of failure.

How many great minds and wise hearts did we never hear from because they weren't accorded the privileges of others—because they couldn't afford to go to college, because they were sick and couldn't afford care, because they were overworked and still not making a livable wage, because they died as a result of unsafe work conditions or the slow death of stealth chemical exposure or the collateral damage of industrial capitalism due to their race, their poverty, or their disability? How many of us are—or will be—collateral damage without even knowing it?

———

For a long time, the patriarchal foundations of industrial capitalism kept Alice's voice from being heard by the wider world. It seemed like nobody, not even Alice, could imagine a world in which she had something of import to say. In the whole of her forty-three years, she only published one item, a strange little letter to the editor, written from London and signed, "INVALID." It was dated July 4, 1890—two years before her death—published in *The Nation*, and later reprinted in the *London Daily News*.* Henry called it her "swan song." Little did he know that her true swan song was still a work in progress.

---

* When an American mother sought for her daughter a home that allowed "plenty of liberty to *scream* through the house," the muffled and disabled Alice, stirred by sudden patriotism, wrote this Independence Day letter.

To the Editor of the Nation:
Sir:

For several years past I have lived in provincial England. Although so far from home, every now and then a transatlantic blast, pure and undefiled, fans to a white heat the fervor of my patriotism.

This morning, most appropriately to the day, a lady from one of our Eastern cities applied to my landlady for apartments. In the process of telling her that she had no rooms to let, the landlady said that there was an invalid in the house, whereupon the lady exclaimed: "In that case perhaps it is just as well that you cannot take us in, for my little girl, who is thirteen, likes to have plenty of liberty to scream *through the house."*

Yours very truly,
INVALID

In the last six weeks of her life, the dying Alice asked Katharine to have the diary typed. Two years later, Katharine had four copies printed, one for herself and one for each of Alice's three surviving brothers, William, Henry, and Robertson. She believed, though Alice never explicitly said it, that the James sister wanted her diary posthumously published. William wrote to Henry that he hoped to see it in print one day. "I am proud of it as a leaf in the family laurel crown."

But Alice's writing languished in obscurity until 1934, when her reflections were published in a book that also included biographies of her lesser-known brothers, Wilky and Robertson, called *Alice James: Her Brothers—Her Journal*.

Thirty years later, Leon Edel edited Alice's first stand-alone publication, *The Diary of Alice James*. Then, in 1980, Jean Strouse published the stunning *Alice James: A Biography*, which is still in print. A year later, Ruth Bernard Yeazell edited an abridged collection of letters, *The Death and Letters of Alice James*, and fifteen years after that Linda Anderson published another collection, *Alice James: Her Life in Letters*.

The swan sings on.

———

To get from Portland to Tasmania, where my brother Jason lives with his family, adds up to more than twenty-four hours of travel, and it is a trip I could not have made as a person with multiple chemical sensitivity and ME/CFS. I'd visualized this journey in vivid detail, from the long, cramped flight to the exotic familial destination, as part of my brain retraining—what Annie Hopper calls a "future position." In allostatic terms, I'd been predicting a different future—one in which I was fully healthy and could fly to Australia—and thus changing biochemical set points.

While I waited at the luggage carousel for my suitcase, my burly, bearded brother, arms crossed casually at his chest, stood chatting with a firefighter who'd flown over to help manage the wildfires that were burning out of control all over Tasmania. We drove to Jason's small town through smoke so thick it obscured the green rolling hills. It was the hottest January on record. These fires, he said, were burning faster and hotter than regular bushfires. Climate change had arrived in Australia; it was no longer possible to deny. The smoke in the air was unrelenting. It smelled apocalyptic.

And still . . . I'd made it. I was on the other side of the world, where people called mosquitoes "mozzies," where pink galah cockatoos flew free around the town, where I could hear a kookaburra laughing, just like I'd sung about in rounds when I was a kid.

I'd barely recovered from the jet lag when I climbed into a car again, this time headed two hours east with Jason; his wife, Melanie; and my teenage niece and nephew, to a ferry that would take us to an island where we would stay for two nights in repurposed nineteenth-century prisoners' barracks. Before the colonial era, for 35,000 years the Puthikwilayti band of the Oyster Bay Nation had made this island their home. Now it was a national park.

As soon as we unloaded our stuff, my fifteen-year-old nephew, Finn—an avid birder who had been to this island before—took me on a hike. Just beyond our barracks, a small mob of grazing kangaroos stood up and watched us pass. Some friendly wombats trundled on by. In the bush, Finn patiently pointed out birds I confessed I could not see.

The next day, we all donned our bathing suits, grabbed our towels, and trekked down to the pier. The water was clear and blue. Finn and my niece, Adele, jumped in from the high pier over and over, and I made jokes with my brother about how I should show them their auntie was brave, and then Finn and I made a deal that if I jumped in, we would swim together to the beach.

I crossed to the edge of the pier and stood for a moment, knees bent, sun shining hot on my skin. And then I jumped.

In a 2007 interview in *The Sun*, author David Korten, who later wrote *Change the Story, Change the Future: A Living Economy for a Living Earth*, suggests that contemporary biologists—and particularly female ones—have published work debunking the Darwinian notion that living systems survive and evolve based solely on ruthless competition. Competition exists, of course, and in humans can prompt innovation, but, says Korten, thriving populations "strive for a dynamic balance between cooperation and competition." He adds, "A degree of competition, particularly competition for excellence, is necessary for vitality. Life's deeper story, however, is one of cooperation."

In fact, according to Dutch historian Rutger Bregman, author of *Humankind: A Hopeful History*, compelling evidence suggests that *Homo sapiens* evolved while other hominins died out not because we were stronger, braver, meaner, or smarter, but because we were more socially oriented. Our sociability allowed us to learn from and support each other, and these traits gave us a leg up on the other hominins. Humans are fundamentally cooperative, and that has been essential to our survival. We need to change the stories we tell about what it means to be human, because the stories we tell become self-fulfilling prophecies.

In his interview in *The Sun*, Korten compares the workings of the human body to a healthful society. We have trillions of cells inside us, he says, and yet,

> All these individual decision-making cells come together in this extraordinary cooperative enterprise that has potential far beyond that of any one cell. . . . For the body to work, each cell needs to maintain its integrity as an independent being, yet be devoted to the health of the whole. So it's constantly balancing the individual interest with the collective interest.

In other words, right down to our very cells, we are products of our relationships—with one another, with ourselves, within our local and national cultures, and as part of our planetary ecosystem.

————

The water smacked the soles of my feet and exploded around me as I plunged into the ocean. I pulled myself up to the air, paddled out of the way, and watched for Finn. His splash scattered into a thousand sparks of light. I could almost see the filaments between them. Droplets on a spider's web.

Together, we swam to shore, and then, as we walked back down the hot pier to fetch our shoes and towels, Finn, just ahead of me, pointed suddenly down into the water: "Stingray!"

The creature, huge and magnificent, soared through the water on its giant winglike fins. We had just swum in those waters, but I wasn't frightened. It felt like a visitation: holy, peaceful. And then the ray slipped into the shadows under the pier and was gone.

Surely the butterfly effect also applies to the flap of a stingray's fins in a cove off the coast of Tasmania. And to the gasp of the fifty-something woman standing above it on the pier, her mouth agape at the sight.

And then something happened to complicate the narrative: I relapsed.

Just a few months before COVID-19 hit, my book deadline five months away, I was at a writing residency on the West Coast and anxious that I wouldn't get the manuscript finished in time. Although by then I'd fully recovered, I was nonetheless prone to viruses, and when I saw a newcomer with her bunched-up tissues and sniffling, I clenched up a little. *Poor woman*, I thought, *to arrive with a cold.*

The next night I found myself standing behind her in line for dinner. I considered stepping away under the pretense of going to wash my hands so that I could move to the back of the line, far behind the writer with the virus. (Now, still in the midst of the pandemic, this instinctual recoil is ingrained in so many of us.) But I reasoned that I was in writers' heaven: surely my immune system was stronger than ever?

It wasn't.

Three days later came the sore throat, and then the fatigue, and then the sneezing and runny nose.

This mild cold ushered in something else, something mysterious and alarming. Even two weeks after returning home, I was inexplicably fatigued, still congested, and then one night in bed I found myself having difficulty breathing. The next day, a Saturday, the clinic scheduled me with a doctor who looked young enough to be fresh out of med school. When he entered the exam room, I was thinking about the ways that doctors dismiss women's complaints and wondering how I needed to behave in order to be taken seriously. Complimenting his ocean view, I opted to assume a friendly yet deferential attitude.

I told him about the difficulty breathing when supine, adding that my ears were plugged and I was clearing my throat a lot and had an unproductive cough and was still fatigued. "I've had walking pneumonia once before," I said, "and I wonder if it's that." I hoped it was. A quick diagnosis. An effective treatment. But he listened to my chest and said he didn't hear any congestion in my lungs. He said he thought it was sleep apnea and recommended a saline nasal spray and a sleep study.

The problem wasn't sleep apnea. I knew what sleep apnea felt like, and besides, it happened when I was awake as well. (By the time the CPAP machine arrived two months later, my breathing had returned to normal, and while the machine may have improved my sleep, it did nothing to help my exhaustion.) Over a period of two weeks I sought the aid of my PCP, a nurse practitioner, and then a physician's assistant at an urgent care clinic. Even these three, although they clearly cared, could offer no answers, no cures.

This was all just too familiar. The puzzling illness. The debilitating fatigue. The dismissive first doctor, the flummoxed subsequent providers.

Relapse. Oh my god, oh my god. Relapse.

I immediately recommenced brain retraining. I quit sugar, dairy, and gluten to give my body the best chance possible to recover. Instead of writing four-plus hours a day, I felt lucky to be able to write one. Then even that was too much: I couldn't lift my arms to the keyboard—not even in bed. Determined to keep making progress, I tried dictating, but my energy continued to deteriorate and soon I couldn't even talk into my computer.

My energy crashed into the negatives. The fatigue pinioned my body and fettered my brain. Forced to set my book aside, I hung shrouds over the shelves that held my research books so I didn't have to look at all that I couldn't do.

Every morning I woke up exhausted. Showering, dressing, brushing my teeth and hair, making and eating breakfast—even when I paced myself, this burst of activity took more energy than my body had in reserve, and by the end of it I was even more fatigued than I'd been when I woke up, and spent the rest of the day resting, replenishing my empty stores. By evening I would often feel just a tiny bit better, but then I would go to sleep and wake up and start the cycle all over again. Frank took over all the chores. He and friends drove me to my appointments. I couldn't even walk the dog.

I was broken. Again.

It's hard for people to understand this if they've always been hale and hearty, but when you have little to no energy, everything costs. Reading a challenging book costs energy. Holding it costs. Sitting upright costs. At my lowest, even talking cost: one sentence cost.

I needed music because the house was too lonely and quiet without it, but everything was too abrasive and jangling. I was so overstimulated, even the violins in a Vivaldi concerto were too shrill. On Pandora I found a musician who blended Native flute with recordings of birdsong and trickling brooks and I made a station, and for months that was all I could bear to listen to.

But at least I had the brain retraining. It had worked before, and it had worked for countless others, so there was no reason it wouldn't work for me again. I knew exactly what I needed to do, and I did it. I figured I could have this thing beat in a couple months. Frank and I still laughed together almost every day. And we hugged more, because we needed it, and because hugging is good for the autonomic nervous system. But by mid-December, I found it harder to stay positive. I began having bouts of despair, unable to get through the brain retraining without breaking into tears; and for the first time in my life, the anxiety was beyond my ability to manage.

I needed a doctor who understood ME/CFS. Stat. Bethany Hays

had retired. I called another functional medicine doctor I knew of in the area who took my insurance, but his receptionist told me that the wait list was so long they'd stopped adding people to it. So I called Sean McCloy, the doctor I'd seen for many years before I started working with Bethany. He was a wonderful doc, but he didn't take insurance, and his fee was $225 an hour. I booked a one-hour appointment for the next week.

How was I going to pay for the healthcare I needed? Since ME/CFS treatment continues to be such uncharted territory, Medicare would cover barely any of it. The acupuncture, energy medicine, supplements, brain retraining coaching, hyperbaric oxygen therapy (HBOT), and other treatments would all have to come out of my pocket. I'd spent more than $2,000 on healthcare in two months, and it appeared that I would need to be spending at least that for several more.

Like many Americans with medical bills they can't afford to pay, I launched a GoFundMe campaign. One hundred and twenty-four friends, family members, and strangers contributed what added up to over $5,000, which paid for the healthcare I needed for four more months. And it did something else: it helped to heal the desperately ill twenty-one-year-old me who had felt so dismissed and abandoned back in 1989.

Sean McCloy is an MD who has worn his dark hair in a ponytail for as long as I've known him. He's got the eager friendliness of a young chocolate Lab; expertise in functional medicine; an open, curious mind; a remarkable ability to type notes while maintaining his connection to his patient; and a gift for accessibly communicating complex science. His office is flooded with natural light. He listened as I first told him the story of my recovery, and I was relieved to find that I didn't have to explain brain retraining to him: he was the only provider who didn't need a mini-tutorial. When I described my relapse, he commiserated with me about the irony that it happened as I was finally making solid progress on the book about my first go-round with the disease. "We have to get you better," he said, "so you can finish that book!"

Looking over the DetoxiGenomic test I took several years earlier under Bethany Hays's care, Sean explained that I have a genetic propensity for ME/CFS. In other words, for me there is an unfortunate undertow toward illness, toward relapses. This reminder brought me an unexpected sense of relief. Here in the United States, we are steeped in a culture that tells us we can—and should—do it all, even when it comes to our diseases. And if we don't, we're failures, our illnesses simply a failure of spirit. If we had just thought more positively or eaten more perfectly or done more yoga, then we wouldn't have gotten sick.

Even if you're aware of this faulty logic and have had years of therapy and are writing a book that refutes it, it's hard not to feel somehow to blame when your body gives way. In the thick of the relapse, my energy meted out in small doses, I was soothed by my doctor's reminder because it meant I could stop flogging myself for not being able to do capitalism right.

I'm not made for this. Perhaps none of us are, not really.

Functional medicine testing revealed that my serotonin, GABA, and dopamine levels were all very low, and unsurprisingly, my cortisol and DHEA were low too. No wonder I felt like crap. The report explained that serotonin and GABA work synergistically to promote optimal sleep, relaxation, positive mood, and a sense of well-being. My low dopamine and related neurotransmitters could be causing at least some of my fatigue, low stamina, and inability to focus. The low cortisol and DHEA were likely also inhibiting my energy and stamina. Sean put me on a targeted supplement program, and within days I started to feel more hopeful and positive and my energy began to creep up. Ultimately, however, I needed to add psychotropics to my regimen to assist with the anxiety and depression.

Of course, psychotropics alone were not going to help me recover from the disabling fatigue. This time, I found a coach from the Gupta Program, Paulien. The foundational tenets and structures of the DNRS and Gupta programs are similar, but each has its own feel, and Gupta's felt gentler to me, and gentler was what I needed. I wanted a coach who could also act as a therapist, helping me to explore the emotional aspects of my illness rather than solely focusing on the function of the brain retraining. Like all Gupta Program and DNRS coaches, Paulien had been through her own journey to recovery; her wisdom was hard-won.

I don't believe we get ill because we have something to learn. All of us have things to learn, not just the ill and suffering. But I do believe that illness creates an *opportunity* to learn and grow that we might not otherwise prioritize.

When I asked Paulien why all the brain retraining hadn't yet done a thing, she pointed out that the last time I did brain retraining, the stakes were much lower. I was capable of working then and had a full, rich life. I was doing the program because I wanted to recover total health. I had little to lose. This time, I was fully disabled and desperate. If the brain retraining didn't work, I might never be able to finish this book or do any of the other things that bring fulfillment to my life. I had returned to a living death, and it terrified me, and this was an enormous stressor, making it harder for the changes I sought to take place.

We were going to need to start by focusing on calming my system. I had to do something antithetical to my way of being in the world: I had to surrender to what was happening to me. I would need to accept and hold my sad part and my anxious part and my overwhelmed part, giving these parts all the love they needed so that they could relax.

When we signed off, I pulled a colored recipe card off my bedside shelf and wrote: *I accept that this is happening right now.* Then I propped it up next to my bed. Somehow I needed to accept this nightmare if I was ever going to get out of it.

My body had put me in lockdown four months before stay-at-home orders went into effect. Then, just as it seemed I was inching my way back toward health, the pandemic struck. My rented hyperbaric oxygen chamber became my safe pod. The coronavirus couldn't get me in there. When I lay down on the cushion and Frank zipped me in and switched on the oxygen and compressor, all the horror and chaos in the world was kept out. I set my Pandora to the Native flute station and put on my noise-canceling headphones.

The questions I had about my body were the same ones I now had for the world. How were we ever going to get out of this? Could we? What if we didn't? I was trapped in my broken body, zipped into my protective chamber, and all around me the world was falling apart.

By February 2022, one in four hundred U.S. residents had died from COVID-19—almost 900,000 people—more than all who died in the four years of the Civil War that raged in Alice's youth. Four months earlier, a systematic review of fifty-seven studies representing over 250,000 unvaccinated COVID patients found that half developed long COVID lasting at least six months. Most common symptoms included neurologic disorders like headaches, difficulty concentrating, and cognitive impairment; pulmonary abnormalities; depression and anxiety; and reduced general functioning, including exercise intolerance. The researchers concluded that long COVID is a multisystem disease and recommended a "holistic clinical framework." The U.S. government's top COVID-19 advisor, Anthony Fauci, was among many noting similarities between long COVID and ME/CFS.

Eighty percent of the patients in the systematic review had been hospitalized with the illness, but for reasons science cannot yet explain, even some asymptomatic people and a percentage with mild cases wind up with long COVID. Early research indicates that the rate of long COVID among fully vaccinated breakthrough cases is about half what it is for infected unvaccinated people. This is good news. But for someone who has so recently been reminded that a mild illness can have disastrous repercussions, these figures are not comforting enough.

In December 2020, Congress allocated $1.15 billion to identify causes and treatments for long COVID. Many who have been living with ME/CFS for years or decades hope that some of what researchers find might also apply to them.

A year later, the Omicron variant arrived, and as of this writing nobody knows for sure if or when or how the pandemic will end.

And yet here I am, so much better but still recovering. While my body has now returned to its former vibrance, I have to remember not to push. And when the fatigue comes, as it sometimes does, I have to remember that even if I accomplish nothing more that day, it's okay. *I'm* okay. If nothing else, I bear, as Alice once wrote, "a certain value as an indestructible quantity."

I don't have it down yet. I'm a work in progress. So are you; so are we all. And I, for one, will keep trying.

Science says: *The body is a machine.*
Advertising says: *The body is a business.*
The body says: *I am a fiesta.*

> —Eduardo Galeano, "Window on the Body"

GRATITUDE

It takes an entire ecosystem to write a book.

Thank you to . . .

My husband, Frank, for anchoring me and making me laugh every day, for cleaning the house when I was too busy writing this book, and for over two decades of dedicated IT support.

My teachers, starting in high school with English teachers Annie Stirling and Don Quarrie, who mentored me; all my professors at the University of New England, who shaped my thinking, an education without which this book would have been very different; writing workshop teachers including Sandra Steingraber, Jane Brox, Steve Almond, and Sarah Braunstein, among many others; past editors, particularly Hattie Fletcher and Jennifer Sahn; clinical supervisor Deb Dana; and storytelling teacher Karen Dietz, who taught me how to be comfortable sharing my stories in front of an audience, as well as Portland Playback Theater, which gave me plenty of opportunity to practice.

Research librarians, including Janice Beal, formerly at the University of New England, for helping me begin my hunt for research and connecting me to Jennifer Tuttle; Roberta "Bobby" Gray, former UNE research librarian; Cadence Atchinson, current UNE research librarian; all the research librarians at the Portland Public Library; and the

Portland Public Library in general for getting me all the books and articles I needed. Praise be to libraries!

Beta readers, so many of them over the years: Jason Anthony, Laura Laing, Elizabeth DeWolfe, Susan Fekety, Wendy Hahn, Tom Mannella, Andrew Johnson, Nicole Chaison, Clare Needham, Alicia Googins, Sarah Winn, Tanya Whiton, Heather Kirn Lanier, and many others have all had a hand in making this book better. Thank you.

Strangers who generously shared their time and expertise: Kimberly Ayers, Mike Belliveau, Jen Brea, Robert Markley, Lucinda Cole, Glory Leu, Stephanie Sellers, Ben Price, Henk Goorhuis, Laken Brooks, Tara Haelle, and David Rosnick. Though they didn't know me, these experts willingly answered my questions and helped deepen my understanding of some important subjects in the book. Any errors are mine alone.

Greek word-maker: Stephen Cole Farrar, for *iatraporiueretia*.

At-hand friend-consultants: Jennifer Tuttle, Elizabeth DeWolfe, Susan Fekety, Bethany Hays, Kathryn Landon-Malone, Cynthia Atkinson, Julie Rehmeyer, Diane Husic, Tina Holt, Catherine Crute, Beth Johnston, Ori Fienberg, and others replied promptly to my Facebook or email queries to help ensure my accuracy. Again, any errors are mine.

Friends: Annie Wadleigh, longtime friend, long-admired writer, and researcher and copyeditor extraordinaire; Sofia Ali-Khan and Emily Maloney, fellow writers and behind-the-scenes cheerleaders; Susan Landry, not just a friend but also the person who taught me how to use Track Changes, which revolutionized my writing process; Jason Anthony and Heather Hardy, for camaraderie; Julie Rehmeyer, for her knowledge, wisdom, and heart; Susan Fekety, for her heartfelt friendship and like-minded beliefs about clinical care; Alex

Marzano-Lesnevich, for their enthusiastic support and helpful feedback; Jennifer Tuttle and Elizabeth DeWolfe, for sharing my passion; Todd and Sharon Pattison, for their generous hospitality and good company; and Deb Gould, my pitch fairy.

Healers: Sean McCloy, Bethany Hays, Joseph Py, Paulien Elzinga, Cynthia Atkinson, Susan Fekety, Edward Bilotti, Jennifer Joy Greaves, Getty Payson, Megan Devine, Mary Johnston, Ken Hamilton, Stephen Beckett, Jenner Greil, Jennifer Daigle, Susan Doughty, Edmund Sears, Derek Libby, Stephen Goldbas, Susan Reed, Laura Meyer, Alexa Gilmore, Michele Kurlanski, Brenda Belanger, Michael Bither, Erin Masterson, Michelle Sirois, and the True North circle.

My therapist peer consultation group, for fifteen-plus years of camaraderie and shared wisdom about relational client care, with special appreciation for my cofounder, Barbara Harvey, and our current members Carolyn Bliss Branson, Carol Leonard, and Deb Feintech.

Residencies: The Virginia Center for the Creative Arts, Yaddo, Hewnoaks Artist Residency, Hedgebrook, Monson Arts, and The Dora Maar House. I am forever grateful for the uninterrupted time, the beautiful spaces, and the camaraderie of fellow artists. Without this support and recognition, I may have given up writing this book.

Hosts: My brother Jason; his wife, Melanie; and their kids, Finn and Adele, for putting me up for a month in their backyard cabin in Tasmania as I wrote about income inequity and the 4-day workweek.

Opportunities: Goldfarb Family Fellowship (VCCA); Bread Loaf-Rona Jaffe Foundation Scholarship in Nonfiction; Maia Williams, Heather Hanley, and the San Miguel Writers' Conference; and the Key West Literary Seminar. Thank you.

Grants: The Barbara Deming/Money for Women Fund, the Canada Council for the Arts, and the Maine Arts Commission. Without these funds I would still be writing this book.

My agent, Mackenzie Brady Watson, for taking a chance on me, and for shepherding me so skillfully and responsively through this process; and her assistant Aemilia Phillips—now an agent in her own right—for her able and enthusiastic teamwork. I am so grateful.

My editor, Karen Rinaldi, for believing in this book, trusting my vision for it, and sharing her expertise.

My line editor, Thomas LeBien of Moon & Company, for helping me cut 35,000 words from this book, and whose shared appreciation for the James family led him to suggest writing an entirely new opening segment.

My copyeditor, Nancy Inglis, for her deft copyediting and for catching a few other errors as well!

The entire Harper Wave team: Thank you.

My Facebook friends, who never failed to answer the call when I was stuck for a word or needed some brainstorming help. And particularly to the Binders, an underground network of Facebook groups dedicated to helping cisgender women, trans, and nonbinary writers get their voices out into the world. I am infinitely grateful to the Binders for helping me find my agent, for answering my many questions over the years, and for the daily support of my Binders Full of Creative Nonfiction check-in group. And to Kit Cudahy, a Facebook friend who, when I posted that I felt stuck about how and where to start the story of Alice James, wrote, "Just talk to her," which turned out to be excellent advice.

All 124 GoFundMe contributors, friends, family, and strangers. Your support covered my out-of-pocket healthcare expenses for four months and helped me get through a very dark time. You helped me finish this book.

People who made soup, picked up groceries, or drove me to appointments when I was so very ill: Frank Turek, Susan Fekety, Anne Elliott, Carolyn Bliss Branson, Jim Alberty, and Annie Wadleigh.

My parents, for always enthusiastically supporting my writing, and my stepmother, Linda, for cheering me on from the sidelines after my father died.

Feminists past, present, and future, in all your glorious waves.

When we work together, we ignite change. Here are some ideas:

1. **Campaign for the separation of corporation and state.** Eliminate corporate personhood and get corporate money out of politics, increase regulation of corporations, break up monopolies. In Joel Bakan's book *The Corporation*, law professor Robert Benson says, "The people mistakenly assume that we have to try to control these giant corporate repeat offenders one toxic spill at a time, one layoff at a time, one human rights violation at a time." But charter revocation laws have "always allowed the attorney general to go to court to simply dissolve a corporation for wrongdoing and sell its assets to others who will operate in the public interest." Learn more at https://www.movetoamend.org/.

2. **Unionize.** And support others attempting to unionize or striking for fair wages and better working conditions.

3. **Agitate for a shorter workweek.** Learn more at https://fourdayweek.com/ and https://www.4dayweek.com/.

4. **Fight for the climate:**

   - **Campaign for a Green Amendment to your state's constitution,** protecting the right to clean air, water, and a stable climate in the same way that it protects the rights to free speech and freedom of religion. Pennsylvania, Montana, and New York have already added this amendment to their constitutions, and there are active movements in seventeen states and counting. Learn more at: https://forthegenerations.org/.

- **Legally establish the right to a livable planet,** as Our Children's Trust is endeavoring to do with its federal lawsuit, *Juliana v. United States*, and in its support for similar actions on the state level. Watch the documentary *Juliana v. United States*, available on streaming services.

- **Legally establish the rights of nature**, as communities are doing all over the United States and the world. Learn more at: https://www.garn.org and https://www.movementrights.org/.

- **Hold your legislators accountable** on municipal, state, and federal levels for supporting legislation that would reduce greenhouse gas emissions by using renewable and zero-emissions power for all the nation's electricity; making transportation, housing, manufacturing, and agriculture more energy-efficient; and creating millions of new jobs in clean energy. The Inflation Reduction Act of 2022 is a start, but it's not enough to stave off the climate crisis.

5. **Work toward passing stronger municipal, state, and federal chemical laws** based on the precautionary principle. Learn more here: https://defendourhealth.org/ and https://www.ewg.org/.

6. **Join a campaign for universal healthcare**. Here are some places to start: Healthcare-NOW, One Payer States, Physicians for a National Health Program.

7. **Fight to establish a Gross National Well-Being index**. Wealth isn't just the amount of money created through exploiting the earth or its people. Wealth includes the health and welfare of people and the integrity of the ecosystem. Learn more here: https://gnhusa.org/.

8. **Push for municipal, state, and federal ranked-choice voting,** just like activists in Maine, New York, Minneapolis, and San Francisco have achieved, so that all Americans, no longer hostage to a two-party system, can freely vote their consciences. Learn more here: https://www.fairvote.org/.

9. **Join the Democratic Socialists of America**. Check out their website for all the ways you can participate, and get involved with your local chapter. Learn more here: https://www.dsausa.org/.

For a selected bibliography, go to www.jenniferlunden.com.

PART I: BEDRIDDEN

1   E. S. Muskie: Maine Senator Edward Muskie, "Earth Day—1970 and 1974," Senate Congressional Record, April 23, 1974, http://abacus.bates.edu/muskie-archives /ajcr/1974/Earth%20Day.shtml.

CHAPTER 1: BANKRUPTCY

3   swimming with friends: Jean Strouse, *Alice James: A Biography* (Cambridge: Harvard University Press, 1999), 73.

3   wrote in her diary: Alice James, *The Diary of Alice James*, ed. Leon Edel (Boston: Northeastern University Press, 1999), 95, entry February 21, 1890, as cited in Strouse, *Alice James*, 81.

5   neurasthenia: The word, translated literally, means "lack of nerve strength." Beard is credited for popularizing the term *neurasthenia* and providing detailed diagnostics, but he was not in fact the first doctor to use it. It can be found in an 1814 medical dictionary and is referenced as early as 1808. Francis G. Gosling, *Before Freud: Neurasthenia and the American Medical Community, 1870–1910* (Urbana: University of Illinois Press, 1987), 26.

8   most of them women: Paul Cheney, personal communication, July 18, 2018.

10   "essence of divine maternity": Strouse, *Alice James*, 26.

10   "she was the keystone of the arch": Richard Warrington Baldwin Lewis, *The Jameses: A Family Narrative* (New York: Farrar, Straus, and Giroux, 1991), 336–37.

11   In addition to debilitating fatigue: Anthony Komaroff and Dedra Buchwald, "Symptoms and Signs of Chronic Fatigue Syndrome," *Reviews of Infectious Diseases* 13, suppl. 1 (1991): S8–S11, doi: 10.1093/clinids/13.Supplement_1.S8.

11   the syndrome was the butt of jokes: Hillary Johnson, *Osler's Web: Inside the Labyrinth of the Chronic Fatigue Syndrome Epidemic* (Lincoln, NE: Author's Guild Backinprint.com, 2006), 153–54.

11   "a new disease which supposedly ravaged": Johnson, *Osler's Web*, 136; "Chronic Fatigue Possibly Related to Epstein-Barr Virus—Nevada," *Morbidity and Mortality*

Weekly Report 35, no. 21 (May 30, 1986), http://www.cdc.gov/mmwr/preview /mmwrhtml/00000740.htm.

11   "whether the cause is biological or emotional": Johnson, *Osler's Web*, 210.

11   "It's a real fad": Johnson, *Osler's Web*, 232.

12   "just don't want to drive their BMW": Johnson, *Osler's Web*, 171.

16   "to go at any expense of health": Strouse, *Alice James*, 68.

16   "your neuralgia or whatever you made believe": Strouse, *Alice James*, 69.

17   No other illness had ever scored so low: Johnson, *Osler's Web*, 256–57, 364.

17   even people undergoing chemotherapy scored higher: Jill S. Anderson and Carol Estwing Ferrans, "The Quality of Life of Persons with Chronic Fatigue Syndrome," *Journal of Nervous and Mental Disease* 185, no. 6 (1997): 359–67, doi: 10.1097/00005053-199706000-00001 as cited in Peggy Munson, "The Paradox of Lost Fingerprints: Metaphor and the Shaming of Chronic Fatigue Syndrome," in *Stricken: Voices from the Hidden Epidemic of Chronic Fatigue Syndrome*, ed. Peggy Munson (New York: Haworth Press, 2000), 95–127.

17   "related profound and multiple losses": Anderson and Ferrans, "The Quality of Life," as cited in Munson, "The Paradox of Lost Fingerprints," 95–127.

17   AIDS patients scored higher: Johnson, *Osler's Web*, 364.

17   "if I had to choose between the two illnesses": Nancy J. Klimas, "Readers Ask: A Virus Linked to Chronic Fatigue Syndrome," *Consults* (blog), *New York Times*, October 15, 2009, http://consults.blogs.nytimes.com/2009/10/15/readers-ask-a -virus-linked-to-chronic-fatigue-syndrome/?_r=0.

17   "chronic devastation syndrome": Johnson, *Osler's Web*, 273.

19   In Canada, everyone had health coverage: "Health Care Funding," *Canadian Health Care* (blog), http://www.canadian-healthcare.org/page8.html.

20   health a fundamental human right: Health as a human right was recognized by the World Health Organization in 1946 and in the United Nations' Universal Declaration of Human Rights in 1948. Office of the United Nations High Commissioner for Human Rights and World Health Organization, "The Right to Health," Fact Sheet No. 31, https://www.ohchr.org/sites/default/files/Documents /Publications/Factsheet31.pdf.

23   "sick role": Talcott Parsons, "Illness and the Role of the Physician: A Sociological Perspective," *American Journal of Orthopsychiatry* 21, no. 3 (1951): 452–60, doi: 10.1111/j.1939-0025.1951.tb00003.x.

23   their duty to get well: Parsons, "Illness," 452–60.

25   "one's force is never equal to their good-will": Strouse, *Alice James*, 98.

CHAPTER 2: STILL WATERS

30   "sorely overtaxed": S. Weir Mitchell, *Wear and Tear: Or, Hints for the Overworked* (Walnut Creek, CA: AltaMira Press, 2004, reprint of the Lippincott 1871 edition), 9.

31   "millionaires of nerve-force": Beard was not one of those men. He himself struggled with symptoms of neurasthenia in his youth. George M. Beard, *American Nervousness: Its Causes and Consequences* (New York: G. P. Putnam's Sons, 1881), 9.

31   "nervous bankruptcy": Beard, *American Nervousness*, 9–10.

31   "emotional prodigality": Jean Strouse, *Alice James: A Biography* (Cambridge: Harvard University Press, 1999), 107–8.

31   quell her emotional life: Alice James, *The Diary of Alice James*, ed. Leon Edel (Boston: Northeastern University Press, 1999), 95, entry February 21, 1890, as cited in Strouse, *Alice James*, 81.

32   "geyser of emotions": James, *Diary*, 25, as cited in Strouse, *Alice James*, 238.

32   "busy trying to idle": Strouse, *Alice James*, 140.

32   when Alice "improved": Richard Warrington Baldwin Lewis, *The Jameses: A Family Narrative* (New York: Farrar, Straus and Giroux, 1991).

32   Alice had sewing bees: Strouse, *Alice James*, 132–43.

32   "slow steadiness of her improvement": Strouse, *Alice James*, 140.

32   "If it keeps on at the same rate": Strouse, *Alice James*, 140.

33   "a fight simply between my body and my will": James, *Diary*, 149, entry October 26, 1890, as cited in Strouse, *Alice James*, 118.

34   "perpetual postponement": James, *Diary*, 95, entry February 21, 1880, as cited in Strouse, *Alice James*, 81.

34   not officially recognized by the Social Security Administration: Social Security Administration, 64 CFR 83 (April 30, 1999), http://www.cfids-me.org/disinissues /ssa0499.html.

        "In accordance with 20 CFR 402.35(b)(1), the Commissioner of Social Security gives notice of Social Security Ruling, SSR 99-2p. This Ruling clarifies disability policy for the evaluation and adjudication of disability claims involving Chronic Fatigue Syndrome (CFS). This Ruling explains that, when it is accompanied by appropriate medical signs or laboratory findings, CFS is a medically determinable impairment that can be the basis for a finding of 'disability.'"

34   remains difficult to win a claim: Aaron Hotfelder, "Getting Disability Benefits for Chronic Fatigue Syndrome," https://www.nolo.com/legal-encyclopedia/getting -disability-benefits-chronic-fatigue-syndrome.html.

35   more sensitive to medications: Centers for Disease Control and Prevention, "Monitoring the Use of All Medicines and Supplements," July 12, 2018, https://www .cdc.gov/me-cfs/healthcare-providers/clinical-care-patients-mecfs/monitoring -medication.html.

37   a woman's "aim in life": Strouse, *Alice James*, 45.

37   "Learning and wisdom do not become her": Strouse, *Alice James*, 45.

37   "knock off the head of the benignant pater": Strouse, *Alice James*, 118.

37   birthed the same year as Alice: Strouse, *Alice James*, 88.

38   never joined the feminist movement: Strouse, *Alice James*, 243.

38   "personal power venting itself on no opportunity": Strouse, *Alice James*, 319.

38   "the only solution": Strouse, *Alice James*, 322.

39   "had neurotic science been born.": Strouse, *Alice James*, ix.

41   "the duties of doctor, nurse, and strait-jacket": James, *Diary*, 149, entry October 26, 1890, as cited in Strouse, *Alice James*, 118.

41   Neurasthenia is often confused with hysteria: Maurizio Paciaroni and Julien

Bogousslavsky, "The Borderland with Neurasthenia," *Frontiers of Neurology and Neuroscience* 35 (2014): 149–56, doi: 10.1159/000360055.

41   Hysteria was almost solely a women's disorder: Strouse, *Alice James*, 104.

41   Doctors often blamed "over-education" and emotional expressiveness: Barbara Sicherman, "The Paradox of Prudence: Mental Health in the Gilded Age," *Journal of American History* 62, no. 4 (1976): 895, doi: 10.2307/1903843; S. Weir Mitchell, *Doctor and Patient* (Philadelphia: J. B. Lippincott, 1888), as cited in Ellen L. Bassuk, "The Rest Cure: Repetition or Resolution of Victorian Women's Conflicts?," *The Female Body in Western Culture: Contemporary Perspectives*, ed. Susan Rubin Suleiman (Cambridge: Harvard University Press, 1986), 143.

43   "possess one's soul in silence": James, *Diary*, 95, as cited in Strouse, *Alice James*, 81.

CHAPTER 3: ELEPHANT

44   "the practical problem of life": Jean Strouse, *Alice James: A Biography* (Cambridge: Harvard University Press, 1999), 284.

44   "Psychiatric Diagnoses in Patients": Marcus J. Kruesi, Janet Dale, and Stephen E. Straus, "Psychiatric Diagnoses in Patients Who Have Chronic Fatigue Syndrome," *Journal of Clinical Psychiatry* 50, no. 2 (1989): 53–56.

44   hand to her forehead: Hillary Johnson, *Osler's Web: Inside the Labyrinth of the Chronic Fatigue Syndrome Epidemic* (Lincoln, NE: Author's Guild Backinprint. com, 2006), 287.

44   "affected by a psychiatric illness": National Institutes of Health, "Lifetime History of Psychiatric Illness in People with Chronic Fatigue Syndrome" (1989), as cited in Johnson, *Osler's Web*, 316.

44   press release: National Institutes of Health, "Lifetime History," as cited in Johnson, *Osler's Web*, 316.

44   "no serious underlying disease": Mayo Clinic, *The Mayo Clinic Family Health Book* (New York: William Morrow, 1990), as cited in Johnson, *Osler's Web*, 367.

44   bestseller: Johnson, *Osler's Web*, 367.

47   Johnson, *Osler's Web*, 318–20.

47   depression pre-occurs or co-occurs: Cecil Bradley, letter, *Journal of Clinical Psychiatry*, 1989, as cited in Johnson, *Osler's Web*, 319–20.

47   Multiple sclerosis is another: Gary Franklin et al., "Cognitive Loss in Multiple Sclerosis, Case Reports and Review of the Literature," *Archives of Neurology* 46, no. 2 (1989): 162–67, as cited in Johnson, *Osler's Web*, 311.

47   interleukin-2 in CFS patients: Paul R. Cheney, Susan E. Dorman, and David S. Bell, "Interleukin-2 and the Chronic Fatigue Syndrome," *Annals of Internal Medicine* 110, no. 4 (1989): 321, as cited in Johnson, *Osler's Web*, 321–22.

48   no more depressed or anxious: Ian Hickie et al., "The Psychiatric Status of Patients with the Chronic Fatigue Syndrome," *British Journal of Psychiatry* 156 (1990): 534–40, as cited in Johnson, *Osler's Web*, 404.

48   "not excessively hypochondriacal": Hickie et al. "The Psychiatric Status," 534.

48   an assertion that was patently false: Johnson, *Osler's Web*, 369.

48   immune system dysfunction: "In fact, every scientific study of patients had turned up immune abnormalities, and the CDC, having failed to conduct any research of its own, lacked any data to the contrary," Johnson, *Osler's Web*, 369.

48   natural killer cells: Susan Levine, "Immune System Gone Haywire?," *The CFIDS Chronicle: Special Issue: The Science and Research of CFS* (2006): 28–31, https://www.me-gids.net/nieuwsartikel/science-research-of-cfs-cfids-chronicle-special-issue/; Ekua W. Brenu et al., "Immunological Abnormalities as Potential Biomarkers in Chronic Fatigue Syndrome/Myalgic Encephalomyelitis," *Journal of Translational Medicine* 9 (2011): e81, http://www.translational-medicine.com/content/9/1/81.

48   "Maybe it takes a psychologist": Johnson, *Osler's Web*, 284.

48   unlike people with CFS, the fatigue: David Tuller, "Learning Firsthand About Chronic Fatigue Syndrome," *New York Times*, May 30, 2008, http://www.cfs-aktuell.de/juni08_2.htm.

49   "the person with CFS would give you a list": Tuller, "Learning Firsthand."

49   "in CFS, the adrenal gland is smaller": Nancy Klimas, "The State of CFS Research," *The CFIDS Chronicle: Special Issue: The Science and Research of CFS* (2006), 7.

49   10 percent of patients who contract mononucleosis: Phoenix Rising Team, "Model of Post Infective Fatigue Forming: The Dubbo Studies," *Phoenix Rising*, March 4, 2012, http://phoenixrising.me/research-2/the-dubbo-studies-a-model-of-post-infective-fatigue-emerging/model-of-post-infective-fatigue-forming-the-dubbo-studies; Peter D. White et al., "Incidence, Risk and Prognosis of Acute and Chronic Fatigue Syndromes and Psychiatric Disorders After Glandular Fever," *British Journal of Psychiatry* 173 (1998): 475–81, doi: 10.1192/bjp.173.6.475; Dedra S. Buchwald et al., "Acute Infectious Mononucleosis: Characteristics of Patients Who Report Failure to Recover," *American Journal of Medicine* 109, no. 7 (2000): 531–37, doi: 10.1016/s0002-9343(00)00560-x; Ian Hickie et al., "Post-Infective and Chronic Fatigue Syndromes Precipitated by Viral and Non-Viral Pathogens: Prospective Cohort Study," *BMJ* 333, no. 7568 (2006): 575, doi: 10.1136/bmj.38933.585764.AE.

49   people with certain gene variants: Suzanne Vernon et al., "Preliminary Evidence of Mitochondrial Dysfunction Associated with Post-Infective Fatigue After Acute Infection with Epstein Barr Virus," *BMC Infectious Diseases* 6 (2006): e15, doi: 10.1186/1471-2334-6-15; Suzanne Vernon et al., "Correlation of Psycho-Neuroendocrine-Immune (PNI) Gene Expression with Symptoms of Acute Infectious Mononucleosis," *Brain Research* 1068, no. 1 (2006): 1–6, doi: 10.1016/j.brainres.2005.11.013, as cited in Phoenix Rising, "Model of Post Infective."

49   autonomic nervous system to CFS: Benjamin N. Goertzel et al., "Combinations of Single Nucleotide Polymorphisms in Neuroendocrine Effector and Receptor Genes Predict Chronic Fatigue Syndrome," *Pharmacogenomics* 7, no. 3 (2006): 475–83, doi: 10.2217/14622416.7.3.475, as cited in Vegard B. Wyller, Hege R.

Eriksen, and Kirsti Malterud, "Can Sustained Arousal Explain the Chronic Fatigue Syndrome?," *Behavioral and Brain Functions* 5 (2009): e10, doi: 10.1186/1744-9081-5-10.

50 "a multisystem illness": Erica F. Verrillo, *Chronic Fatigue Syndrome: A Treatment Guide*, 2nd ed. (self-published, 2012), 71.

50 awry in the autonomic nervous systems: Anthony L. Komaroff, "What Causes CFS?," *The CFIDS Chronicle: Special Issue: The Science and Research of CFS* (2006), 25.

50 may be overactivated: Cort Johnson, "Autonomically Speaking," *The CFIDS Chronicle: The Science Issue* (2008), 14.

51 disturbance in the HPA axis: Komaroff, "What Causes CFS?," 25.

51 relatively low levels of cortisol: Komaroff, "What Causes CFS?," 25.

51 "for a period of at least 6 months": Gary P. Holmes et al., "Chronic Fatigue Syndrome: A Working Case Definition," *Annals of Internal Medicine* 108, no. 3 (1988): 387–89, doi: 10.7326/0003-4819-108-3-387.

52 at least eight different case definitions: Mary Dimmock and Matthew Lazell-Fairman, *Thirty Years of Disdain: How HHS and a Group of Psychiatrists Buried ME* (self-published, 2015), 154, https://www.dropbox.com/s/bycueauxmh49z4l / Thirty%20Years%20of%20Disdain%20-%20Background.pdf?dl=0.

52 "too confusing for many nonmedical persons": Gary Holmes, letter to Craig Barshinger, December 7, 1987, as cited in Johnson, *Osler's Web*, 231.

52 "It's difficult to imagine": Johnson, *Osler's Web*, 231.

53 "only a small amount of evidence": Julie Rehmeyer, personal communication, January 1, 2017.

53 the role of "shirkers": Johnson, *Osler's Web*, 219.

53 "chronic thirst syndrome": Johnson, *Osler's Web*, 219.

53 moments of near paralysis: Julie Rehmeyer, *Through the Shadowlands: A Science Writer's Odyssey into an Illness Science Doesn't Understand* (New York: Rodale, 2017), 31.

53 Sophia Mirza: Investigating Officer, "Report of the Investigation into the Complaints of Mrs. Wilson for Brighton and Hove City Council," October 25, 2007, http://www.sophiaandme.org.uk/ssd/(26)251007-p1+p2-p27.html.

54 to die from CFS: Criona Wilson, Comment, "Report of the Investigation into the Complaints of Mrs. Wilson for Brighton and Hove City Council," October 25, 2007, 22–25, http://www.investinme.org/Article-050%20Sophia%20Wilson%2001 .htm, as cited in Dimmock and Lazell-Fairman, *Thirty Years*; Rowan Hooper, "First Official UK Death from Chronic Fatigue Syndrome," *New Scientist*, June 16, 2006, https://www.newscientist.com/article/dn9342-first-official-uk-death -from-chronic-fatigue-syndrome/.

54 "chronic fatigue and immune dysfunction syndrome": Johnson, *Osler's Web*, 228.

54 "patient's self-absorption": Elaine Showalter, *Hystories: Hysterical Epidemics and Modern Media* (New York: Columbia University Press, 1997), 124.

54 "Florence Nightingale Disease": Leonard A. Jason et al., "Evaluating Attributions for an Illness Based Upon the Name: Chronic Fatigue Syndrome, Myalgic En-

cephalopathy and Florence Nightingale Disease," *American Journal of Community Psychology* 30, no. 1 (2002): 133–48, doi: 10.1023/A:1014328319297, as cited in Peggy Munson, "Introduction," *Stricken: Voices from the Hidden Epidemic of Chronic Fatigue Syndrome*, ed. Peggy Munson (New York: Haworth Press, 2000), 13.

55   "don't like malingerers": Johnson, *Osler's Web*, 311.

55   "badge of success": Arthur Kleinman and Stephen Straus, "Introduction," in *Chronic Fatigue Syndrome*, ed. Gregory R. Bock and Julie Whelan (London: Wiley, 1993), 3, as quoted in Showalter, *Hystories*, 116.

55   people with less money: Johnson, *Osler's Web*, 639–40.

55   "financial ability": Johnson, *Osler's Web*, 640.

55   "hits the lower classes harder": Johnson, *Osler's Web*, 640.

56   yuppies of the Victorian era: Francis G. Gosling, *Before Freud: Neurasthenia and the American Medical Community, 1870–1910* (Urbana: University of Illinois Press, 1987), xxi.

56   "The march of scientific progress": Gosling, *Before Freud*, 94.

56   across the economic spectrum: Gosling, *Before Freud*, 184–85.

56   the ones who could afford to see them: Gosling, *Before Freud*, 16.

56   "professional men most like themselves": Gosling, *Before Freud*, 160.

56   "their diagnoses reflected their opinions": Gosling, *Before Freud*, 54. The research from *Before Freud* was first published in Francis George Gosling and Joyce M. Ray, "The Right to Be Sick: American Physicians and Nervous Patients, 1885–1910," *Journal of Social History* 20, no. 2 (1986), 251–67, doi: 10.1353/jsh/20.2.251.

57   among laborers "sexual excess": Gosling, *Before Freud*, 55.

57   more women than men: Solve ME/CFS Initiative, "About the Disease," https://solvecfs.org/me-cfs-long-covid/about-the-disease/.

57   women's concerns are more often dismissed: Shari Munch, "Gender-Biased Diagnosing of Women's Medical Complaints: Contributions of Feminist Thought, 1970–1995," *Women & Health* 40, no. 1 (2004): 101–21, doi: 10.1300/J013v40n01_06.

57   identified heart disease in 41 percent fewer women: Gabrielle R. Chiaramonte and Roland Friend, "Medical Students' and Residents' Gender Bias in the Diagnosis, Treatment, and Interpretation of CHD Symptoms," *Health Psychology* 25, no. 3 (2006): 255–66, doi: 10.1037/0278-6133.25.3.255, as cited in Maya Dusenbery, "Is Medicine's Gender Bias Killing Young Women?," *Pacific Standard*, March 23, 2015, http://www.psmag.com/health-and-behavior/is-medicines-gender-bias-killing-young-women.

57   while men's symptoms are perceived as organic: Chiaramonte and Friend, "Gender Bias," as cited in Dusenbery, "Is Medicine's Gender Bias?"

58   unable to work at all: Meghan O'Rourke, "A New Name, and Wider Recognition, for Chronic Fatigue Syndrome," *New Yorker*, February 27, 2015, https://www.newyorker.com/tech/annals-of-technology/chronic-fatigue-syndrome-iom-report.

58   economic hardship: Jill S. Anderson and Carol Estwing Ferrans, "The Quality of

Life of Persons with Chronic Fatigue Syndrome," *Journal of Nervous and Mental Disease* 185, no. 6 (1997): 359–67, doi: 10.1097/00005053-199706000-00001, as cited in Peggy Munson, "The Paradox of Lost Fingerprints: Metaphor and the Shaming of Chronic Fatigue Syndrome," in *Stricken: Voices from the Hidden Epidemic of Chronic Fatigue Syndrome*, ed. Peggy Munson (New York: Haworth Press, 2000), 95–127.

58   "marked feelings of isolation": Anderson and Ferrans, "The Quality of Life"

58   Only 5 percent: R. Cairns and M. Hotopf, "A Systematic Review Describing the Prognosis of Chronic Fatigue Syndrome," *Occupational Medicine* 55, no. 1 (2005): 20–31, doi: 10.1093/occmed/kqi013.

58   medical expenditures and lost productivity: Kenneth J. Reynolds et al., "The Economic Impact of Chronic Fatigue Syndrome," *Cost Effectiveness and Resource Allocation* 2, no. 4 (2004), doi: 10.1186/1478-7547-2-4.

59   "(PTSD)-like syndrome": Munson, "Introduction," in *Stricken*, 8–9.

60   $407,000 to fund ME/CFS research: Johnson, *Osler's Web*, 238.

60   "watching it disappear": Johnson, *Osler's Web*, 264.

60   "I asked them where the money was": Johnson, *Osler's Web*, 371.

60   granted just $683,000: Johnson, *Osler's Web*, 454.

60   "the division's golden goose": Johnson, *Osler's Web*, 455.

60   led to an independent audit: Office of Inspector General, Department of Health and Human Services, "Audit of Costs Charged to the Chronic Fatigue Syndrome Program at the Centers for Disease Control and Prevention," May 1999, https://oig.hhs.gov/oas/reports/region4/49804226.pdf.

61   PACE trial: Peter D. White et al., "Comparison of Adaptive Pacing Therapy, Cognitive Behaviour Therapy, Graded Exercise Therapy, and Specialist Medical Care for Chronic Fatigue Syndrome (PACE): A Randomised Trial," *The Lancet* 377, no. 9768 (2011): 823–36, critiqued by David Tuller, "Trial by Error: The Troubling Case of the PACE Chronic Fatigue Syndrome Study," *Virology* (blog), October 21, 2015, https://www.virology.ws/2015/10/21/trial-by-error-i/.

61   "got back to normal": Julie Rehmeyer, "Hope for Chronic Fatigue Syndrome," *Slate*, November 13, 2015, https://slate.com/technology/2015/11/chronic-fatigue-pace-trial-is-flawed-should-be-reanalyzed.html.

61   claimed that 22 percent: Rehmeyer, "Hope for Chronic Fatigue."

61   a sweeping critique: Tuller, "Trial by Error," part 2.

62   modest gain pales in comparison: Tuller, "Trial by Error."

62   CDC adopted the PACE: Julie Rehmeyer, "Bad Science Misled Millions with Chronic Fatigue Syndrome. Here's How We Fought Back," *Stat*, September 21, 2016, https://www.statnews.com/2016/09/21/chronic-fatigue-syndrome-pace-trial/.

62   "the PACE trial is the most convincing evidence": Julie Rehmeyer, personal communication, January 1, 2017.

62   CDC has since removed: Centers for Disease Control and Prevention, "Treatment," January 28, 2021, https://www.cdc.gov/me-cfs/treatment/index.html.

63   2.5 million Americans: Centers for Disease Control and Prevention, "Myalgic

Encephalomyelitis/Chronic Fatigue Syndrome (ME/CFS)," June 1, 2022, https://www.cdc.gov/me-cfs/.

63   budget for hay fever: National Institutes of Health, "Estimates of Funding for Various Research, Condition, and Disease Categories (RCDC)," May 16, 2022, https://report.nih.gov/categorical_spending.aspx.

63   and cancer: National Institutes of Health, "Estimates of Funding."

63   undiagnosed: Leonard Jason, "Defining CFS: Diagnostic Criteria and Case Definition" (paper presented at CFIDS Association webinar, April 14, 2010).

63   "can inhibit a patient's motivation": Dana J. Brimmer, "U.S. Healthcare Providers' Knowledge, Attitudes, Beliefs, and Perceptions Concerning Chronic Fatigue Syndrome (CDC-Sponsored Survey)," *BMC Primary Care* 11 (2010): 28, doi: 10.1186/1471-2296-11-28, as cited in Mary Dimmock and Matthew Lazell-Fairman, *Thirty Years of Disdain: How HHS and a Group of Psychiatrists Buried ME* (self-published, 2015), 154, 74–75, https://www.dropbox.com/s/bycueauxm h49z4l/.Thirty%20Years%20of%20Disdain%20-%20Background.pdf?dl=0.

63   "Diagnosis elicits the belief": Marcus J. H. Huibers and Simon Wessely, "The Act of Diagnosis: Pros and Cons of Labelling Chronic Fatigue Syndrome," *Psychological Medicine* 36, no. 7 (2006): 895–900, as cited in Dimmock and Lazell-Fairman, *Thirty Years*, 74–75.

64   "All great avalanches": Johnson, *Osler's Web*, 675–76.

64   "serious, chronic, complex and systemic disease": David Cox, "Is Chronic Fatigue Syndrome Finally Being Taken Seriously?," *The Guardian*, April 4, 2016, 3, https://www.theguardian.com/lifeandstyle/2016/apr/04/chronic-fatigue-syndrome-cfs-taken-seriously.

CHAPTER 4: TERRITORIES

65   planet as a living—and female—organism: Carolyn Merchant, *The Death of Nature: Women, Ecology and the Scientific Revolution* (New York: HarperOne, 1990), xvi.

65   celestial machine: Rupert Sheldrake, *Science Set Free: 10 Paths to New Discovery* (New York: Deepak Chopra Books, 2012), 30.

65   He was a sickly child: Russell Shorto, *Descartes' Bones: A Skeletal History of the Conflict Between Faith and Reason* (New York: Doubleday, 2008), 3.

65   "I think, therefore I am": Descartes first wrote this statement in *Discourse on Method* (1637).

66   "even if the body did not exist": Sheldrake, *Science Set Free*, 293.

66   would have studied Kepler: Ronald S. Fishman, "The Study of the Wonderful: The First Topographical Mapping of Vision in the Brain," *JAMA Opthamology* 126, no. 12 (2008): 1767–73, doi: 10.1001/archopht.126.12.1767.

67   "man's serious, objective work of controlling nature": Richard Watson, *Cogito, Ergo Sum: The Life of René Descartes* (Boston: David R. Godine, Publisher, 2002), 17.

67   medical colonialism: Arthur W. Frank, *The Wounded Storyteller: Body, Illness, and Ethics*, 2nd ed. (Chicago: University of Chicago Press, 2013), 10.

67   surrender themselves to the care of a doctor: Talcott Parsons, *Action Theory and the Human Condition* (New York: Free Press, 1978), chapters 1–3, as cited in Frank, *The Wounded Storyteller,* 5–6.

67   "wisest ask the fewest questions": S. Weir Mitchell, *Doctor and Patient* (Philadelphia: J. B. Lippincott, 1888), as cited in Nancy Cervetti, *S. Weir Mitchell: 1829–1914: Philadelphia's Literary Physician* (University Park, PA: Pennsylvania State University Press), 142.

67   "knowledge that can be verified as objective": David B. Morris, *Illness and Culture in the Postmodern Age* (Berkeley: University of California Press, 1998), 37–38.

68   "reduced to an object being repaired": Ivan Illich, *Medical Nemesis: The Expropriation of Health* (New York: Bantam Books, 1977), as cited in Marc Renaud, "On the Structural Constraints to State Intervention in Health," *The Cultural Crisis of Modern Medicine,* ed. John Ehrenreich (New York: Monthly Review Press, 1978), 109.

68   health is compromised when emotions are suppressed: "Since emotional expression is always tied to a specific flow of peptides in the body, the chronic suppression of emotions results in a massive disturbance of the psychosomatic network," Candace Pert, *Molecules of Emotion: Why You Feel the Way You Feel* (New York: Scribner, 1997), 192; James W. Pennebaker and Sandra K. Beall, "Confronting a Traumatic Event: Toward an Understanding of Inhibition and Disease," *Journal of Abnormal Psychology* 95, no. 3 (1986): 274–81, doi: 10.1037/0021-843X.95.3.274; and see all of Bessel van der Kolk, MD, *The Body Keeps the Score: Brain, Mind, and Body in the Healing of Trauma* (New York: Penguin, 2014).

68   "bottled lightning": Jean Strouse, *Alice James: A Biography* (Cambridge: Harvard University Press, 1999), 238.

68   golden spike: The story of the Golden Spike is an American myth akin to the myth of George Washington cutting down a cherry tree. There were in fact a number of ceremonial spikes, and these were gently tapped into the predrilled holes, but the final spike was an ordinary iron spike. In fact, many reporters wrote their "eyewitness accounts" before the event took place. J. N. Bowman, "Driving the Last Spike at Promontory, 1869," *California Historical Society Quarterly* 36, no. 2 (1957): 96–106, doi: 10.2307/2515112; J. N. Bowman, "Driving the Last Spike at Promontory, 1869 (Concluded)," *California Historical Society Quarterly* 36, no. 3 (September 1957): 263–74, doi: 10.2307/25155136.

69   his gynecological experiments: Sarah Zhang, "The Surgeon Who Experimented on Slaves," *The Atlantic,* April 18, 2018, https://www.theatlantic.com/health /archive/2018/04/j-marion-sims/558248/.

69   "a new and important territory": J. Marion Sims, *The Story of My Life,* ed. H. Marion Sims (New York: D. Appleton, 1885), 231, as cited in Ben Barker-Benfield, "The Spermatic Economy: A Nineteenth Century View of Sexuality," *Feminist Studies* 1, no. 1 (1972), 63, doi: 10.2307/3180106.

69   "has not dared willingly to tread": Robert Battey, "Normal Ovariotomy," *Atlanta Medical and Surgical Journal* 11 (1873), as cited in Barker-Benfield, "The Spermatic

Economy," 64. Barker-Benfield makes the interesting aside that Battey's use of the phrase *consecrated ground* evokes, tellingly, the burial of dead bodies.

70   *"built a woman around it"*: Hillary M. Lips, *Sex and Gender: An Introduction*, 6th ed. (New York: McGraw-Hill Publishing Company, 2008).

70   "man has been born of woman": Augustus Kinsley Gardner, *Conjugal Sins Against the Laws of Life and Health* (New York: J. S. Redfield, 1870), in Barker-Benfield, "The Spermatic Economy," 63.

70   also called "desexing": Barker-Benfield, "The Spermatic Economy," 60.

70   "that we may make them tractable": Dr. David Gilliam, "Oophorectomy for the Insanity and Epilepsy of the Female: A Plea for Its More General Adoption," *Transactions of the American Association of Obstetricians and Gynecologists* 9 (1896), as cited in Barker-Benfield, "The Spermatic Economy," 61.

71   would now be considered organic complaints: Richard Webster, *Why Freud Was Wrong: Sin, Science, and Psychoanalysis* (New York: Basic Books, 1995), 163.

71   misdiagnosed as hysteria: Richard Webster, "Freud, Charcot and Hysteria: Lost in the Labyrinth," https://www.richardwebster.org/freudandcharcot.html; Webster, *Why Freud Was Wrong*, 157.

71   adds endometriosis and autoimmune disorders: Maya Dusenbery, *Doing Harm: The Truth About How Bad Medicine and Lazy Science Leave Women Dismissed, Misdiagnosed, and Sick* (New York: HarperOne, 2018), 140, 383.

71   exaggerated the success of his treatments: Webster, "Freud, Charcot and Hysteria," 9.

72   Even before Freud: Francis G. Gosling, *Before Freud: Neurasthenia and the American Medical Community, 1870–1910* (Urbana: University of Illinois Press, 1987), 168.

72   "ending the more holistic approach to health care": Gosling, *Before Freud*, 139.

72   outbreaks of illnesses with similar: Byron Hyde and J. Gordon Parish, "A Bibliography of M.E./CFS Epidemics," in *The Clinical and Scientific Basis of Myalgic Encephalomyelitis/Chronic Fatigue Syndrome*, eds. Byron M. Hyde, Jay Goldstein, and Paul Levine (Ogdensburg, NY: Nightingale Research Foundation, 1992), 176–88.

72   between the 1934 epidemic: Hyde and Parish, "A Bibliography of M.E./CFS Epidemics."

72   in the late 1970s: Erica F. Verrillo, *Chronic Fatigue Syndrome: A Treatment Guide*, 2nd ed. (self-published, 2012), 22.

72   upswing of patients: Verrillo, *Chronic Fatigue Syndrome*, 23.

73   "obedience to his decrees": S. Weir Mitchell, *Fat and Blood*, 2nd ed. (Philadelphia: J. B. Lippincott, 1878), 54–55, as quoted in Cervetti, *S. Weir Mitchell*, 111–12.

73   "a rather bitter medicine": Mitchell, *Fat and Blood*, 39, as cited in Barbara Ehrenreich and Deirdre English, *For Her Own Good: 150 Years of the Experts' Advice to Women*, 2nd ed. (New York: Doubleday, 1989), 136.

73   "moral medication": Mitchell, *Fat and Blood*, 39–40, as cited in Cervetti, *S. Weir Mitchell*, 245.

73   organized a women's luncheon club: Strouse, *Alice James*, 177.

74 "would be quite superfluous": Strouse, *Alice James*, 177.

74 "recurrence of her old troubles": Strouse, *Alice James*, 183.

74 suicidality: Strouse, *Alice James*, 186.

74 "a passive part in life": Strouse, *Alice James*, 189.

74 "was left high and dry": Strouse, *Alice James*, 189.

74 "much believed-in joy of mere existence": Alice James, August 9, 1879, *Alice James: Her Life in Letters*, ed. Linda Anderson (Bristol, England: Thoemmes Press, 1996), 104.

74 Strouse implied a manipulative aspect: Strouse, *Alice James*, 183.

74 "tyrannical helplessness": Strouse, *Alice James*, 242.

75 women had more financial power: Silvia Federici, *Caliban and the Witch: Women, the Body and Primitive Accumulation*, 2nd rev. ed. (New York: Autonomedia, 2014), as cited in Eula Biss, *Having and Being Had* (New York: Riverhead Books, 2020), 108.

75 "women worked in hundreds of professions": Federici, *Caliban and the Witch*, as cited in Biss, *Having and Being Had*, 108.

75 lost the right: Federici, *Caliban and the Witch*, as cited in Biss, *Having and Being Had*, 108.

75 "a machine to produce more workers": Federici, *Caliban and the Witch*, 12.

75 Those punished as witches: Biss, *Having and Being Had*, 108; Ehrenreich and English, *For Her Own Good*, 35.

76 "part of the same process": Federici, *Caliban and the Witch*, as cited in Biss, *Having and Being Had*, 107.

76 relegated to the domestic realm: Greta Nettleton, *The Quack's Daughter: A True Story About the Private Life of a Victorian College Girl*, rev. ed. (Iowa City: University of Iowa Press, 2014).

76 "masculine, and imminently more salable": Ehrenreich and English, *For Her Own Good*, 45–47.

76 Mary Putnam Jacobi: Cervetti, *S. Weir Mitchell*, 2.

76 "the man who does not know sick women": Mitchell, *Doctor and Patient*, as quoted in Cervetti, *S. Weir Mitchell*, 119.

77 "childlike acquiescence": Mitchell, *Fat and Blood*, as cited in Cervetti, *S. Weir Mitchell*, 112.

77 to reclaim their manly vigor: Jennifer S. Tuttle, "Rewriting the West Cure: Charlotte Perkins Gilman, Owen Wister, and the Sexual Politics of Neurasthenia," *The Mixed Legacy of Charlotte Perkins Gilman*, eds. Catherine J. Golden and Joanna Schneider Zangrando (Newark: University of Delaware Press, 2000), 104–5. Tuttle was publicly presenting her research on the "West Cure" at the same time that Barbara Will coined the term in print, in "The Nervous Origins of the American Western," *American Literature* 70, no. 2 (1998): 293–316.

77 the "Camp Cure": Mitchell, *Doctor and Patient*, 155.

78 "wisely directed mental activity": Strouse, *Alice James*, 172.

78 Alice described to her friend Sara Darwin as: Strouse, *Alice James*, 83.

78 "it is what I most care about just now": Strouse, *Alice James*, 176.

78 "I am becoming ardently matrimonial": Strouse, *Alice James*, 164.

78   the clearly besotted Alice: Strouse, *Alice James*, 191.

79   women were rarely included in medical studies: Dusenbery, *Doing Harm*, 3.

79   put a fetus at risk: Dusenbery, *Doing Harm*, 30–32.

79   even to contract different diseases: Dusenbery, *Doing Harm*, 23–59.

79   women made up only 37 percent of the sample: Stacie E. Geller, Marci Goldstein Adams, and Molly Carnes, "Adherence to Federal Guidelines for Reporting of Sex and Race/Ethnicity in Clinical Trials," *Journal of Women's Health* 15, no. 10 (2006): 1123–31, doi: 10.1089/jwh.2006.15.1123.

79   A 2011 update: Stacie E. Geller et al., "Inclusion, Analysis, and Reporting of Sex and Race/Ethnicity in Clinical Trials: Have We Made Progress?," *Journal of Women's Health* 20, no. 3 (2011): 315–20, https://www.doi.org/10.1089/jwh.2010.2469.

79   fell to 24 percent in drug trials: Geller, Adams, and Carnes, "Adherence to Federal Guidelines."

79   adverse drug reaction: Heather P. Whitley and Wesley Lindsey, "Sex-Based Differences in Drug Activity," *American Family Physician* 80, no. 11 (2009): 1254–58, as cited in Dusenbery, *Doing Harm*, 44.

79   did not break results down by sex: Geller, Adams, and Carnes, "Adherence to Federal Guidelines."

79   suffer worse side effects: Melinda Wenner Moyer, "Women Report Worse Side Effects After a Covid Vaccine," *New York Times*, March 8, 2021, https://www.nytimes.com/2021/03/08/health/vaccine-side-effects-women-men.html.

79   peculiar theory: Frederick Crews, *Freud: The Making of an Illusion* (New York: Metropolitan Books, 2017), 423–24.

80   surgical intervention: Crews, *Freud*, 459.

80   cocaine-addicted Freud: Crews, *Freud*, 456–57.

81   "So this is the strong sex": Crews, *Freud*, 475.

81   "rapidly moving toward a bad ending": Crews, *Freud*, 476.

81   Eckstein survived her ordeal: Crews, *Freud*, 477.

81   "certain young doctor": Crews, *Freud*, 478.

81   "an unconscious intent of longing to entice me": Crews, *Freud*, 479.

81   "accusing a mutilated patient": Crews, *Freud*, 479–80.

82   would support his diagnosis: Crews, *Freud*, 483.

82   "he blew up": Crews, *Freud*, 483.

82   "remained abnormal": Jeffrey Moussaieff Masson, *The Assault on Truth: Freud's Suppression of the Seduction Theory* (New York: Pocket Books, 1998), 255.

82   that Alice suffered from endometriosis: Nancy Hedrick, "Alice James and Endometriosis," *Psychiatric Services*, 52, no. 8 (2001): 1106–107, doi: 10.1176/appi .ps.52.8.1106; Mary Lou Ballweg, "Blaming the Victim: The Psychologizing of Endometriosis," *Obstetrics and Gynecology Clinics of North America* 24, no. 2 (1997): 441–53, doi: 10.1016/s0889-8545(05)70312-0.

83   "disproportionate and persistent thoughts": American Psychiatric Association, *Diagnostic and Statistical Manual of Mental Disorders*, 5th ed. (Washington DC: American Psychiatric Association, 2013).

83   eventually found to have an organic basis: Charles Ford, Wayne Katon, and Mack Lipkin Jr., "Managing Somatization and Hypochondriasis," *Patient Care* 27, no. 2 (1993): 31–44, as cited in Ballweg, "Blaming the Victim," 446.

83   later found to have organic illnesses: Koyama et al., "Avoiding Diagnostic Errors in Psychosomatic Medicine: A Case Series Study," *BioPsychoSocial Medicine* 12 (2018): e4, doi: 10.1186/s13030-018-0122-3.

83   "I have had sixteen periods": Alice James, *The Death and Letters of Alice James: Selected Correspondence*, ed. Ruth Bernard Yeazell (Boston: Exact Change, 1997), 123, as cited in Strouse, *Alice James*, 237.

83   could be another clue: Hedrick, "Alice James," 1106–107.

84   the second illness was either ME/CFS: Salynn Boyles, "Endometriosis Linked to Other Disease," WebMD, September 26, 2002, https://www.webmd.com/women/endometriosis/news/20020926/endometriosis-linked-to-other-diseases.

84   "modern women's conflict over her role": Ballweg, "Blaming the Victim," 447.

84   "than those held by trained mental health professionals": Dusenbery, *Doing Harm*, 148.

84   "mental health professionals were often the first": Charles W. Schmidt, "Questions Persist: Environmental Factors in Autoimmune Disease," *Environmental Health Perspectives* 119, no. 6 (2011), doi: 10.1289/ehp.119-a248, as cited in Dusenbery, *Doing Harm*, 148.

84   misdiagnosed as "psychological cases": Judith Green, Jennifer Romei, and Benjamin H. Natelson, "Stigma and Chronic Fatigue Syndrome," *Journal of Chronic Fatigue Syndrome* 5, no. 2 (1999): 63–75, doi: 10.1300/J092v05n02_04, as cited in Munson, "The Paradox of Lost Fingerprints," 112.

84   paper published in *American Family Physician*: N. Rasmussen and R. Avant, "Somatization Disorder in Family Practice," *American Family Physician* 40, no. 2 (1989): 206–14.

85   "somatization allows patients to avoid blaming themselves": Ballweg, "Blaming the Victim," 446.

85   "The converse is surely worth considering": Ballweg, "Blaming the Victim," 446.

85   iatraporiueretia: I coined this word with the help of Stephen Cole Farrar, a specialist in classical Greek.

86   Strouse revealed: Allison Silver, "Writing the Good Life," *New York Times*, November 8, 1981, https://www.nytimes.com/1981/11/08/books/writing-the-good-life.html.

86   "manipulated from beyond the grave": Silver, "Writing the Good Life."

87   "I dare to be busy": Strouse, *Alice James*, 171.

87   "denoted failure and waste": Strouse, *Alice James*, 291–92.

CHAPTER 5: MINEFIELD

93   also meet the major criteria for ME/CFS: Nicholas Ashford and Claudia Miller, *Chemical Exposures: Low Levels and High Stakes*, 2nd ed. (New York: Van Nostrand Reinhold, 1998), 229.

93   one of the most prominent complaints: Ashford and Miller, *Chemical Exposures*, 229.

93   chemical weapons experimentation: Marie-Monique Robin, "Our Daily Poison: How Chemicals Have Contaminated the Food Chain," *Truthout*, November 30, 2014, https://truthout.org/articles/our-daily-poison-how-chemicals-have-contaminated -the-food-chain/.

93   pesticides can also damage our nervous systems: Erica F. Verrillo, *Chronic Fatigue Syndrome: A Treatment Guide*, 2nd ed. (self-published, 2012), 56.

93   "may be similar, if not identical": Dedra Buchwald and Deborah Garrity, "Comparison of Patients with Chronic Fatigue Syndrome, Fibromyalgia, and Multiple Chemical Sensitivities," *Archives of Internal Medicine* 154, no. 18 (1994): 2049–53, https://pubmed.ncbi.nlm.nih.gov/8092909, as cited in Ashford and Miller, *Chemical Exposures*, 229.

93   as many as 67 percent: Buchwald and Garrity found that 53 to 67 percent of people with CFS were sensitive to chemicals, "Comparison of Patients," as cited in Ashford and Miller, *Chemical Exposures*, 229.

94   health issues when exposed to fragranced products: Anne Steinemann, "International Prevalence of Chemical Sensitivity, Co-Prevalences with Asthma and Autism, and Effects from Fragranced Consumer Products," *Air Quality, Atmosphere & Health* 12, no. 12 (2019): 519–27, doi: 10.1007/s11869-019-00672-1.

94   Chemical sensitivity afflicts 57 percent of Americans with: Steinemann, "International Prevalence."

94   contained an average of 17 VOCs: Steinemann et al., "Fragranced Consumer Products."

94   VOCs permeate the brain: Marina Schauffler, "Everyday Chemical Fragrances May Be Hazardous to Health," *Maine Sunday Telegram*, September 7, 2014, S2.

97   air fresheners a barrier to accessing: Steinemann, "International Prevalence."

97   formaldehyde and benzene: American Cancer Society, "Benzene and Cancer Risk," https://www.cancer.org/cancer/cancer-causes/benzene.html.

97   fragranced products typically emit hazardous chemicals: Steinemann et al., "Fragranced Consumer Products."

97   *secondhand scents*: Anne Steinemann, "Ten Questions Concerning Air Fresheners and Indoor Build Environments," *Building and Environment* 111 (2017): 280, doi: 10.1016/j.buildenv.2016.11.009.

97   manufacturers are not required to disclose: Steinemann et al., "Fragranced Consumer Products."

104   "she had my full permission to end her life": Jean Strouse, *Alice James: A Biography* (Cambridge: Harvard University Press, 1999), 186.

106   leaching into my body: Jennifer Lunden, "The Mercury in Your Mouth," *Portland Phoenix*, February 27, 2004, https://www.toxicteeth.org/natCamp_stateGovt_NH _Feb04.aspx.

CHAPTER 6: OUR DOMESTIC POISONS

111 olfactory bulb: Stuart Firestein, "From Nose to Brain: The Neurology of Smell," *Big Think*, January 13, 2011, http://bigthink.com/videos/from-nose-to-brain-the-neurology-of-smell.

111 access point for chemicals: Iris R. Bell, Claudia S. Miller, and Gary E. Schwartz, "An Olfactory-Limbic Model of Multiple Chemical Sensitivity Syndrome: Possible Relationships to Kindling and Affective Spectrum Disorders," *Biological Psychiatry* 32, no. 3 (1992): 218–42, doi: 10.1016/0006-3223(92)90105-9.

111 have been diagnosed with MCS: Anne C. Steinemann et al., "Fragranced Consumer Products: Chemicals Emitted, Ingredients Unlisted," *Environmental Impact Assessment Review* 31, no. 3 (2011): 328–33, doi: 10.1016/j.eiar.2010.08.002, Table 22.

111 chemical sensitivities rose by over 200 percent: Anne Steinemann, "National Prevalence and Effects of Multiple Chemical Sensitivities," *Journal of Occupational and Environmental Medicine* 60, no. 3 (2018): e152–e156, doi: 10.1097/JOM.0000000000001272.

113 "Death by Wallpaper": Joshua Glenn, "Death by Wallpaper," *Boston Globe*, June 22, 2003, D3.

113 "brilliant green arsenic-and-copper compound": Glenn, "Death by Wallpaper," D3.

113 papers Morris designed contained arsenic: Andrew A. Meharg, *Venomous Earth: How Arsenic Caused the World's Worst Mass Poisoning* (New York: Macmillan, 2005), 78.

115 novels that influenced: See Christina Scull and Wayne G. Hammond, *The J. R. R. Tolkien Companion & Guide*, 2nd ed. (New York: HarperCollins, 2017), 816; "He was at once captivated by the seeming eccentricities of the prose of Freeman and William Morris. He read them as one would read a thesaurus and made a garner of words," James Joyce, *Stephen Hero* (London: Jonathan Cape Ltd., 1944), 19.

115 "is superb and beautiful": Pamela Todd, *William Morris and the Arts and Crafts Home* (San Francisco: Chronicle Books, 2005), 10.

116 "Is money to be gathered?": From his lecture *Against the Age*, cited in Meharg, *Venomous Earth*, 146.

116 dirty little secret: Meharg, *Venomous Earth*, 135.

117 drives her to distraction: Charlotte Perkins Gilman, "The Yellow Wallpaper," ed. Ann J. Lane, *The Charlotte Perkins Gilman Reader: "The Yellow Wallpaper" and Other Fiction* (New York: Pantheon Books, 1980), 5.

117 "things in that wallpaper": Gilman, "The Yellow Wallpaper," 11.

117 "distasteful design and color": Heather Kirk Thomas, "'[A] Kind of 'Debased Romanesque' with *Delirium Tremens*': Late-Victorian Wall Coverings and Charlotte Perkins Gilman's 'The Yellow Wall-Paper,'" in *The Mixed Legacy of Charlotte Perkins Gilman*, eds. Catherine J. Golden and Joanna Schneider Zangrando (Newark: University of Delaware Press, 2000), 196.

117 tainted a variety of colors: Meharg, *Venomous Earth*, 69; Lucinda Hawksley, *Bitten by Witch Fever: Wallpaper and Arsenic in the Victorian Home* (London: Thames & London, 2016).

117 "Our Best Bedroom": [Robert Chambers?], "Our Best Bedroom," *Chambers's Journal of Popular Literature, Science and Arts* 18 (July–December 1862): 165–72. Most likely it was by copublisher Robert Chambers, who wrote many of the articles in *Chambers's Journal* and was the anonymous author of the potentially scandalous evolutionist treatise *Vestiges of the Natural History of Creation*, as cited in Peter W. J. Bartrip, "How Green Was My Valance? Environmental Arsenic Poisoning and the Victorian Domestic Ideal," *English Historical Review* 111, no. 433 (1994): 891–913, 899–900, doi: 10.1093/ehr/CXI.433.891. This story can be viewed on the author's website, https://jenniferlunden.com/.

118 Devon Great Consols: Meharg, *Venomous Earth*, 139.

119 used the dividends: Meharg, *Venomous Earth*, 143.

119 paper the nursery: Todd, *William Morris*, 39.

119 Arsenic, originally a waste product: Meharg, *Venomous Earth*, 131.

119 many new uses for arsenic: Meharg, *Venomous Earth*, 135.

119 top hat: Meharg, *Venomous Earth*, 144.

119 Morris's uncle Thomas was the resident director: Meharg, *Venomous Earth*, 141–43.

120 girls as young as eight: Patrick O'Sullivan, "Devon Great Consols and William Morris," *Report and Transactions: Devonshire Association for the Advancement of Science, Literature, and Art* 145 (June 2013), 186.

120 too sick to work: Meharg, *Venomous Earth*, 141–43.

120 crawl their pastures on their knees: Meharg, *Venomous Earth*, 132.

120 Morris resigned his directorship: Florence S. Boos and Patrick O'Sullivan, "Morris and Devon Great Consols," *The Journal of William Morris Studies* 19, no. 4 (2012): 22, https://morrissociety.org/document/vol-19-no-4-p-011-39-morris-and-devon -great-consols/.

120 his socialism and his environmentalism: O'Sullivan, "Devon Great Consols," 145, 182.

121 shall take pleasure in his work: Emma Lazarus, "A Day in Surrey with William Morris," *The Century* 32 (May 1886–October 1886): 392.

121 "cheerful, uncramped industry": Lazarus, "A Day in Surrey," 394.

121 "entirely free from arsenic": Meharg, *Venomous Earth*, 81.

122 population tripled: Bill Bryson, *At Home: A Short History of Private Life* (New York: Anchor Books, 2011), 256.

122 nation's wealth rose: Bryson, *At Home*, 256.

123 "mere feeders of machines": Henry George, *Social Problems* (Chicago: Belford, Clarke & Co., 1883), as cited in Alan Trachtenberg, *The Incorporation of America: Culture and Society in the Gilded Age* (New York: Hill and Wang, 1982), 43.

123 explained neurasthenia by comparing: George M. Beard, *American Nervousness: Its Causes and Consequences* (New York: G. P. Putnam's Sons, 1881), 12, 98.

123 "the cry of the system": Beard, *American Nervousness*, as cited in Trachtenberg, *The Incorporation of America*, 47.

124 Scheele's green and emerald green: Meharg, *Venomous Earth*, 84.

124 bonbons and other candies: Meharg, *Venomous Earth*, 84–88.

125   warn people away from the toxic papers: Bartrip, "How Green Was My Valance,"
      900.

125   *memento mori*: Bartrip, "How Green Was My Valance," 901.

125   vocal advocates for reform: Meharg, *Venomous Earth, Venomous Earth*, 68; Bartrip,
      "How Green Was My Valance," 902.

125   *Our Domestic Poisons*: Henry Carr, *Our Domestic Poisons; or the Poisonous Effects
      of Certain Dyes and Colours Used in Domestic Fabrics* (London, 1879), as cited in
      Bartrip, "How Green Was My Valance," 906.

126   "bitten by the witch fever": Meharg, *Venomous Earth*, 81–82; Hawksley, *Bitten by
      Witch Fever*.

126   France had banned arsenic: State Board of Health of Massachusetts, *On the Evil
      Effects of the Use of Arsenic in Certain Green Colors* (Boston: Wright & Potter, 1872),
      19.

126   manufacturers insisted: Bartrip, "How Green Was My Valance," 900.

127   "the histories of numerous instances": State Board of Health of Massachusetts, *On
      the Evil Effects*, 37.

127   a third harbored dangerous amounts: Hawksley, *Bitten by Witch Fever*, 159.

127   arsenic present in the urine of 43 percent: James J. Putnam, "The Frequency with
      Which Arsenic Is Found in the Urine; With Notes on Some New Cases of Poi-
      soning from Wall-Paper and Fabrics," *Boston Medical and Surgical Journal* 122
      (1890): 421–24, doi: 10.1056/NEJM189005011221803.

127   a movement to legislate arsenical wallpapers: James C. Whorton, *Before Silent
      Spring: Pesticides and Public Health in Pre-DDT America* (Princeton, NJ: Princeton
      University Press, 1974), 41–43.

127   Four attempts at legislation: Frederick C. Shattuck, "Some Remarks on Arsenical
      Poisoning, with Special Reference to Its Domestic Sources," *The Medical and Surgical
      Journal* 122 (June 3, 1893): 544. https://archive.org/stream/101745682.nlm.nih
      .gov/101745682_djvu.txt.

127   "a mass of evidence": State Board of Health of Massachusetts, *On the Evil Effects*,
      37.

127   legislators were loath to impose regulations: State Board of Health of Massachu-
      setts, *On the Evil Effects*, 57.

127   *Shadows from the Walls of Death*: M. B. Church, "Sanitary Ceiling and Walls," *Sci-
      ence: A Weekly Newspaper of All the Arts and Sciences* 13 (June 28, 1889): 334.

127   poisoned by paging through it: Robert Kedzie, *Shadows from the Walls of Death*
      (Lansing, MI: W. S. George & Co., Printers and Binders, 1874). The suggestion
      that a woman was poisoned by thumbing through a copy is from Shattuck, "Some
      Remarks," 544.

128   argued again for regulation: Shattuck, "Some Remarks," 545.

128   not true: Shattuck, "Some Remarks," 544.

128   didn't pass till 1900: Whorton, *Before Silent Spring*, 42.

128   converting into a volatile gas: Meharg, *Venomous Earth*, 69–71.

129   fell into obscurity: W. M. Kenna, "The Quantitative Determination of Arsenic in

Wall- and Kindergarten Papers by the Berzelius-Marsh Test; With a Discussion of Poisoning by Arsenical Wall-Papers," (master's thesis, Yale School of Medicine, 1892).

129 dust, mechanically disengaged: State Board of Health of Massachusetts, *On the Evil Effects*, 49.

129 identified the gas as trimethylarsine: Meharg, *Venomous Earth*, 71.

129 "A yellow smell": Gilman, "The Yellow Wallpaper," 15.

129 a representative list: State Board of Health of Massachusetts, *On the Evil Effects*, 18–57; James J. Putnam, "On Chronic Arsenic Poisoning, Especially from Wall-Paper, Based on the Analyses of Twenty-Five Cases in Which Arsenic Was Found in the Urine," *Boston Medical and Surgical Journal* 120 (1889): 235–37, doi: 10.1056/NEJM188903071201002; Putnam, "The Frequency"; Charles Robert Sanger, "On Chronic Arsenical Poisoning from Wall Papers and Fabrics," *Proceedings of the American Academy of Arts and Sciences* 29, no. 8 (1893): 148–77, doi: 10.2307/20020554; Shattuck, "Some Remarks," 540–46, as cited in Jennifer Lunden, "'There Are Things in That Paper That Nobody Knows but Me': An Alternative Reading of Neurasthenia," *Charlotte Perkins Gilman: New Texts, New Contexts*, eds. Jennifer S. Tuttle and Carol Farley Kessler (Columbus: Ohio State University Press, 2011).

130 Excessive fatigue from slight exertion: Francis G. Gosling, *Before Freud: Neurasthenia and the American Medical Community, 1870–1910* (Urbana: University of Illinois Press, 1987), 79–80.

130 "baffle all medical skill": Alfred Swaine Taylor, *Medical Jurisprudence* (London: John Churchill, 1861), as cited in Meharg, *Venomous Earth*, 83.

130 "anomalous character" of the symptoms: State Board of Health of Massachusetts, *On the Evil Effects*, 48.

130 "is to another an active poison": State Board of Health of Massachusetts, *On the Evil Effects*, 52.

131 "may then be more susceptible": Shattuck, "Some Remarks," 544.

131 came to the conclusion that trimethylarsine: William R. Cullen and Ronald Bentley, "The Toxicity of Trimethylarsine: An Urban Myth," *Journal of Environmental Monitoring* 7, no. 1 (2005): 11–15, doi: 10.1039/b413752n.

131 "Exposure to various mold products": Institute of Medicine of the National Academies, *Damp Indoor Spaces and Health* (Washington, DC: National Academies Press, 2004), as cited in Cullen, "The Toxicity of Trimethylarsine," 11–15.

132 "could have been a sensitive indicator": Andrew Meharg, personal correspondence, March 27, 2019.

132 "arsine is highly toxic": Andrew Meharg, personal correspondence, March 27, 2019.

132 telltale garlicky odor: Centers for Disease Control and Prevention, "Facts About Arsine," April 4, 2018, https://emergency.cdc.gov/agent/arsine/facts.asp.

132 studied for use in chemical warfare: CDC, "Facts About Arsine."

132 carbon monoxide (CO) poisoning: Albert Donnay, "Carbon Monoxide as an

Unrecognized Cause of Neurasthenia: A History," in *Carbon Monoxide Toxicity*, ed. David G. Penney (Boca Raton, FL: CRC Press, 2000), 239.

132   contained 4 to 6 percent carbon monoxide: Albert Donnay, "Prologue: And the Call Was Coming from the Basement," *This American Life*, October 27, 2007, https://www.thisamericanlife.org/319/and-the-call-was-coming-from-the -basement; Albert Donnay, "A True Tale of a Truly Haunted House," Ghostvillage, http://www.ghostvillage.com/resources/2004/resources_10312004.shtml.

132   and other volatile organic compounds: Albert Donnay, "On the Recognition of Multiple Chemical Sensitivity in Medical Literature and Government Policy," *International Journal of Toxicology* 18, no. 6 (1999): 383–92, doi: 10.1080/1091581 99225099; Donnay, "Carbon Monoxide," 244.

132   Leaks in gas lines and fixtures: Donnay, "Carbon Monoxide," 244.

132   "A True Tale of a Truly Haunted House": W. H. Wilmer, "Effects of Carbon Mon- oxid [sic] Upon the Eye," *American Journal of Ophthalmology* 4, no. 2 (1921), as cited in Donnay, "A True Tale."

134   detailed description of the carbon monoxide poisoning: Donnay, "Carbon Monoxide."

134   "entire organism reacts with unnecessary readiness": William Osler, *The Principles and Practice of Medicine* (New York: D. Appleton and Co., 1892), as cited in Don- nay, "Carbon Monoxide," 240.

134   "marked variation": Donnay, "Carbon Monoxide," 246–47.

135   cosmetics often contained dangerous toxicants: Kathy Peiss, *Hope in a Jar: The Making of America's Beauty Culture* (New York: Metropolitan Books, 1998).

CHAPTER 7: OUR DOMESTIC POISONS, REDUX

136   19,000 television ads a year: Debra J. Holt et al., *Children's Exposure to TV Advertising in 1977 and 2004: Information for the Obesity Debate*, Federal Trade Commission Bureau of Economics Staff Report, June 1, 2007, 49. https://www.ftc.gov/sites /default/files/documents/reports/childrens-exposure-television-advertising-1977 -and-2004-information-obesity-debate-bureau-economics/cabebw.pdf.

138   "relatively low mammalian toxicity": Agency for Toxic Substances and Disease Registry, *Toxicological Profile for Pyrethrins and Pyrethroids* (Atlanta: U.S. Depart- ment of Health and Human Services, Agency for Toxic Substances and Disease Registry, Public Health Service, 2003), 13, https://www.atsdr.cdc.gov/toxprofiles /tp155.pdf.

138   "unacceptable to any rational person": M. Adrian Gross to Douglas D. Campt, Memorandum "Re: Safety of Permethrin," as cited in Beyond Pesticides, "Perme- thrin," *ChemicalWatch Factsheet*, https://www.beyondpesticides.org/assets/media /documents/ pesticides/factsheets/permethrin.pdf.

138   EPA's new standard allowed: Eliot Marshall, "EPA's High-Risk Carcinogen Policy," *Science* 218 (Dec. 3, 1982): 975, https://www.science.org/doi/abs/10.1126/science .6897126.

138   to approve permethrin for residential use: Environmental Protection Agency,

"Permethrin Facts," August 2009, https://www3.epa.gov/pesticides/chem_search /reg_actions/reregistration/fs_PC-109701_1-Aug-09.pdf.

138 "possible human carcinogen": Beyond Pesticides, "Permethrin"; EPA, "Permethrin Facts."

138 "likely" human carcinogen: EPA, "Permethrin Facts."

138 still on the market: Paolo Boffetta and Vimi Desai, "Exposure to Permethrin and Cancer Risk: A Systematic Review," *Critical Reviews in Toxicology* 48, no. 6 (2018): 433–42, doi: 10.1080/10408444.2018.1439449.

139 "significant neurobehavioral deficits": A. Abdel-Rahman et al., "Neurological Deficits Induced by Malathion, DEET, and Permethrin, Alone or in Combination in Adult Rats," *Journal of Toxicology and Environmental Health, Part A* 67, no. 4 (2004): 331–56, doi: 10.1080/15287390490273569.

139 "increased sensitivity to external stimuli": A. S. Bloom, C. G. Staatz, and T. Dieringer, "Pyrethroid Effects on Operant Responding and Feeding," *Neurobehavioral Toxicology and Teratology* 5, no. 3 (1983): 321–24.

139 impact on immune function: Brandi L. Blaylock et al., "Suppression of Cellular Immune Responses in BALB/c Mice Following Oral Exposure to Permethrin," *Bulletin of Environmental Contamination and Toxicology* 54, no. 5 (1995): 768–74, doi: 10.1007/BF00206111; Nina Grosman and Friedhelm Diel, "Influence of Pyrethroids and Piperonyl Butoxide on the Ca(2+)-ATPase Activity of Rat Brain Synaptosomes and Leukocyte Membranes," *International Immunopharmacology* 5, no. 2 (2005): 263–70, doi: 10.1016/j.intimp.2004.09.030; Korawuth Punareewattana et al., "Topical Permethrin Exposure Inhibits Antibody Production and Macrophage Function in C57B1/6N Mice," *Food and Chemical Toxicology* 39, no. 2 (2001): 133–39, doi: 10.1016/S0278-6915(00)00116-2.

139 risk of breast cancer: Joan Garey and Mary S. Wolff, "Estrogenic and Antiprogestagenic Activities of Pyrethroid Insecticides," *Biochemical and Biophysical Research Communications* 251, no. 3 (1998): 855–59, doi: 10.1006/bbrc.1998.9569; Vera Go et al., "Estrogenic Potential of Certain Pyrethroid Compounds in the MCF-7 Human Breast Carcinoma Cell Line," *Environmental Health Perspectives* 107, no. 3 (1999): 173–77, doi: 10.1289/ehp.99107173; Kavita Kasat, Vera Go, and Beatriz G. T. Pogo, "Effects of Pyrethroid Insecticides and Estrogen on WNT10B Proto-Oncogene Expression," *Environment International* 28, no. 5 (2008): 429–32, doi: 10.1016/S0160-4120(02)00072-7.

139 actually *more* likely than high doses: Kasat, "Effects of Pyrethroid."

139 "more vulnerable to toxicant injury": Jeffrey S. Gillette and Jeffrey R. Bloomquist, "Differential Up-Regulation of Striatal Dopamine Transporter and Alpha-Synuclein by the Pyrethroid Insecticide Permethrin," *Toxicology and Applied Pharmacology* 192, no. 3 (2003): 287–93, doi: 10.1016/S0041-008X(03)00326-0.

140 Multiple doses of toxicants, however: Peter Radetsky, *Allergic to the Twentieth Century: The Explosion in Environmental Allergies—From Sick Buildings to Multiple Chemical Sensitivity* (Boston: Little, Brown, 1997), 226.

140 can damage the blood-brain barrier: Radetsky, *Allergic to the Twentieth Century*, 226.

140 William Henry Perkin: Frederick Alfred Mason, "The Influence of Research on the Development of the Coal-Tar Dye Industry, Part I," *Science Progress in the Twentieth Century (1906–1916)* 10, no. 38 (1915): 237–55, https://www.jstor.org /stable/43427950.

140 quinine, was hard to obtain: Colin Schultz, "In Ancient Rome, Purple Dye Was Made from Snails," *Smithsonian Magazine,* October 10, 2013, https://www .smithsonianmag.com/smart-news/in-ancient-rome-purple-dye-was-made -from-snails-1239931/.

140 "strangely beautiful color": Simon Garfield, *Mauve: How One Man Invented a Color That Changed the World* (New York: W. W. Norton, 2001), 81.

140 glandular mucus of snails: Schultz, "In Ancient Rome."

140 indigo, madder, and other plants: Kenneth Geiser, *Materials Matter: Toward a Sustainable Materials Policy* (Cambridge, MA: MIT Press, 2001), 23.

141 canal turned a different color each week: Garfield, *Mauve,* 81.

141 faded terribly: Garfield, *Mauve,* 52, 81.

141 glue making: Paul D. Blanc, *How Everyday Products Make People Sick: Toxins at Home and in the Workplace* (Berkeley: University of California Press, 2007), 55.

141 in seventy-eight popular sunscreens: Brittany Leitner, "A Report Found the Carcinogen Benzene in 78 Popular Sunscreens," *Shape,* May 27, 2021, https://www .shape.com/lifestyle/beauty-style/carcinogen-benzene-sunscreen.

141 all emit benzene: Janet Gray et al., "State of the Evidence 2017: An Update on the Connection Between Breast Cancer and the Environment," *Environmental Health* 16, no. 94 (2017), https://doi.org/10.1186/s12940-017-0287-4.

142 in hair products and cleaning supplies: Jennifer Lunden, "Exposed: The Mammogram Myth and the Pinkwashing of America," *Orion,* September/October 2013, https://orionmagazine.org/article/exposed/.

142 an ingredient in pesticides: Gray, *State of the Evidence.*

142 almost all food and beverage cans: Lunden, "Exposed"; Environmental Working Group, "EWG Assessment of EPA Draft Human Health Risk Assessment for the Teflon Chemical PFOA," November 7, 2007, https://www.ewg.org/research /ewg-assessment-epa-draft-human-health-risk-assessment-teflon-chemical-pfoa; and to see the plastic lining inside a can, check out Gary Manners's Aug. 7, 2019 "Kick the Cans" in his column "Beery," in *Mainer:* https://mainernews.com/beery/.

142 in perfumes and other scented products: Gray, *State of the Evidence.*

142 effects on human health: Zhanyun Wang et al., "Toward a Global Understanding of Chemical Pollution: A First Comprehensive Analysis of National and Regional Chemical Inventories," *Environmental Science and Technology* 54, no. 5 (2020): 2575–84, doi: 10.1021/acs.est.9b06379.

142 by-products of oil and natural gas: Geiser, *Materials Matter,* 43.

142 chemical industry mushroomed: Michael P. Wilson and Megan R. Schwarzman, "Toward a New U.S. Chemicals Policy: Rebuilding the Foundation to Advance New Science, Green Chemistry, and Environmental Health," *Environmental Health Perspectives* 117, no. 8 (2009): 1202–209, doi: 10.1289/ehp.0800404.

142 $486-billion-a-year industry: American Chemistry Council, "U.S. Chemical Production Expands in July," August 24, 2021, Cision PR Newswire, https://www.prnewswire.com/news-releases/us-chemical-production-expands-in-july-301361919.html.

144 "petrochemical problem": Nicholas A. Ashford and Claudia S. Miller, *Chemical Exposures: Low Levels and High Stakes*, 2nd ed. (New York: Van Nostrand Reinhold, 1998), 19.

144 progressively sick, then stuporous: Theron G. Randolph, *Human Ecology and Susceptibility to the Chemical Environment* (1962; Springfield, IL: Charles C Thomas, Publisher, 1976), 13.

144 "suspect hysteria": Randolph, *Human Ecology*, 19.

145 forty years before Dr. Randolph's discovery: Blanc, *How Everyday Products*, 56.

146 benzene exposure and aplastic anemia: Blanc, *How Everyday Products*, 61.

146 safe concentration for benzene is zero: Kristen Lombardi and Jared Bennett, "A Dozen Dirty Documents," Center for Public Integrity, December 5, 2014, https://publicintegrity.org/environment/a-dozen-dirty-documents/; American Petroleum Institute, *API Toxicological Review, Benzene, September 1948*, Agency for Toxic Substances and Disease Registry, Department of Health and Human Services, https://fixourfuel.com/wp-content/uploads/2016/05/API-Benzene-Toxicology-Review-2.pdf.

146 known human carcinogen: Blanc, *How Everyday Products*, 86.

146 The chemical was not regulated: Blanc, *How Everyday Products*, 75.

146 *body burden*: Environmental Working Group, "Body Burden: The Pollution in Newborns," July 14, 2005, https://www.ewg.org/research/body-burden-pollution-newborns.

146 higher levels in indoor air: Ashford and Miller, *Chemical Exposures*, 14; Lance A. Wallace et al., "The TEAM Study: Personal Exposures to Toxic Substances in Air, Drinking Water, and Breath of 400 Residents of New Jersey, North Carolina, and North Dakota," *Environmental Research* 43, no. 2 (1987): 297, doi: 10.1016/S0013-9351(87)80030-0.

147 and seemingly inexplicable symptoms: Ashford and Miller, *Chemical Exposures*, 16.

CHAPTER 8: SPIN

148 Environmental Protection Agency: Jack Lewis, "The Birth of EPA," *EPA Journal* (November 1985): 3, http://www2.epa.gov/aboutepa/birth-epa.

148 stacked the agency's upper administration: Michelle Murphy, *Sick Building Syndrome and the Problem of Uncertainty: Environmental Politics, Technoscience, and Women Workers* (Durham, NC: Duke University Press, 2006), 117.

149 "devising false cover for Agency policies": National Treasury Employees Union, Chapter 280, "The Official History of NTEU, Chapter 280: Seventeen Years of Public Service at the EPA," April 9, 2001, http://www/nteu280.org/history.htm in Murphy, *Sick Building Syndrome*, 119.

149   "doing things harmful to the environment": National Treasury Employees Union,
      Chapter 280, "Why We Need a Code of Professional Ethics," August 25, 1999,
      http://www/nteu280.org/issues/nteu-20%professional%20Ethics.htm as cited in
      Murphy, *Sick Building Syndrome*, 119.

149   "expert at those manipulations": Murphy, *Sick Building Syndrome*, 120.

150   in its own building: Daniel Grossman, "EPA Hauls the Toxics Out on the Carpet,"
      In These Times, June 22–July 5, 1988, 5.

150   poorly ventilated Waterside Mall: George J. Benda, "Chapter 3: EPA Headquarters,"
      Indoor Air Quality Case Studies Reference Guide (Lilburn, GA: Fairmont Press,
      1998), 26.

150   worked for the Superfund program: Alison Johnson, *Amputated Lives: Coping with
      Chemical Sensitivity* (Brunswick, ME: Cumberland Press, 2008), 173.

150   Over eight hundred employees: This is a conservative estimate. EPA officials put
      the number at 880, or 24 percent, of the 3,700 employees. *The Indoor Air News*, a
      union publication, reported that 40 percent of EPA employees were made ill by
      1989, as cited in David Steinman, "The Architecture of Illness: Millions of Workers
      Are 'Sick of Work,'" Fall 1993, https://www.environmentalhealth.ca/fall93sick.html.

150   Like replaceable parts: According to Bobbie Lively-Diebold, in Johnson, *Ampu-
      tated Lives*, 176.

150   need to organize: Johnson, *Amputated Lives*, 174.

151   and the union: Murphy, *Sick Building Syndrome*, 124.

151   Reading that flyer was the first time: Sarah Pratt, "Every Breath She Takes," *Spin*,
      12, December 1996.

151   dark jokes: Kirby Biggs, former EPA Superfund analyst, personal conversation,
      July 30, 2012.

151   standards normally applied to outdoor sites: Benda, "Chapter 3."

151   suspected corrupted results: Murphy, *Sick Building Syndrome*, 124.

151   "ill after 15 minutes inside Waterside": *Testimony on the Indoor Air Quality Act of
      1989 Before the US House of Representatives Committee on Science, Space, and Tech-
      nology, Subcommittee on Natural Resources, Agriculture, Research and Environment*,
      101st Congress (July 20, 1989); National Federation of Federal Employees, Local
      2050 and American Federation of Government Employees, Local 3331, *Indoor Air
      Quality and Work Environment Study: EPA Headquarters Buildings*, Supplement to
      Volume 1: Additional Employee Adverse Health Effects Information, Novem-
      ber 20, 1989.

151   EPA attorney James Handley, who developed: Johnson, *Amputated Lives*, 118–27.

151   guaranteeing an inaccurate reading: Arthur Day to Joseph S. Carra, Memorandum
      on "Indoor Air Problems at EPA Headquarters," in *Indoor Air Quality and Work
      Environment Study: EPA Headquarters Buildings, Supplement to Volume 1: Additional
      Employee Adverse Health Effects Information*, November 20, 1989, 8–9.

151   employees later learned: Benda, "Chapter 3."

152   "chief sources appeared to be ordinary consumer products": Wayne R. Ott and
      John W. Roberts, "Everyday Exposure to Toxic Pollutants," *Scientific American*,

February 1998, https://www.scientificamerican.com/article/everyday-exposure-to-toxic-pollutan/.

152 airborne toxicants: Lance Wallace, "The TEAM Studies," *EPA Journal* 19, no. 4 (1993): 23–24, https://www.epaalumni.org/userdata/pdf/1993-10-12-400008E1.PDF.

152 causing more cancer than: Pratt, "Every Breath She Takes."

152 unique position to challenge the results: Johnson, *Amputated Lives*, 260; David Steinman, "The Architecture of Illness: Millions of Workers Are 'Sick of Work,'" *Update* (Fall 1993), 2, http://www.environmentalhealth.ca/fall93sick.html.

153 "formula for a gas chamber": Johnson, *Amputated Lives*, 122.

153 comatose or dead: Johnson, *Amputated Lives*, 125.

154 like a series of small strokes: Johnson, *Amputated Lives*, 125.

154 "off the record": Cindy Duehring, "Carpet . . . Part One: EPA Stalls and Industry Hedges While Consumers Remain at Risk," *Informed Consent* 1, no. 1 (November/December 1993): 8, https://www.holisticmed.com/carpet/tc1.txt.

154 unions finally halted the carpet installation: Benda, "Chapter 3," 26.

154 carpet in other EPA buildings: Lynn Lawson, *Staying Well in a Toxic World: Understanding Multiple Chemical Sensitivities, Chemical Injuries, and Sick Building Syndrome, a New Millennium Update* (Evanston, IL: Lynnword Press, 2000), 171.

154 claimed that the carpet posed no problems: Duehring, "Carpet . . . Part One," 8.

154 initiate the lawsuit: Joanne Bahura et al., Appellants/Cross-Appellees v. S.E.W Investors et al., Appellees/Cross-Appellants, District of Columbia Court of Appeals, Hon. Rufus G. King, III, Trial Judge, Argued October 4, 1999, 2.

154 jury awarded the plaintiffs damages: *Bahura v. S.E.W. Investors*, 25.

155 evidence of toxic encephalopathy: *Bahura v. S.E.W. Investors*, 37.

156 symptoms were perhaps being triggered: Duehring, "Carpet . . . Part One."

157 the manufacturer was being disingenuous: Duehring, "Carpet . . . Part One."

157 "spokespeople for the safety of carpet": Duehring, "Carpet . . . Part One."

158 CRI suggested this answer: Duehring, "Carpet . . . Part One."

158 Bernie Sanders (I-VT) said: Duehring, "Carpet . . . Part One."

158 In 2021 several whistleblowers: Sharon Lerner, "Leaked Audio Shows Pressure to Overrule Scientists in 'Hair-on-Fire' Cases," *The Intercept*, August 4, 2021, https://theintercept.com/2021/08/04/epa-hair-on-fire-chemicals-leaked-audio/.

158 altered without their knowledge: Sharon Lerner, "Whistleblowers Expose Corruption in EPA Chemical Safety Office," *The Intercept*, July 2, 2021, https://theintercept.com/2021/07/02/epa-chemical-safety-corruption-whistleblowers/.

159 "override everything": Lerner, "Leaked Audio."

159 number of chemicals they approve: Sharon Lerner, "New Evidence of Corruption at EPA Chemicals Division," *The Intercept*, September 18, 2021, https://theintercept.com/2021/09/18/epa-corruption-harmful-chemicals-testing/.

159 jobs at those very corporations: Sharon Lerner, "The Department of Yes," *The Intercept*, June 30, 2021, https://theintercept.com/2021/06/30/epa-pesticides-exposure-opp/.

159　waiving 972 toxicity tests: Lerner, "The Department of Yes."

159　threw a party: Lerner, "The Department of Yes."

159　pesticides that were banned in other countries: Nathan Donley, "The USA Lags Behind Other Agricultural Nations in Banning Harmful Pesticides," *Environmental Health* 18, no. 1 (2019): 44, doi: 10.1186/s12940-019-0488-0, as cited in Lerner, "The Department of Yes."

159　EPA colluded with Monsanto to cover up: Lerner, "The Department of Yes."

160　hormone disrupters: Environmental Working Group, "Cheatsheet: Phthalates," https://www.ewg.org/enviroblog/2008/05/cheatsheet-phthalates.

160　genital abnormalities in baby boys: Marina Schauffler, "Everyday Chemical Fragrances May Be Hazardous to Health," *Maine Sunday Telegram*, September 7, 2014, S2.

160　lower sperm counts: Centers for Disease Control and Prevention, "Phthalates Factsheet," April 5, 2021, https://www.cdc.gov/biomonitoring/Phthalates_FactSheet .html.

160　breast cancer, and higher weight: Breast Cancer Prevention Partners, "Phthalates," 2021, https://www.bcpp.org/resource/phthalates/.

160　phthalate exposure is widespread: CDC, "Phthalates Factsheet."

160　PBDEs had reached significant levels: Tom Laskawy, "Flame Retardants Could Affect Our Bodies for Generations," *Grist*, May 24, 2012, https://grist.org/green -home/flame-retardants-and-farm-chemicals-could-affect-our-bodies-for -generations/.

160　links to cancer, thyroid disruption: Gerald Markowitz and David Rosner, "Your Body Is a Corporate Test Tube," BillMoyers.com, April 29, 2013, https://billmoyers .com/2013/04/29/your-body-is-a-corporate-test-tube/.

160　fetal defects, and reproductive problems: Laskawy, "Flame Retardants."

160　PBDEs aren't even effective: Nicholas Kristof, "Are You Safe on That Sofa?," *New York Times*, May 19, 2012, https://www.nytimes.com/2012/05/20/opinion/sunday /kristof-are-you-safe-on-that-sofa.html?_r=1.

160　free of flame retardants: Elizabeth Grossman, "Banned in Europe, Safe in the U.S.," *Ensia*, June 9, 2014, https://ensia.com/features/banned-in-europe-safe-in -the-u-s/.

160　also found in checkout receipts: Gwen Ranniger, "How Is BPA Bad for My Health?," *Environmental Health News*, April 20, 2020, https://www.ehn.org/bpa -pollution-2645493129/bpa-science-in-the-news.

160　Even low doses of BPA are linked: Environmental Working Group, "BPA," https:// www.ewg.org/areas-focus/toxic-chemicals/bpa.

161　Formaldehyde, a known carcinogen: Nicholas Kristoff, "The Cancer Lobby," *New York Times*, October 6, 2012, https://www.nytimes.com/2012/10/07/opinion/sunday /kristof-the-cancer-lobby.html.

161　accumulates in people's bodies: Markowitz and Rosner, "Your Body."

161　almost all homes had formaldehyde concentrations exceeding guidelines: Kristoff, "The Cancer Lobby."

161   common in cosmetics, nail polish, and: Grossman, "Banned in Europe."

161   better known as PFAS: National Institute for Occupational Safety and Health, "Per- and Polyfluoroalkyl Substances (PFAS)," July 7, 2021, https://www.cdc.gov /niosh/topics/pfas/default.html.

161   these chemicals are found in: Environmental Working Group, "What Are PFAS Chemicals?," March 2022, https://www.ewg.org/pfaschemicals/what-are-forever -chemicals.html.

161   drinking PFAS-tainted water: Environmental Working Group, "What Are PFAS Chemicals?"

161   even unborn babies: Rob Bilott, "The Poison Found in Everyone, Even Unborn Babies—and Who Is Responsible for It," *The Guardian*, December 17, 2020, https://www.theguardian.com/commentisfree/2020/dec/17/dark-waters-pfas -ticking-chemical-time-bomb-in-your-blood.

161   Studies link the chemicals to: Environmental Working Group, "What Are PFAS Chemicals?"

161   hazardous substances: Dino Grandoni, "EPA Finally Moves to Label Some 'Forever Chemicals' as Hazardous," *Washington Post*, August 26, 2022, https://www .washingtonpost.com/climate-environment/2022/08/26/forever-chemicals-epa -cleanup-rule/.

161   all are on the rise: Ellen Ruppel Shell, "Does Civilization Cause Asthma?," *Atlantic Monthly*, May 2000, 90 (asthma); Lawson, *Staying Well*, 51 (autism and learning disabilities); Roger D. Hodge, "Findings," *Harper's Magazine* (October 2004), 104 (Alzheimer's and Parkinson's); Theo Colborn, Dianne Dumanoski, and John Peterson Myers, *Our Stolen Future* (New York: Dutton, 1996), 9 (sterility); Mayo Clinic, "Increased Incidence of Migraine Headaches," *ScienceDaily* (October 25, 1999), http://www.sciencedaily.com/releases/1999/10/991025075957.htm (migraines); Dan Fagin and Marianne Lavelle, *Toxic Deception: How the Chemical Industry Manipulates Science, Bends the Law, and Endangers Your Health* (Monroe, ME: Common Courage Press, 1999), xv–xvi (cancers); Sandra Steingraber, *Living Downstream: A Scientist's Personal Investigation of Cancer and the Environment* (New York: Vintage Books, 1998), 40–43 (cancers).

162   "to create the illusion of controversy about MCS": Ann McCampbell, "Multiple Chemical Sensitivities Under Siege," *Townsend Letter*, no. 210 (January 2001): 20–27, https://annmccampbellmd.com/publicationswritings/publication-1/.

162   *Idiopathic* simply means "of unknown etiology," but: Ashford and Miller, *Chemical Exposures*, 284, as cited in McCampbell, "Multiple Chemical Sensitivities."

162   "'smoker's cough' to 'idiopathic respiratory paroxysms'": McCampbell, "Multiple Chemical Sensitivities."

162   successful in shutting the event down: McCampbell, "Multiple Chemical Sensitivities."

163   "an anti-MCS conference": "Annals of Multiple Chemical Sensitivities: State-of -the-Science Symposium," *Regulatory Toxicology and Pharmacology* 24, no. 1 (2006), doi: 10.1006/rtph.1996.0096, as cited by McCampbell, "Multiple Chemical Sensitivities."

163   "a peculiar manifestation of our technophobic and chemophobic society": Peter
      Montagne, "Cigarette Science at Johns Hopkins," *Rachel's Environment and Health
      Weekly*, no. 464, October 19, 1995, 2.

163   to lawyers defending corporations in product liability lawsuits: Montagne, "Ciga-
      rette Science," 2.

163   deny benefits for the diagnosis of chemical sensitivities: McCampbell, "Multiple
      Chemical Sensitivities."

163   arseniophobia: "The Danger from Arsenic," *Medical Record*, May 23, 1891, 599–
      600, as cited in James C. Whorton, *Before Silent Spring: Pesticides and Public Health
      in Pre-DDT America* (Princeton, NJ: Princeton University Press, 1975), 59.

163   "Boston fad": "Arsenic in Paper and Clothing," *New York Times*, April 6, 1891,
      http://query.nytimes.com/mem/archive-free/pdf?res=9902E6DE163AE533A
      25756C0A9629C94609ED7CF.

164   American Council on Science and Health: American Council on Science and
      Health, "About American Council on Science and Health," http://acsh.org/about
      -acsh/.

164   donors "comprise a who's-who of energy, agriculture, cosmetics": Andy Kroll
      and Jeremy Schulman, "Leaked Documents Reveal the Secret Finances of a
      Pro-Industry Science Group," *Mother Jones*, October 28, 2013, http://www
      .motherjones.com/politics/2013/10/american-council-science-health-leaked
      -documents-fundraising.

164   did prison time for defrauding: Kroll and Schulman, "Leaked Documents."

164   an ACSH scientific advisor: American Council on Science and Health, "Our
      Team," http://acsh.org/about-acsh/scientific-advisors/.

PART III: THE AMERICAN WAY OF STRESS

165   "a dangerous amount of friction": S. Weir Mitchell, *Wear and Tear: Or, Hints for the
      Overworked* (Walnut Creek, CA: AltaMira Press, 2004, reprint of the Lippincott
      1871 edition), 21.

166   "NO TIME: the chronic complaint": Deborah Campbell, "In Praise of Radical
      Leisure (in Seven Parts)," *Adbusters*, May/June 2003, as cited in Ann Japenga, "The
      Siesta Cure," *Utne*, February 2004, http://www.annjapenga.com/Images/articles
      /wSiesta.pdf. Reprinted with permission.

CHAPTER 9: CLOCKWORK

168   link stress with suppression of the immune response: Sheldon Cohen, David A.
      J. Tyrrell, and Andrew P. Smith, "Psychological Stress and Susceptibility to the
      Common Cold," *New England Journal of Medicine* 325 (1991): 606–12, https://doi
      .org/10.1056/NEJM199108293250903.

168   revealed immune dysregulation in people under stress: Tracy B. Herbert and
      Sheldon Cohen, "Stress and Immunity in Humans: A Meta-Analytic Review,"

Psychosomatic Medicine 55, no. 4 (1993): 364–79, doi: 10.1097/00006842-199307000 -00004; Eric P. Zorrilla et al., "The Relationship of Depression and Stressors to Immunological Assays: A Meta-Analytic Review," *Brain, Behavior, and Immunity* 15, no. 3 (2001): 199–226, doi: 10.1006/brbi.2000.0597.

168   more likely to succumb to the common cold: Robert M. Sapolsky, *Why Zebras Don't Get Ulcers*, 3rd ed. (New York: Times Books, 2004), 167.

169   "the body's metabolic banks": Sapolsky, *Why Zebras*, 428.

169   "strong internal locus of control": B. K. Houston, "Control Over Stress, Locus of Control, and Response to Stress," *Journal of Personality and Social Psychology* 21, no. 2 (1972): 249, doi: 10.1037/h0032328, as cited in Sapolsky, *Why Zebras*, 303.

169   they could not overcome them: American Psychological Association, *Stress in America: The Impact of Discrimination, Stress in America Survey* (Washington, DC: American Psychological Association, 2016), https://www.apa.org/news/press /releases/stress/2015/impact-of-discrimination.pdf.

169   "feel harried too much of the time": Juliet Schor, "Less Work, More Living," *Yes!*, September 2, 2011, 1.

169   higher average levels of stress than men: American Psychological Association, *Stress in America.*

169   stress level 5 percent greater than those with higher incomes: American Psychological Association, *Stress in America.*

169   Stress was also notably higher for: American Psychological Association, *Stress in America.*

170   money and work as significant sources of stress: American Psychological Association, *Stress in America.*

170   Before capitalism, Europe was largely "timeless": Juliet B. Schor, *The Overworked American: The Unexpected Decline of Leisure* (New York: Basic Books, 1991), 137.

170   *Werkglocken*, or "work clocks": Schor, *The Overworked American*, 49.

170   time became "currency . . . not passed but spent": Schor, *The Overworked American*, 50.

170   "'an objective force within which [they] were imprisoned.'": Schor, *The Overworked American*, 50.

170   *"Time itself had become a commodity"*: Schor, *The Overworked American*, 139.

171   "William's panacea for all ills": *Alice James: Her Life in Letters*, ed. Linda Anderson (Bristol, England: Thoemmes Press, 1996), 104–7, as cited in Jean Strouse, *Alice James: A Biography* (Cambridge: Harvard University Press, 1999), 194. Interestingly, Sigmund Freud and Carl Jung visited the cabin's owner, Dr. James Jackson Putnam, there in September 1909.

171   "the sportive midge who found me quite the loveliest": *Alice James: Her Life in Letters*, 104–7, as cited in Strouse, *Alice James*, 194.

171   "weaker in body than I expected": Strouse, *Alice James*, 198.

171   long walks with Katharine: Strouse, *Alice James*, 199.

172   "The railroad had eclipsed the sun": Rebecca Solnit, *River of Shadows: Eadweard Muybridge and the Technological Wild West* (New York: Penguin, 2003), 61–62.

172 "different degrees of doze": David K. Randall, *Dreamland: Adventures in the Strange Science of Sleep* (New York: W. W. Norton, 2012), 40.

172 "to domesticate light": Randall, *Dreamland*, 38.

173 time wasn't measured by minutes and hours: Schor, *The Overworked American*, 44–47.

173 from feudalism to capitalism: Silvia Federici, *Caliban and the Witch: Women, the Body and Primitive Accumulation*, 2nd rev. ed. (New York: Autonomedia, 2014), 9.

173 the imperative to reign over nature: Carolyn Merchant, *The Death of Nature: Women, Ecology, and the Scientific Revolution* (San Francisco: Harper & Row, 1980), 9.

173 long fight to reduce their workdays to ten hours: Schor, *The Overworked American*, 72.

174 "for the cultivation of their mind and for self improvement": John Rogers et al., ed., *A Documentary History of American Industrial Society*, vol. 5 (Cleveland: A. H. Clark, 1910), 80, as cited in Benjamin Kline Hunnicutt, *Free Time: The Forgotten American Dream* (Philadelphia: Temple University Press, 2013), 6.

174 became major players in the struggle: Schor, *The Overworked American*, 72.

174 "utilize the forces of the animal nature and passions": Jonathan Baxter Harrison, *Certain Dangerous Tendencies in American Life* (Boston: Houghton, Osgood and Company, 1880), as cited in Alan Trachtenberg, *The Incorporation of America: Culture and Society in the Gilded Age* (New York: Hill and Wang, 1982), 148.

174 Americans worked fewer than forty hours a week: Schor, "Less Work," 2.

174 began working harder and longer for less: Schor, *The Overworked American*, 80–81.

174 union members earn 13 percent more: John Schmitt, Elise Gould, and Josh Bivens, "America's Slow-Motion Wage Crisis: Four Decades of Slow and Unequal Growth," Economic Policy Institute, September 13, 2018, https://www.epi.org /publication/americas-slow-motion-wage-crisis-four-decades-of-slow-and -unequal-growth-2/.

174 now dropped to just 10 percent: Matthew Desmond, "Capitalism," in *The 1619 Project: A New Origin Story*, eds. Nikole Hannah-Jones, Caitlin Roper, Ilena Silverman, and Jake Silverstein (New York: One World, 2021), 182.

174 number of major strikes and lockouts has plummeted: U.S. Bureau of Labor Statistics, "Major Work Stoppages (Annual) News Release," February 23, 2022, https:// www.bls.gov/web/wkstp/annual-listing.htm.

175 in Iceland 90 percent of wage and salary workers belong: Desmond, "Capitalism," 182.

175 widening chasm between rich and poor: Schmitt, Gould, and Bivens, "America's Slow-Motion Wage Crisis."

175 only industrialized country that hasn't legislated guaranteed paid vacation days: Katie Johnston, "Nearly 1 in 4 US Workers Go Without Paid Time Off," *Boston Globe*, August 14, 2014, https://www.bostonglobe.com/business/2014/08/13/one -few-countries-that-doesn-mandate-paid-vacation-time/eqodEqumohPyca5k t6hrZO/story.html.

175 a paltry sum when compared: Zack Guzman, "This Chart Shows How Far Behind

America Is in Paid Time Off Compared to the Rest of the World," CNBC, August 15, 2018, https://www.cnbc.com/2018/08/15/statista-how-far-behind-us-is-in-paid-time-off-compared-to-the-world.html.

175 we are generally not more productive: David Rosnick and Mark Weisbrot, "Are Shorter Work Hours Good for the Environment? A Comparison of U.S. and European Energy Consumption," *Center for Economic and Policy Research*, December 2006, http://cepr.net/documents/publications/energy_2006_12.pdf.

175 "work an unusually high number of hours for the country's level of productivity": Rosnick and Weisbrot, "Are Shorter Work Hours."

175 "here, among this robust and sanguine people": Alice James, *The Diary of Alice James*, ed. Leon Edel (Boston: Northeastern University Press, 1999), 36, as cited by Strouse, 233.

176 "fervently radical": Strouse, *Alice James*, 277.

176 putting in 124 more hours per year: Maurie Backman, "Here's How Many Hours the Average American Works per Year," The Motley Fool, December 17, 2017, https://www.fool.com/careers/2017/12/17/heres-how-many-hours-the-average-american-works-pe.aspx.

176 50 hours or more a week: "The Six-Hour Workday," *Online Masters* (blog), July 29, 2022, https://onlinemasters.ohio.edu/blog/benefits-of-a-shorter-work-week/.

176 Eighteen percent work over 60: "The Six-Hour Workday."

176 work almost 8 percent more hours: Economic Policy Institute, "Examination of Work Hours Reveals Two Labor Markets," February 22, 2018, https://www.epi.org/press/examination-of-work-hours-reveals-two-labor-markets/.

176 a $62.2 billion bonanza: U.S. Travel Association, "State of American Vacation 2018," May 8, 2018, https://www.ustravel.org/research/state-american-vacation-2018.

176 "and how often you go to the bathroom": Erin Griffith, "Why Are Young People Pretending to Love Work?" *New York Times*, January 26, 2019, https://www.nytimes.com/2019/01/26/business/against-hustle-culture-rise-and-grind-tgim.html.

176 Elon Musk: Griffith, "Why Are Young People."

177 the correct number of hours: Griffith, "Why Are Young People."

177 working 70 hours per week produced little more: John Pencavel, "The Productivity of Working Hours," IZA Discussion Paper 8129, April 2014, https://docs.iza.org/dp8129.pdf

177 "hymns to the virtues of relentless work": Griffith, "Why Are Young People."

177 "assumption that the only value we have": Griffith, "Why Are Young People."

177 "Cathedral of Perpetual Hustle": Griffith, "Why Are Young People."

177 "an antidemocratic force": Mark Slouka, "Quitting the Paint Factory: On the Virtues of Idleness," *Harper's Magazine*, November 2004, 58.

177 people had everything they needed: Anjula Razdan, "Take Your Time," *Utne*, January–February 2005, 60, https://www.utne.com/mind-and-body/take-your-time.

178 advertising had become a major industry: Stuart Ewen, *Captains of Consciousness:*

Advertising and the Social Roots of the Consumer Culture (New York: Basic Books, 2001), 32.

178 "the engineering of consent": Edward Bernays, *Propaganda* (originally published in 1928; Ig Publishing, 2004).

178 advertising sells a standard of normalcy: Ewen, *Captains of Consciousness*, 54.

179 free time in America has dropped by almost 40 percent: Schor, *The Overworked American*, 22; "Americans Today Have Less Free Time, Study Says," *Public Relations Society of America* (blog), December 8, 2008, https://apps.prsa.org/SearchResults /view/7722/105/Americans_today_have_less_free_time_study_says#.Yy5GWy -B30o.

179 people who had deliberately cut back their hours: Schor, "Less Work."

179 decrease their work hours by 1 percent may reduce their energy use: Jonas Nässén and Jörgen Larsson, "Would Shorter Working Time Reduce Greenhouse Gas Emissions? An Analysis of Time Use and Consumption in Swedish Households," *Environment and Planning C: Politics and Space* 33, no. 4 (2015): 726–45, doi: 10.1068/c12239.

179 if Americans pared back work hours to match those of Western European countries: Rosnick and Weisbrot, "Are Shorter Work Hours."

180 "considerably smaller ecological and carbon footprints": Kyle W. Knight, Eugene A. Rosa, and Juliet B. Schor, "Could Working Less Reduce Pressure on the Environment? A Cross-National Panel Analysis of OECD Countries, 1970–2007," *Global Environmental Change* 23, no. 4 (2013): 691–700, doi: 10.1016/j .gloenvcha.2013.02.017, as cited in Schor, "Less Work," 3.

180 federal minimum wage has not budged since 2009: Drew Desilver, "5 Facts About the Minimum Wage," Pew Research Center FactTank, January 4, 2017, https:// www.pewresearch.org/fact-tank/2017/01/04/5-facts-about-the-minimum-wage/.

180 has lost more than twenty-seven percent of its buying power: Maurie Backman, "Minimum Wage Earners Have Lost More Than 27% of Their Buying Power Due to Inflation," *The Ascent*, July 25, 2022, https://www.fool.com/the-ascent /personal-finance/articles/minimum-wage-earners-have-lost-more-than-27-of -their-buying-power-due-to-inflation/.

180 Raising the minimum wage: Schor, *The Overworked American*, 151.

180 economist John Maynard Keynes predicted: Lisa Evans, "Why We Still Don't Have a Four-Day Workweek," Fast Company, September 8, 2014, https://www .fastcompany.com/3035279/why-we-still-dont-have-a-four-day-workweek.

180 by working just 10 hours a week: G. E. Miller, "The U.S. Is the Most Overworked Developed Nation in the World," 20 Something Finance, January 30, 2022, https://20somethingfinance.com/american-hours-worked-productivity-vacation/.

180 wages haven't kept up with productivity: Lawrence Mishel, "Growing Inequalities, Reflecting Growing Employer Power, Have Generated a Productivity-Pay Gap Since 1979," *Economic Policy Institute* (blog), September 2, 2021, https://www .epi.org/blog/growing-inequalities-reflecting-growing-employer-power-have

-generated-a-productivity-pay-gap-since-1979-productivity-has-grown-3-5-times
-as-much-as-pay-for-the-typical-worker/.

180 than any other industrialized country: Razdan, "Take Your Time," 60.

180 all while we get less in: Samuel P. Huntington, *Who Are We? The Challenges to America's National Identity* (New York: Simon & Schuster, 2004).

181 experienced stress "a lot of the day": Niraj Chokshi, "Americans Are Among the Most Stressed People in the World, Poll Finds," *New York Times*, April 25, 2019, https://www.nytimes.com/2019/04/25/us/americans-stressful.html.

181 20 percent higher than the global average: Chokshi, "Americans Are Among."

181 "rat race is exacerbated": "Why Is Everybody So Busy?," *The Economist*, December 20, 2014, 7.

181 job-related stress is estimated to cost American companies: "Financial Costs of Job Stress," 2009, Stress@Work, https://www.uml.edu/research/cph-new/worker /stress-at-work/financial-costs.aspx.

181 "leading to burnout": Gary Drevitch, "Worn Out," *Psychology Today*, May 2, 2016, 48, https://www.psychologytoday.com/us/articles/201605/worn-out.

181 healthcare expenditures are nearly 50 percent greater: "Financial Costs of Job Stress."

181 enjoying their lives, they actually perform better: 4-Day Week Campaign, "A 4-Day Work Week Is Coming," 2022, https://www.4dayweek.co.uk/.

182 chose the path with more free time: Schor, *The Overworked American*, 148.

182 84 cents to every man's dollar: Amanda Barroso and Anna Brown, "Gender Pay Gap in U.S. Held Steady in 2020," Pew Research Center, May 25, 2021, https:// www.pewresearch.org/fact-tank/2021/05/25/gender-pay-gap-facts/.

182 women still do three times as much housework: Danielle Kurtzleben, "Charts: How American Men and Women Spend Their Time," *US News and World Report*, June 24, 2013, https://www.usnews.com/news/articles/2013/06/24/charts-how -american-men-and-women-spend-their-time.

182 "imposed ever-more exacting practices on American women": Schor, *The Over-worked American*, 97.

183 principles of scientific management for the home: Nancy Giges, "Lillian Moller Gilbreth,"The American Society of Mechanical Engineers, April 30, 2012, https:// www.asme.org/career-education/articles/management-professional-practice /lillian-moller-gilbreth.

183 "Housework was functional for capitalism": Schor, *The Overworked American*, 97.

183 "By Their Floors Shall Ye Judge Them": Schor, *The Overworked American*, 97.

183 "Norms of cleanliness rose": Schor, *The Overworked American*, 8.

183 "the material embodiment of a task": Barbara Ehrenreich and Deirdre English, *For Her Own Good: Two Centuries of the Experts' Advice to Women*, 2nd Anchor Books ed. (New York: Anchor Books, 1989), 179.

184 four-day workweeks can actually *boost* efficiency: Schor, *The Overworked American*, 154–56; Liz Alderman, "In Sweden, an Experiment Turns Shorter Workdays

into Bigger Gains," *New York Times*, May 20, 2016, https://www.nytimes.com /2016/05/21/business/international/in-sweden-an-experiment-turns-shorter -workdays-into-bigger-gains.html?module=inline; Evans, "Why We Still Don't Have a Four-Day Workweek."

184 and a boost in profits: Alex Kjerulf, "How Toyota Gothenburg Moved to a 30-Hour Workweek and Boosted Profits and Customer Satisfaction," January 6, 2016, https://positivesharing.com/2016/01/toyota-gothenburg-30-hour-work-week/.

184 took fewer sick days: Alderman, "In Sweden, an Experiment."

184 workweeks were cut by four to five hours: Briony Harris, "Working Fewer Hours Makes You More Efficient. Here's the Proof," *Brink*, August 2, 2018, https:// www.brinknews.com/working-fewer-hours-makes-you-more-efficient-heres-the -proof/.

184 first European country to implement a four-day workweek: Antonia Noori Farzan, "Spain Will Experiment with Four-Day Workweek, a First for Europe," *Washington Post*, March 15, 2021, https://www.washingtonpost.com/world/2021/03/15 /spain-four-day-workweek/.

184 "productivity rose": Schor, *The Overworked American*, 157.

184 seven to nine hours experts recommend: Jeffrey M. Jones, "In U.S., 40% Get Less Than Recommended Amount of Sleep," *Gallup News*, December 19, 2013, https:// news.gallup.com/poll/166553/less-recommended-amount-sleep.aspx.

186 seemingly disparate disciplines of biology and psychology: Sapolsky, *Why Zebras*, 305.

CHAPTER 10: LOAD

187 a "life-long occupation of 'improving'": Letter to Alice Howe Gibbens James (William's wife), 5 February 1890, in Alice James, *The Death and Letters of Alice James: Selected Correspondence*, ed. Ruth Bernard Yeazell (Boston: Exact Change, 1997), 189.

188 long-term stress can cause: American Institute of Stress, "What Is Stress?," 2020, https://www.stress.org/daily-life.

188 Stress in America survey: American Psychological Association, *Stress in America: The Impact of Discrimination, Stress in America Survey* (Washington, DC: American Psychological Association, 2016), https://www.apa.org/news/press/releases /stress/2015/impact-of-discrimination.pdf.

188 consume 65 percent of the world's psychotropic drugs: David Barsamian, "Capitalism and Its Discontents: Richard Wolff on What Went Wrong," *The Sun*, February 2012, https://www.thesunmagazine.org/issues/434/capitalism-and-its -discontents, 8.

189 stress emergency: Robert M. Sapolsky, *Why Zebras Don't Get Ulcers*, 3rd ed. (New York: Times Books, 2004), 11.

189   stress makes it harder to fight illness: Pamela Young, "The Biology of Stress," *The CFIDS Chronicle: The Science Issue* (Winter 2007): 10–11, https://solvecfs.org/wp-content/uploads/2013/10/stress4.pdf.

189   fatigue can result: Sapolsky, *Why Zebras,* 13.

190   in his 2005 paper about allostasis: Bruce S. McEwen, "Stressed or Stressed Out: What Is the Difference?," *Journal of Psychiatry & Neuroscience* 30, no. 5 (2005): 315–18, https://www.ncbi.nlm.nih.gov/pmc/articles/PMC1197275/.

192   21 percent say they're not: American Psychological Association, *Stress in America.*

193   Adverse Childhood Experiences (ACE) study: Vincent J. Felitti et al., "Relationship of Childhood Abuse and Household Dysfunction to Many of the Leading Causes of Death in Adults. The Adverse Childhood Experiences (ACE) Study," *American Journal of Preventive Medicine* 14, no. 4 (1998): 245–58, doi: 10.1016/s0749-3797(98)00017-8; Donna Jackson Nakazawa, "Childhood, Disrupted," *Aeon,* July 7, 2015, https://aeon.co/essays/how-bad-experiences-in-childhood-lead-to-adult-illness.

193   ten-point questionnaire: National Council of Juvenile and Family Court Judges, "Finding Your Ace Score," 2022, https://www.ncjfcj.org/wp-content/uploads/2006/10/Finding-Your-Ace-Score.pdf.

193   ACE score of 4 are twice as likely: Shanta R. Dube et al., "Growing Up with Parental Alcohol Abuse: Exposure to Childhood Abuse, Neglect, and Household Dysfunction," *Child Abuse and Neglect* 25, no. 12 (2001): 1627–40, doi: 10.1016/S0145-2134(01)00293-9, as cited in Donna Jackson Nakazawa, *Childhood Disrupted: How Your Biography Becomes Your Biology, and How You Can Heal* (New York: Atria, 2015), 14; Nakazawa, "Childhood, Disrupted."

193   autoimmune disease rises by 20 percent for every point: Shanta R. Dube et al., "Cumulative Childhood Stress and Autoimmune Diseases in Adults," *Psychosomatic Medicine* 71, no. 2 (February 2009): 243–50, doi: 10.1097/PSY.0b13e3181907888, as cited in Nakazawa, *Childhood Disrupted,* 97; Nakazawa, "Childhood, Disrupted."

194   risk of depression is 460 percent higher: Nakazawa, *Childhood Disrupted,* 14–15; Nakazawa, "Childhood, Disrupted,"

194   The higher the ACE score: Nakazawa, "Childhood, Disrupted."

194   ACE score of 6 or higher: Nakazawa, "Childhood, Disrupted."

194   increased risk for ME/CFS: Christine Heim et al., "Early Adverse Experience and Risk for Chronic Fatigue Syndrome: Results from a Population-Based Study," *Archives of General Psychiatry* 63, no. 11 (2006): 1258–66, doi: 10.1001/archpsyc.63.11.1258; Christine Heim et al., "Childhood Trauma and Risk for Chronic Fatigue Syndrome: Association with Neuroendocrine Dysfunction," *Archives of General Psychiatry* 66, no. 1 (2009): 72–80, doi: 10.1001/archgenpsychiatry.2008.508.

194   implicated in the pathophysiology of CFS: Heim et al., "Childhood Trauma," 72–80.

194   many adult diseases should be viewed as developmental disorders: Jack P. Shonkoff
      et al., "The Lifelong Effects of Early Childhood Adversity and Toxic Stress," *Pedi-
      atrics* 129, no. 1 (2012): e232–e246, doi: 10.1542/peds.2011-2663.

195   "psychobiological theory of everything": Nakazawa, "Childhood, Disrupted."

195   an emotional buffer against external stressors: Allan N. Schore, *Affect Regulation
      and the Origin of the Self: The Neurobiology of Emotional Development* (Hillsdale,
      NJ: Lawrence Erlbaum Associates, 1994), 142, as cited in Gabor Maté, "Addiction:
      Childhood Trauma, Stress and the Biology of Addiction," *Journal of Restorative
      Medicine* 1, no. 1 (2012): 56–63, https://restorativemedicine.org/journal/addiction
      -childhood-trauma-stress-and-the-biology-of-addiction/.

195   increases the child's sensitivity to stressors: Maté, "Addiction."

195   "asking and listening . . . was itself a very powerful": Marcelle Pick, "It's Not in
      Your Head, It's in Your Body," *HuffPost*, August 24, 2013, https://www.huffpost
      .com/entry/adverse-childhood-experiences_n_3489949.

196   emergency room visits dropped by 11 percent: Anne Hallward, MD, "Child Abuse
      and Physical Health 25 Years Later with Vincent Felitti," *Safe Space Radio*, April
      15, 2013, https://safespaceradio.com/child-abuse-and-physical-health-25-years
      -later/, as cited in Pick, "It's Not in Your Head."

196   low socioeconomic status: Sapolsky, *Why Zebras*, 366.

196   the United States was one of the most egalitarian: David Barsamian, "Capitalism and
      Its Discontents: Richard Wolff on What Went Wrong," *The Sun*, February 2012, 8,
      https://www.thesunmagazine.org/issues/434/capitalism-and-its-discontents.

196   disparity between rich and poor: American Psychological Association, *Stress in
      America: Paying with Our Health*, February 4, 2015, https://www.apa.org/news
      /press/releases/stress/2014/stress-report.pdf, 3.

196   diseases that correlate most strongly with low socioeconomic status: Sapolsky, *Why
      Zebras*, 366–67.

196   These include: Sapolsky, *Why Zebras*, 373.

196   greater a country's income inequality: Richard Wilkinson and Kate Pickett, *The
      Spirit Level: Why Greater Equality Makes Societies Stronger* (New York: Bloomsbury
      Press, 2010), as cited in Sapolsky, *Why Zebras*, 375.

196   not only the poor but the wealthy, too: Wilkinson and Pickett, *The Spirit Level*, as
      cited in Sapolsky, *Why Zebras*, 378.

CHAPTER 11: GILT

202   golden toilet: Nancy Spector, "Maurizio Cattelan's Golden Toilet in the Time of
      Trump," August 17, 2017, https://www.guggenheim.org/blogs/checklist/maurizio
      -cattelans-golden-toilet-in-the-time-of-trump.

203   "government of the corporation": Jack Beatty, "The Dark Side of the Gilded Age,"
      The Atlantic, June 2007, https://www.theatlantic.com/magazine/archive/2007/06
      /the-dark-side-of-the-gilded-age/306012/.

203   Between 1860 and 1900 the top 2 percent owned: George Brown Tindall and

David E. Shi, *America: A Narrative History*, 9th ed., vol. 2 (New York: W. W. Norton, 2012).

203 crush the union and bully his workers: Newsroom, "Carnegie Was 'Brutal Boss Who Exploited His Workforce,'" *The Scotsman*, July 17, 2005, https://www.scotsman.com/news/carnegie-was-brutal-boss-who-exploited-his-workforce-2513190.

203 "If we will not endure a king": Eric Holder, "Attorney General Eric Holder Speaks at the Sherman Act Award Ceremony," News, United States Department of Justice, April 20, 2010, https://www.justice.gov/opa/speech/attorney-general-eric-holder-speaks-sherman-act-award-ceremony.

204 dismantled Rockefeller's Standard Oil: History.Com Editors, "John D. Rockefeller," October 9, 2019, https://www.history.com/topics/early-20th-century-us/john-d-rockefeller.

204 lopsided ways that it has interpreted and enforced antitrust law: William O. Douglas, *An Almanac of Liberty* (New York: Doubleday & Company, 1954), 189.

205 "lax enforcement of anti-trust laws": Joseph E. Stiglitz, "Of the 1%, by the 1%, for the 1%," *Vanity Fair*, March 31, 2011, https://www.vanityfair.com/news/2011/05/top-one-percent-201105.

205 tax cuts have favored the rich: Paul Krugman, "We Are the 99.9%," *New York Times*, November 24, 2011, https://www.nytimes.com/2011/11/25/opinion/we-are-the-99-9.html.

205 reduced taxes for wealthy Americans: Larry M. Bartels, *Unequal Democracy: The Political Economy of the New Gilded Age*, 2nd ed. (Princeton, NJ: Princeton University Press, 2016), 5.

205 top 1 percent would pay $111 billion less: David Leonhardt, "$111 Billion in Tax Cuts for the Top 1%," *New York Times*, July 11, 2018, https://www.nytimes.com/2018/07/11/opinion/trump-republicans-tax-cuts-inequality.html.

205 "kept in office by money from the top 1 percent": Stiglitz, "Of the 1%."

205 wages for regular Americans have stagnated: Dave Gilson and Carolyn Perot, "It's the Inequality, Stupid," *Mother Jones*, March/April 2011, https://www.motherjones.com/politics/2011/02/income-inequality-in-america-chart-graph/.

205 paycheck to paycheck: Emmie Martin, "The Government Shutdown Spotlights a Bigger Issue: 78% of US Workers Live Paycheck to Paycheck," CNBC, https://www.cnbc.com/2019/01/09/shutdown-highlights-that-4-in-5-us-workers-live-paycheck-to-paycheck.html.

205 1 percent take home about 19 percent of the income: Elise Gould and Josh Bivens, "Top 1 Percent Receive Record High Share of Total U.S. Income," *Working Economics Blog*, Economic Policy Institute, September 12, 2013, https://www.epi.org/blog/top-1-percent-receive-record-high-share-2/.

205 household debt: Nomi Prins, "Survival of the Richest: All Are Equal, Except Those Who Aren't," *Tom Dispatch* (blog), February 26, 2019, https://truthout.org/articles/survival-of-the-richest-all-are-equal-except-those-who-arent/.

206 disagree with the principles of capitalism: Max Ehrenfreund, "A Majority of Millennials Now Reject Capitalism, Poll Shows," *Washington Post*, April 26, 2016,

https://www.washingtonpost.com/news/wonk/wp/2016/04/26/a-majority-of
-millennials-now-reject-capitalism-poll-shows/.

206 slavery has been encoded in our founding documents: Matthew Desmond, "Capitalism," in *The 1619 Project: A New Origin Story*, eds. Nikole Hannah-Jones, Caitlin Roper, Ilena Silverman, and Jake Silverstein (New York: One World, 2021), 167–69.

206 assessed the market value of enslaved people: Desmond, "Capitalism," 178–79; Matthew Desmond, "In Order to Understand the Brutality of American Capitalism, You Have to Start on the Plantation," *The New York Times Magazine*, August 14, 2019, https://www.nytimes.com/interactive/2019/08/14/magazine/slavery -capitalism.html.

206 "built by the enslaved": Mehrsa Baradaran, "The Limits of Banking Regulation," *The New York Times Magazine*, August 14, 2019, https://www.nytimes.com/interactive /2019/08/14/magazine/slavery-capitalism.html.

206 co-opting the Fourteenth Amendment: Adam Winkler, "'Corporations Are People' Is Built on an Incredible 19th-Century Lie," *The Atlantic*, March 5, 2018, https:// www.theatlantic.com/business/archive/2018/03/corporations-people-adam -winkler/554852/.

207 "to embrace artificial persons": Winkler, "'Corporations Are People.'"

207 made a pivotal discovery: Adam Winkler, *We the Corporations: How American Businesses Won Their Civil Rights* (New York: Liveright Publishing Company, 2018), 135–36.

207 that the drafters intended: Winkler, "'Corporations Are People.'"

208 robber barons of our day: Stacy Mitchell, Interview by Tracy Frisch, "Unfair Advantage: Stacy Mitchell on How Amazon Undermines Local Economies," *The Sun*, November 2018, 8.

208 third-richest person: Allison Morrow, "An Indian Tycoon Just Ousted Jeff Bezos as the World's Second-Richest Person," CNN Business, September 18, 2022, https:// www.cnn.com/2022/09/16/economy/worlds-richest-person-musk-adani-bezos.

208 so that the other company can't compete: Mitchell, Interview by Frisch, "Unfair Advantage," 7.

209 paid $0 in U.S. federal income tax: Andrew Davis, "Why Amazon Paid No 2018 US Federal Income Tax," April 4, 2019, https://www.cnbc.com/2019/04/03/why -amazon-paid-no-federal-income-tax.html.

209 European Commission slapped Google: Ivana Kottasová, "EU Slaps Google with Record $2.7 Billion Fine," CNN Business, June 27, 2017, https://money.cnn.com /2017/06/27/technology/business/google-eu-antitrust-fine/index.html.

209 Federal Trade Commission made the opposite: Edward Wyatt, "A Victory for Google as F.T.C. Takes No Formal Steps," *New York Times*, January 3, 2013, https://www.nytimes.com/2013/01/04/technology/google-agrees-to-changes-in -search-ending-us-antitrust-inquiry.html.

209 antitrust violations, but a judge threw the case out: Cecilia Kang, "States Say They Will Appeal the Dismissal of Their Facebook Antitrust Suit," *New York Times*,

July 28, 2021, https://www.nytimes.com/2021/07/28/technology/state-facebook-antitrust-lawsuit.html.

209 report recommended strengthening antitrust laws: Subcommitte on Antitrust Commerical and Administrative Law, Committee on the Judiciary, 116th Congress, *Investigation of Competition in Digital Markets, Majority Staff Report and Recommendations* (2020), https://fm.cnbc.com/applications/cnbc.com/resources/editorialfiles/2020/10/06/investigation_of_competition_in_digital_markets_majority_staff_report_and_recommendations.pdf.

209 "the workers are in service to the machines": Mitchell, Interview by Frisch, "Unfair Advantage," 12.

210 first successful campaign to unionize: Alina Selyukh, "Chris Smalls Started Amazon's 1st Union. He's Now Heard from Workers at 50 Warehouses," *Morning Edition*, April 6, 2022, https://www.npr.org/2022/04/06/1091130929/chris-smalls-amazon-union-50-warehouses.

210 approval of unions is the highest it's been: Katie Schoolov, "Amazon's First U.S. Union Faces an Uphill Battle After Historic Win at Staten Island Warehouse," CNBC, July 21, 2022, https://www.cnbc.com/2022/07/21/how-chris-smalls-formed-amazons-first-us-union-and-whats-next.html.

210 corporations started to post lobbyists: Joel Bakan, *The Corporation: The Pathological Pursuit of Profit and Power* (New York: Free Press, 2004), 102–3.

211 "business/government relationship is a symbiotic": Bakan, *The Corporation*, 107.

211 "government officials who were formerly top executives": Bakan, *The Corporation*, 188, footnote.

211 to fight federal environmental regulations: Brady Dennis and Steven Mufson, "Thousands of Emails Detail EPA Head's Close Ties to Fossil Fuel Industry," *Washington Post*, February 22, 2017, https://www.washingtonpost.com/news/energy-environment/wp/2017/02/22/oklahoma-attorney-generals-office-releases-7500-pages-of-emails-between-scott-pruitt-and-fossil-fuel-industry/.

211 former coal industry lobbyist: Jeff Turentine, "Who Is Andrew Wheeler? (And Why You Should Be Afraid of Him)," *On Earth*, April 13, 2018, https://www.nrdc.org/onearth/who-andrew-wheeler-and-why-you-should-be-afraid-him.

211 American Petroleum Institute: Erik Baptist, [LinkedIn page], LinkedIn, (n.d.), retrieved from https://www.linkedin.com/in/erik-baptist-2378a22b/.

211 previously Monsanto's: Michael R. Taylor, "Employment History," Open Secrets, 2022, https://www.opensecrets.org/revolving/rev_summary.php?id=20919.

211 160 former lobbyists serving under: Nadja Popovich, Livia Albeck-Ripka, and Kendra Pierre-Louis, "The Trump Administration Rolled Back More Than 100 Environmental Rules. Here's the Full List," *New York Times*, January 20, 2021, https://www.nytimes.com/interactive/2020/climate/trump-environment-rollbacks-list.html.

212 "persons with no moral conscience": Howard Zinn in Joel Bakan, writer, and Mark Achbar and Jennifer Abbott, dir., *The Corporation*, 2003, https://www.youtube.com/watch?v=xHrhqtY2khc.

212 "no *body* to incarcerate": Robert Monks was paraphrasing Edward Thurlow, Lord Chancellor of Great Britain from 1778 to 1783, who said, "Corporations have neither bodies to be punished, nor souls to be condemned; they therefore do as they like." Robert Monks in Bakan, *The Corporation.*

212 ignited due to a cost-saving decision: Bakan, *The Corporation*, 62; Andrew Pollack, "$4.9 Billion Jury Verdict in G.M. Fuel Tank Case," *New York Times*, July 10, 1999, https://www.nytimes.com/1999/07/10/us/4.9-billion-jury-verdict-in-gm-fuel-tank-case.html.

213 "hallmark of good corporate behavior": Bakan, *The Corporation*, 63–64.

213 "An externality": Bakan, *The Corporation.*

214 "externalize the cost onto the community": Bakan, *The Corporation*,198, footnote.

214 releasing toxic chemicals into a river: Dan Fagin, "Toms River: Pollution and Its Cancerous Wake," *GreenBiz*, July 18, 2015, https://www.greenbiz.com/article/toms-river-pollution-and-its-cancerous-wake.

214 hiding the dangers to fetuses: As head of the EPA, Scott Pruitt lifted the ban on chlorpyrifos. Amy Roost, "What Has Been Making My Kids So Sick?," *Dame*, October 4, 2018, https://www.damemagazine.com/2018/10/04/what-has-been-making-my-kids-so-sick/.

214 lying to physicians about the addictiveness: "Purdue Pharma Used Deceptive Sales Tactic for Oxycontin After Settlement, Ex-Sales Rep Says," June 21, 2018, https://www.cbsnews.com/news/oxycontin-purdue-pharma-former-sales-representative-deceptive-sales-psuedoaddiction/.

214 *cunning* and *ruthless*: "Notes on the Robert Hare Psychopathy Checklist—Revised," 2021, https://www.decision-making-confidence.com/hare-psychopathy-checklist.html.

214 "corporate persons—institutional psychopaths": Bakan, *The Corporation*, 110.

215 replicate an aristocracy: Sarah Churchwell, Interview by Brandon Tensley, "How the American Dream Went from Meaning Equality to Meaning Capitalism," *Pacific Standard*, March 1, 2019, https://psmag.com/ideas/how-the-american-dream-went-from-meaning-equality-to-meaning-capitalism-sarah-churchwell.

216 the American dream was repackaged: Anna Diamond, "The Original Meanings of the 'American Dream' and 'America First' Were Starkly Different from How We Use Them Today," *Smithsonian Magazine*, October 2018, https://www.smithsonianmag.com/history/behold-america-american-dream-slogan-book-sarah-churchwell-180970311/.

216 only ranks sixteenth: John F. Helliwell et al., "Happiness, Benevolence, and Trust During COVID-19 and Beyond, *World Happiness Report*, 2022, https://worldhappiness.report/ed/2022/happiness-benevolence-and-trust-during-covid-19-and-beyond/.

216 happiness starts to decline: Daniel Kahneman and Angus Deaton, "High Income Improves Evaluation of Life but Not Emotional Well-Being," *Proceedings of the National Academy of Sciences* 107, no. 38 (2010): 16489–26493, doi: 10.1073/pnas.1011492107; Andrew T. Jebb et al., "Happiness, Income Satiation and Turn-

ing Points Around the World," *Nature Human Behaviour* 2, no. 1 (2018): 33–38, doi: 10.1038/s41562-017-0277-0.

216 were happiest: Jebb et al., "Happiness," 33–38. I based this number on Jebb et al.'s data for positive and negative affect and excluded their data for life evaluation, because that is more likely to be based on cognitive comparisons with others.

216 people in most of the country: Of course, some cities, like New York and San Francisco, have a higher cost of living, and these figures, which are averages for all of North America, might not be adequate in some places.

217 happiness quotient holds true for nations, too: Richard Layard, *Happiness: Lessons from a New Science* (New York: Penguin Books, 2005), 33.

217 happiness has stagnated: Layard, *Happiness,* 51.

217 "Gross National Happiness": Tashi Dorji, "The Story of a King, a Poor Country, and a Rich Idea," *Earth Journalism Network,* June 15, 2012, https://earthjournalism.net//stories/6468.

217 defining a measurement of happiness: Jigmi Y. Thinley and Janette Hartz-Karp, "National Progress, Sustainability and Higher Goals: The Case of Bhutan's Gross National Happiness," *Sustainable Earth* 2 (2019): e11, doi: 10.1186/s42055-019-0022-9.

217 first carbon-neutral country: Tshering Tobgay, "The First Carbon Neutral Country in the World," TED, April 1, 2016, https://www.youtube.com/watch?v=7Lc_dlVrg5M.

217 even has universal healthcare: Silver Donald Cameron, "Bhutan: The Pursuit of Gross National Happiness," TEDxHalifax, July 20, 2011, https://www.youtube.com/watch?v=1CLJwYW6-Ao.

218 "create the conditions for happiness": Jody Rosen, "Bhutan: A Higher State of Being," *New York Times,* October 30, 2014, https://www.nytimes.com/2014/10/30/t-magazine/bhutan-bicycle-gross-national-happiness.html.

218 last country in the world to get TV: Cameron, "Bhutan: The Pursuit of Gross National Happiness."

218 its impact on the culture: Cathy Scott-Clark and Adrian Levy, "Fast Forward into Trouble," *The Guardian,* June 13, 2003, https://www.theguardian.com/theguardian/2003/jun/14/weekend7.weekend2.

218 Suicide rates: "Concern over Bhutan Suicide Rate," BBC News, July 1, 2009, http://news.bbc.co.uk/2/hi/south_asia/8128227.stm.

219 new economic paradigm: Bhutan, "Defining a New Economic Paradigm: The Report of the High-Level Meeting on Wellbeing and Happiness," Sustainable Development Goals Knowledge Platform, 2012, https://sustainabledevelopment.un.org/ index.php?page=view&type=400&nr=617&menu=35.

219 first World Happiness Report: John F. Helliwell, Richard Layard, and Jeffrey Sachs, eds., "World Happiness Report," 2012, https://worldhappiness.report/ed/2012/.

219 Canadian Index of Wellbeing: Canadian Index of Wellbeing, "Wellbeing as the Lens for Decision-Making in Canada," 2021, https://uwaterloo.ca/canadian-index-wellbeing/.

219 New Zealand became the first: Charlotte Graham-McLay, "New Zealand's Next Liberal Milestone: A Budget Guided by 'Well-Being,'" *New York Times,* May 22, 2019, https://www.nytimes.com/2019/05/22/world/asia/new-zealand-wellbeing -budget.html.

219 Key National Indicator System: The State of the USA, "History," http://www .stateoftheusa.org/about/history/.

219 "a very pale tint": Jean Strouse, *Alice James: A Biography* (Cambridge: Harvard University Press, 1999), 267.

219 "over every little public event here": *Alice James: Her Life in Letters,* ed. Linda Anderson (Bristol, England: Thoemmes Press, 1996), 193, as cited in Strouse, *Alice James,* 276.

220 "tipping point phenomena": Luke Kemp, "Are We On the Road to Civilisation Collapse?," BBC Future, February 18, 2019, https://www.bbc.com/future /article/20190218-are-we-on-the-road-to-civilisation-collapse.

220 depletion of conventional crude oil: Daniel J. Murphy and Charles A. S. Hall, "Energy Return on Investment, Peak Oil, and the End of Economic Growth," *Annals of the New York Academy of Sciences* 1219 (2011): 52–72, doi: 10.1111/j.1749 -6632.2010.05940.x.

220 the CO_2 in our atmosphere: "Daily CO_2," CO_2-Earth, https://www.co2.earth/daily -co2.

220 greenhouse gases: Maya Wei-Haas, "How America Stacks Up When It Comes to Greenhouse Gas Emissions," *Smithsonian Magazine,* June 2, 2017, https://www .smithsonianmag.com/smart-news/how-America-stacks-up-greenhouse-gas -emissions-180963560/.

220 greatest responsibility for climate change: Umair Irfan, "Why the US Bears the Most Responsibility for Climate Change, in One Chart," *Vox,* December 4, 2019, https://www.vox.com/energy-and-environment/2019/4/24/18512804/climate -change-united-states-china-emissions.

220 Global temperatures are climbing: NASA, "How Do We Know Climate Change Is Real?," August 24, 2022, https://climate.nasa.gov/evidence/.

221 at the expense of the best interests of society: Mike Gismondi, "*Radical Transformation: Oligarchy, Collapse, and the Crisis of Civilization* (2017). Interview with Kevin MacKay," March 2018, https://www.researchgate.net/publication /323653399_Radical_Transformation_Oligarchy_Collapse_and_the_Crisis_of _Civilization_2017_Interview_with_Kevin_MacKay_By_Mike_Gismondi _Athabasca_University_August_2017.

PART IV: FIRST, DO NO HARM

223 "think about our illnesses": David B. Morris, *Illness and Culture in the Postmodern Age* (Berkeley: University of California Press, 1998), 273. Reprinted with permission.

224 "supposed to be the rules": William James, "The Hidden Self," *Scribner's,* March 1890, 361–73, https://en.wikisource.org/wiki/The_Hidden_Self.

CHAPTER 12: ASYLUM

225 "curing their patients, etc.": Letter to William James, December 23, 1884, *Alice James: Her Life in Letters*, ed. Linda Anderson (Bristol, England: Thoemmes Press, 1996), 126.

225 push doctors: Roni Caryn Rabin, "15-Minute Doctor Visits Take a Toll on Patient–Physician Relationships," *PBS NewsHour*, April 21, 2014, https://www.pbs.org/newshour/health/need-15-minutes-doctors-time.

226 "technicians on an assembly line": Sandeep Jauhar, *Doctored: The Disillusionment of an American Physician* (New York: Farrar, Straus, and Giroux, 2014), as cited in Meghan O'Rourke, "Doctors Tell All—and It's Bad," *The Atlantic*, November 2014, https://www.theatlantic.com/magazine/archive/2014/11/doctors-tell-all-and-its-bad/380785//.

226 doctors interrupt their patients: David Von Drehle, "Medicine Is About to Get Personal," *Time Magazine*, December 22, 2014, https://time.com/3643841/medicine-gets-personal/.

226 whether the patient felt truly heard: Martin J. Bass et al., "The Physician's Actions and the Outcome of Illness in Family Practice," *Journal of Family Practice* 23, no. 1 (1986): 43–47, as cited in Howard Brody with Daralyn Brody, *The Placebo Response: How You Can Release The Body's Inner Pharmacy for Better Health* (New York: Cliff Street Books, 2000), 4–5; The Headache Study Group of the University of Western Ontario, "Predictors of Outcome in Headache Patients Presenting to Family Physicians—A One Year Prospective Study," *Headache Journal* 26, no. 6 (1986): 285–94, as cited in Brody with Brody, *The Placebo Response*, 4–5.

226 "Some friends and I started talking": Christina Baldwin and Ann Linnea, *The Circle Way: A Leader in Every Chair* (San Francisco: Berrett-Koehler Publishers, 2010).

227 "reverent participatory relationship": Kathryn Landon-Malone, personal communication, April 7, 2011.

227 In 2019, the U.S. GDP: World Population Review, "GDP Ranked by Country 2022," 2022, http://worldpopulationreview.com/countries/countries-by-gdp/.

228 spend 48 percent of their crop revenue: Gary Schnitkey and Sarah Sellars, "Growth Rates of Fertilizer, Pesticide, and Seed Costs Over Time," *FarmdocDaily* 6: 130, 1–4, July 12, 2016, https://farmdocdaily.illinois.edu/wp-content/uploads/2016/07/fdd120716.pdf.

228 more connected to nature: "How Nature Is Good for Our Health and Happiness," BBCEarth, http://www.bbc.com/earth/story/20160420-how-nature-is-good-for-our-health-and-happiness.

228 leaving them more prone to disease: Liza Gross, "Pesticides Are Harming Bees in Literally Every Possible Way," *Wired*, January 24, 2019, https://www.wired.com/story/pesticides-are-harming-bees-in-literally-every-possible-way/; Erick V. S. Motta, Kasie Raymann, and Nancy A. Moran, "Glyphosate Perturbs the Gut Microbiota of Honeybees," *Proceedings of the National Academy of Sciences* 115, no. 41 (October 9, 2018), https://www.pnas.org/content/115/41/10305.

229   systems biology: Institute for Systems Biology, "What Is Systems Biology," December 12, 2019, https://systemsbiology.org/about/what-is-systems-biology/.

230   responsible for 90 percent of healthcare expenditures: Centers for Disease Control and Prevention, "Health and Economic Costs of Chronic Diseases," Autumn 10, 2022, https://www.cdc.gov/chronicdisease/about/costs/index.htm#ref1.

230   puzzle of human disease: Nitin K. Ahuja, "The Body Is Not a Machine," *Aeon*, November 11, 2021, https://aeon.co/essays/how-ecological-thinking-fills-the-gaps-in-biomedicine.

230   make the problem worse: Christina Reimer et al., "Proton-Pump Inhibitor Therapy Induces Acid-Related Symptoms in Healthy Volunteers After Withdrawal of Therapy," *Gastroenterology* 137, no. 1 (2009): 80–87, doi: 10.1053/j.gastro.2009.03.058, as cited in Richard Knox, "Study: Heartburn Drugs Can Cause More Heartburn," NPR, September 6, 2009, https://www.npr.org/templates/story/story.php?storyId =112564382.

231   can cause further problems: Susan Fekety, RN, MSN, CNM (ret), personal communication, August 7, 2019.

231   transcend anatomical boundaries: David S. Jones and Sheila Quinn, *Reversing the Chronic Disease Trend: Six Steps to Better Wellness*, The Institute for Functional Medicine, 2017, https://docplayer.net/202172149-Reversing-the-chronic-disease-trend -six-steps-to-better-wellness-by-david-s-jones-md-and-sheila-quinn.html.

232   equal to the task: Jean Strouse, *Alice James: A Biography* (Cambridge: Harvard University Press, 1999), 206.

232   that November, Alice collapsed: Strouse, *Alice James*, 207.

232   "something lying back of her nervousness": Strouse, *Alice James*, 207.

232   "nervous people who are not insane": Mary Norton Bradford, "Adams-Nervine Asylum," *Boston Globe*, April 18, 1887, https://www.jphs.org/victorian-era/adams -nervine-asylum-boston-globe-article.html.

233   on a case-by-case basis: Bradford, "Adams-Nervine Asylum,"

233   the treasurer: Strouse, *Alice James*, 222.

233   strain and fatigue of quintessential feminine functions: Strouse, *Alice James*, 223.

233   galvanic electrical currents: Strouse, *Alice James*, 225.

233   designed to feel homelike: Candace Jenkins and Judith McDonald, "Adams-Nervine Asylum: National Register Nomination Form," June 1, 1982, https://www .jphs.org/victorian-era/adams-nervine-asylum-national-register-nomination -form.html.

233   newly papered walls: Strouse, *Alice James*, 222.

233   again doing poorly: Strouse, *Alice James*, 225–26.

233   consumptive sister, Louisa: Strouse, *Alice James*, 226–27.

234   neurologist named William B. Neftel: Strouse, *Alice James*, 227.

234   "quite as if I had been transformed": Strouse, *Alice James*, 228.

234   based on their income: Elisabeth Rosenthal, *An American Sickness: How Healthcare Became Big Business and How You Can Take It Back* (New York: Penguin Press, 2017), 59.

234   ensuring patients' bills were paid: Rosenthal, *An American Sickness*, 16–17.

234 One of the first insurers: Rosenthal, *An American Sickness*, 17.

235 for-profit plans: Rosenthal, *An American Sickness*, 17.

235 board of directors voted to allow: Rosenthal, *An American Sickness*, 18.

235 average medical loss ratio: Rosenthal, *An American Sickness*, 19.

235 300 times what their average employee earned: Evan Sweeney and Mike Stankiewicz, "Health Insurance CEOs Earned $342.6M in 2017," *FierceHealthcare*, May 7, 2018, https://www.fiercehealthcare.com/payer/ceo-pay-2017-342 -million-unitedhealth-molina-cigna-aetna.

235 annual salaries for the heads: Sweeney and Stankiewicz, "Health Insurance CEOs."

235 requiring insurance companies: Rosenthal, *An American Sickness*, 19–20.

235 Medicare spends: Rosenthal, *An American Sickness*, 20.

235 greater motivation to make big payouts: Rosenthal, *An American Sickness*, 20.

235 rates keep going up: Sara R. Collins and David C. Radley, "The Cost of Employer Insurance Is a Growing Burden for Middle-Income Families," The Commonwealth Fund, December 7, 2018, https://www.commonwealthfund.org/publications /issue-briefs/2018/dec/cost-employer-insurance-growing-burden-middle -income-families.

236 only one without universal healthcare: Stephen Lendman, "America the Only Developed Country Without Universal Healthcare," *Global Research*, July 9, 2017, https://www.globalresearch.ca/america-the-only-developed-country-without -universal-healthcare/5598311 and http://factmyth.com/factoids/the-us-is-the -only-very-highly-developed-country-without-universal-healthcare/.

236 spend twice as much on healthcare: Rosenthal, *An American Sickness*, 3.

236 dead last on overall performance: Eric C. Schneider et al., "Mirror, Mirror 2021: Reflecting Poorly," The Commonwealth Fund, August 4, 2021, https://www .commonwealthfund.org/publications/fund-reports/2021/aug/mirror-mirror -2021-reflecting-poorly.

236 half of all U.S. bankruptcies: David U. Himmelstein et al., "Medical Bankruptcy: Still Common Despite the Affordable Care Act," *American Journal of Public Health* 109, no. 3 (March 2019), http://www.pnhp.org/docs/AJPHBankruptcy2019.pdf.

236 250,000 GoFundMe campaigns: Himmelstein et al., "Medical Bankruptcy."

236 $3 trillion a year on healthcare: Rosenthal, *An American Sickness*, 3.

236 subdomain of timeliness: Schneider et al., "Mirror, Mirror 2021."

236 ranking dead last: Schneider et al., "Mirror, Mirror 2021."

236 incomplete and fragmented coverage: Schneider et al., "Mirror, Mirror 2021."

236 Lost productivity due to illness costs: Integrated Benefits Institute, "Poor Health Cost US Employers $530 Billion and 1.4 Billion Work Days of Absence and Impaired Performance According to Integrated Benefits Institute," November 15, 2018, https://www.ibiweb.org/poor-health-costs-us-employers-530-billion-and -1-4-billion-work-days-of-absence-and-impaired-performance/.

237 leaky gut: Marcelo Campos, "Leaky Gut: What Is It, and What Does It Mean for You?," *Harvard Health Blog*, November 16, 2021, https://www.health.harvard.edu /blog/ leaky-gut-what-is-it-and-what-does-it-mean-for-you-2017092212451.

238 due to lack of health insurance: Andrew P. Wilper et al., "Health Insurance and Mortality in US Adults," *American Journal of Public Health* 99, no. 12 (2009): 2289–95, https://www.ncbi.nlm.nih.gov/pmc/articles/PMC2775760/.

238 completely uninsured: Wilper et al., "Health Insurance."

238 shrunk to 28.9 million: Jennifer Tolbert, Kendal Orgera, and Anthony Damico, "Key Facts About the Uninsured Population," November 6, 2020, Kaiser Family Foundation, https://www.kff.org/uninsured/fact-sheet/key-facts-about-the-uninsured-population/.

239 postpone or forgo necessary care: Tolbert, Orgera, and Damico, "Key Facts."

239 less likely to receive preventive care: Tolbert, Orgera, and Damico, "Key Facts."

239 can't afford to take their meds as prescribed: Tami Luhby, "One-Third of Uninsured Can't Afford to Take Drugs as Prescribed, Says Government Report," CNN Health, March 19, 2019, https://www.cnn.com/2019/03/19/health/drug-costs.

239 cut back on their meds: Luhby, "One-Third."

239 more likely to wind up in the hospital: Tolbert, Orgera, and Damico, "Key Facts."

239 not adequately covered: Sara R. Collins, Munira Z. Gunia, and Michelle M. Doty, "How Well Does Insurance Coverage Protect Consumers from Health Care Costs: Findings from the Commonwealth Fund Biennial Health Insurance Survey, 2016," The Commonwealth Fund, October 18, 2017, https://www.commonwealthfund.org/publications/issue-briefs/2017/oct/how-well-does-insurance-coverage-protect-consumers-health-care.

239 not getting needed care: Collins, Gunia, and Doty, "How Well Does Insurance Coverage Protect Consumers from Health Care Costs."

240 largest healthcare payer in the United States: Centers for Medicare and Medicaid Services, "CMS Roadmaps Overview," 2008, https://www.cms.gov/medicare/quality-initiatives-patient-assessment-instruments/qualityinitiativesgeninfo/downloads/ roadmapoverview_oea_1-16.pdf.

240 quarter of all healthcare expenditures: Tevi D. Troy, "How the Government as a Payer Shapes the Health Care Marketplace," American Health Policy Institute, 2015, http://www.americanhealthpolicy.org/Content/documents/resources/Government_as_Payer_12012015.pdf.

240 "in charge of determining fair value and payment": Rosenthal, *An American Sickness*, 63.

240 "often wildly inaccurate": Rosenthal, *An American Sickness*, 64.

240 estimates were longer than actual times: Rosenthal, *An American Sickness*, 64.

240 as much as double: Rosenthal, *An American Sickness*, 64.

240 "making six times as much money": David von Drehle, "Medicine Is About to Get Personal," *Time*, December 22, 2014, https://time.com/3643841/medicine-gets-personal/.

241 "whether they should be done at all": Katy Butler, "What Broke My Father's Heart," *New York Times*, June 18, 2010, https://www.nytimes.com/2010/06/20/magazine/20pacemaker-t.html.

241 lower mortality rates: Robert L. Phillips Jr. and Andrew W. Bazemore, "Primary

Care and Why It Matters for U.S. Health System Reform," *Health Affairs* 29, no. 5 (2010): 806–10, doi: 10.1377/hlthaff.2010.0020.

241 unnecessary treatments: Phillips and Bazemore, "Primary Care."

241 Countries with strong primary care: Barbara Starfield et al., "Contribution of Primary Care to Health Systems and Health," *Milbank Quarterly* 83, no. 3 (2005): 457–502, https://www.ncbi.nlm.nih.gov/pmc/articles/PMC2690145/#b62.

241 it is at the lowest level: Von Drehle, "Medicine Is About to Get Personal."

241 shortage of primary care doctors: Beth Duff-Brown, "More Primary Care Physicians Leads to Longer Life Spans," *Stanford Medicine News Center*, February 18, 2019, https://med.stanford.edu/news/all-news/2019/02/more-primary-care -physicians-lead-to-longer-life-spans.html.

242 updated analysis: William H. Shrank, Teresa L. Rogstad, and Natasha Parekh, "Waste in the US Health Care System: Estimated Costs and Potential for Savings," *JAMA* 322, no. 15 (2019): 1501–509, doi: 10.1001/jama.2019.13978.

242 doctors are more likely to perform unnecessary procedures when: Heather Lyu et al., "Overtreatment in the United States," *PLoS One* 12, no. 9 (2017): e0181970, doi: 10.1371/journal.pone.0181970.

242 vary widely between hospitals: Emily Oshima Lee and Ezekiel J. Emanuel, "Shared Decision Making to Improve Care and Reduce Costs," *New England Journal of Medicine* 368, no. 1 (2013): 6–8, doi: 10.1056/NEJMp1209500, as cited in Heidi Julavits, "Diagnose This! How to Be Your Own Best Doctor," *Harper's*, April 2014.

242 "on the basis of financial incentives": Julavits, "Diagnose This."

242 informed decision-making: Clarence H. Braddock III et al., "Informed Decision Making in Outpatient Practice: Time to Get Back to Basics," *JAMA* 282, no. 24 (1999): 2313–20, https://jamanetwork.com/journals/jama/fullarticle/192233.

242 aligned with their values: Dawn Stacey et al., "Decision Aids to Help People Facing Health Treatment or Screening Decisions," *Cochrane Database Systematic Review*, April 12, 2017, https://www.cochranelibrary.com/cdsr/doi/10.1002/14651858. CD001431.pub5/full.

242 shared decision-making: Lee and Emanuel, "Shared Decision Making."

242 Choosing Wisely campaign: Daniel Wolfson, John Santa, and Lorie Slass, "Engaging Physicians and Consumers in Conversations About Treatment Overuse and Waste: A Short History of the Choosing Wisely Campaign," *Academic Medicine* 89, no. 7 (2014): 990–95, doi: 10.1097/ACM.0000000000000270.

245 multiple insurers is intrinsically more complex and costly: Irene Papanicolas, Liana R. Woskie, and Ashish Jha, "Health Care Spending in the United States and Other High-Income Countries," *JAMA* 319, no. 10 (2018): 1024–39, doi: 10.1001 /jama.2018.1150.

245 to collect deductibles and copayments: Austin Frakt, "The Astonishingly High Administrative Costs of U.S. Health Care," *New York Times*, July 16, 2018, https:// www.nytimes.com/2018/07/16/upshot/costs-health-care-us.html.

245 time spent on insurance billing: Papanicolas, Woskie, and Jha, "Health Care Spending."

245   to cover billing-related activities: Julie Ann Sakowski et al., "Peering into the Black
      Box: Billing and Insurance Activities in a Medical Group," *Health Affairs* 28, no.
      suppl. 1 (2009), doi: 10.1377/hlthaff.28.4.w544, as cited in Frakt, "The Astonish-
      ingly High."

245   American practices spend almost four times more: Dante Morra et al., "US Phy-
      sician Practices Versus Canadians: Spending Nearly Four Times as Much Money
      Interacting with Payers," *Health Affairs*, 30, no. 8 (2011): 1443–50, doi: 10.1377
      /hlthaff.2010.0893, as cited in Frakt, "The Astonishingly High."

245   enough to cover every single uninsured American: Gregory Warner, "The Battle of
      the Billing Codes," *Marketplace,* April 10, 2012, https://www.marketplace.org/2012
      /04/10/battle-over-billing-codes/.

246   "in a *very* knocked up condition": Strouse, *Alice James,* 235.

246   "have printed into a small pamphlet": Alice James, *The Death and Letters of Alice
      James: Selected Correspondence*, ed. Ruth Bernard Yeazell (Berkeley: University of
      California Press, 1981), 102, as cited in Strouse, *Alice James,* 235.

247   "their *only* interest being diagnosis": James, *The Death,* 107.

247   move in with Alice: Strouse, *Alice James,* 240.

247   rich social life: Strouse, *Alice James,* 253.

CHAPTER 13: BEDLAM

248   spent more money to influence lawmakers: Open Secrets, "Industry Profile: Pharma-
      ceuticals/Health Products," https://www.opensecrets.org/lobby/indusclient.php?id
      =H04&year=2018.

248   of the next industry: Open Secrets, https://www.opensecrets.org/lobby/top.php?
      showYear=2018&indexType=i.

248   donations to congressional candidates: Open Secrets, https://www.opensecrets.
      org/industries/summary.php?ind=H04++.

248   allow drug companies to set their own prices: Annie Waldman, "Big Pharma Qui-
      etly Enlists Leading Professors to Justify $1,000-Per-Day Drugs," *ProPublica*,
      February 23, 2017, https://www.propublica.org/article/big-pharma-quietly-enlists
      -leading-professors-to-justify-1000-per-day-drugs.

248   for the very same drugs: Irene Papanicolas, Liana R. Woskie, and Ashish Jha,
      "Health Care Spending in the United States and Other High-Income Countries,"
      JAMA 319, no. 10 (2018): 1024–39, doi: 10.1001/jama.2018.1150.

248   prescription drugs account for almost 11 percent: Organisation for Economic
      Co-operation and Development, "Pharmaceutical Spending," 2021, https://data
      .oecd.org/healthres/pharmaceutical-spending.htm; Stephen Heffler et al., "Health
      Spending Growth Up in 1999: Faster Growth Expected in the Future," *Health
      Affairs* 20, no. 2 (2001): 193–203, doi: 10.1377/hlthaff.20.2.193.

249   biggest source of healthcare overspending: Ezekiel J. Emanuel, "Big Pharma's
      Go-To Defense of Soaring Drug Prices Doesn't Add Up," *The Atlantic,* March

23, 2019, https://www.theatlantic.com/health/archive/2019/03/drug-prices-high-cost-research-and-development/585253/.

249 Name-brand drugs: Waldman, "Big Pharma Quietly Enlists."

249 their prices doubled: Waldman, "Big Pharma Quietly Enlists."

249 three times what they spent in 2000: Matej Mikulic, "Prescription Drug Expenditure in the United States from 1960 to 2020," Statistica, July 27, 2022, https://www.statista.com/statistics/184914/prescription-drug-expenditures-in-the-us-since-1960/.

249 most lucrative sectors: Waldman, "Big Pharma Quietly Enlists."

249 $19 in marketing: Donald W. Light and Joel R. Lexchin, "Pharmaceutical Research and Development: What Do We Get for All That Money?," *BMJ* 345 (2012): e4348, doi: 10.1136/bmj.e4348.

249 Charlotte Perkins Gilman was prescribed: Nancy Cervetti, *S. Weir Mitchell: 1829–1914: Philadelphia's Literary Physician* (University Park, PA: Pennsylvania State University Press), 152.

250 a painkiller or a stimulant: Gosling, *Before Freud,* 116–17.

250 "great distress of the heart": Jean Strouse, *Alice James: A Biography* (Cambridge: Harvard University Press, 1999), 235.

250 Doctors prescribed: Francis G. Gosling, *Before Freud: Neurasthenia and the American Medical Community, 1870–1910* (Urbana: University of Illinois Press, 1987), 116–17.

250 "impossible to estimate the damage": Gosling, *Before Freud,* 116–17.

251 IFS process: IFS Institute, "What Is Internal Family Systems?," 2022, https://ifs-institute.com/.

252 "funded by the [pharmaceutical] industry": Richard Smith, "Medical Journals Are an Extension of the Marketing Arm of Pharmaceutical Companies," *PLoS Medicine* 2, no. 5 (2005): e138, doi: 10.1371/journal.pmed.0020138.

252 "Journals have devolved": Richard Horton, "The Dawn of McScience," *The New York Review of Books,* March 11, 2004, https://www.nybooks.com/articles/2004/03/11/the-dawn-of-mcscience/, as cited in Smith, "Medical Journals."

252 researchers can manipulate data: Smith, "Medical Journals."

253 suppressing unfavorable results: Ben Goldacre, "Health Care's Trick Coin," *New York Times,* February 1, 2013, https://www.nytimes.com/2013/02/02/opinion/health-cares-trick-coin.html.

253 ignored the requirements: Andrew P. Prayle, Matthew N. Hurley, and Alan R. Smyth, "Compliance with Mandatory Reporting of Clinical Trial Results on ClinicalTrials.gov: Cross Sectional Study," *BMJ,* no. 344 (2012): d7373, doi: 10.1136/bmj.d7373, as cited in Goldacre, "Health Care's Trick Coin."

254 "we don't know which half is which": Harvard Medical School, "Past Deans of the Faculty of Medicine," 2022, https://hms.harvard.edu/about-hms/facts-figures/past-deans-faculty-medicine.

255 "misleading, exaggerated, and often flat-out wrong": David H. Freedman, "Lies,

Damned Lies, and Medical Science," *The Atlantic*, November 2010, https://www.theatlantic.com/magazine/archive/2010/11/lies-damned-lies-and-medical-science/308269/.

255 "Why Most Published Research Findings Are False": John P.A. Ioannidis, "Why Most Published Research Findings Are False," *PLoS Medicine* 19, no. 8 (2005): e1004085, doi: 10.1371/journal.pmed.0020124, as cited in Freedman, "Lies, Damned Lies, and Medical Science."

255 41 percent were wrong or significantly exaggerated: Freedman, "Lies, Damned Lies, and Medical Science"; Snigdha Prakash and Vikki Valentine, "Timeline: The Rise and Fall of Vioxx," NPR, November 10, 2007, https://www.npr.org/2007/11/10/5470430/timeline-the-rise-and-fall-of-vioxx.

255 generally persist for years: Freedman, "Lies, Damned Lies, and Medical Science," 8.

256 Vioxx, for instance: Elisabeth Rosenthal, *An American Sickness: How Healthcare Became Big Business and How You Can Take It Back* (New York: Penguin Press, 2017), 100.

256 lifesaver for its maker, Merck: Gardiner Harris, "F.D.A. Official Admits 'Lapses' on Vioxx," *New York Times*, March 2, 2005, https://www.nytimes.com/2005/03/02/politics/fda-official-admits-lapses-on-vioxx.html.

256 a blockbuster: David Brown, "Maker of Vioxx Is Accused of Deception," *Washington Post*, April 16, 2008, http://www.washingtonpost.com/wp-dyn/content/article/2008/04/15/AR2008041502086.html.

256 arranging ghostwriters for industry-backed studies: Joseph S. Ross et al., "Guest Authorship and Ghostwriting in Publications Related to Rofecoxib: A Case Study of Industry Documents from Rofecoxib Litigation," *JAMA* 299, no. 15 (2008): 1800–12, http://psychrights.org/research/digest/Science4Sale/Vioxx (JAMA2008).pdf, as cited in Amanda Gardner, "Key Vioxx Research Was Written by Merck, Documents Allege," *Washington Post*, April 15, 2008, http://www.washingtonpost.com/wp-dyn/content/article/2008/04/15/AR2008041502014.html.

256 caused an estimated 88,000 heart attacks: Prakash and Valentine, "Timeline," as cited in Rosenthal, *An American Sickness*, 100.

256 paid a fine: Rosenthal, *An American Sickness*, 100.

256 $4.85 billion to settle 27,000 lawsuits: Alex Berenson, "Merck Agrees to Settle Vioxx Suits for $4.85 Billion," *New York Times*, November 9, 2007, https://www.nytimes.com/2007/11/09/business/09merck.html.

257 of the thirty-two panel members, ten had financial ties: Marcia Angell, "Big Pharma, Bad Medicine," *Boston Review*, May 1, 2010, http://bostonreview.net/angell-big-pharma-bad-medicine.

257 eventually pulled from the market: ProCon.org, "FDA-Approved Prescription Drugs Later Pulled from the Market," December 1, 2021, https://prescriptiondrugs.procon.org/view.resource.php?resourceID=005528.

257 "only work in 30 or 50 percent": Steve Connor, "Glaxo Chief: Our Drugs Do

Not Work on Most Patients," *The Independent*, December 8, 2003, https://www
.independent.co.uk/news/science/glaxo-chief-our-drugs-do-not-work-most
-patients-5508670.html.

258 accelerated approval (AA) protocol: Rosenthal, *An American Sickness*, 98–99.

258 no mechanism to revoke FDA approval: Rosenthal, *An American Sickness*, 99.

259 "did not extend life": Rosenthal, *An American Sickness*, 99.

259 "over the objections of FDA safety reviewers": Alicia Mundy, "Risk Management:
The FDA's Deference to Drug Companies Is Bad for America's Health," *Harper's*,
September 2004.

259 known risks of brain swelling and hemorrhage: Aaron S. Kesselheim and Jerry
Avorn, "The F.D.A. Has Reached a New Low," *New York Times*, June 15, 2021,
https://www.nytimes.com/2021/06/15/opinion/alzheimers-drug-aducanumab
-fda.html.

259 "Congress is getting paid to not hold pharma accountable": Adriana Belmonte,
"FDA Medical Adviser: 'Congress Is Owned by Pharma,'" Yahoo! Finance,
March 13, 2019, https://finance.yahoo.com/news/congress-big-pharma-money
-123757664.html.

259 conflict of interest in members of FDA advisory boards: Charles Piller and Jia You,
"Hidden Conflicts? Pharma Payments to FDA Advisers After Drug Approvals
Spark Ethical Concerns," *Science*, July 5, 2018, https://www.sciencemag.org/news
/2018/07/hidden-conflicts-pharma-payments-fda-advisers-after-drug-approvals
-spark-ethical.

260 "play nice with these companies": Piller and You, "Hidden Conflicts?"

260 even approving one additional drug after the fraudulent activities: Charles Seife
and Rob Garver, "FDA Approved New Drug Despite Ongoing Investigations of
Lab Misconduct," *ProPublica*, April 22, 2013, http://www.propublica.org/article
/fda-approved-new-drug-despite-ongoing-investigation-of-lab-misconduct.

260 "educating" doctors: Lindsey Tanner, "US Medical Marketing Reaches $30 Bil-
lion, Drug Ads Top Surge," AP News, January 8, 2019, https://apnews.com/article
/f44a7baa710d458ca50edd66affc1b91.

260 industry-sponsored educational sessions: Kirsten E. Austad, Jerry Avorn, and
Aaron S. Kesselheim, "Medical Students' Exposure to and Attitudes About the
Pharmaceutical Industry: A Systematic Review," *PLoS Medical* 8, no. 5 (May
2011): e1001037, https://www.ncbi.nlm.nih.gov/pmc/articles/PMC3101205/.

260 90 percent of students in clinical rotation received: Austad, Avorn, and Kesselheim,
"Medical Students' Exposure."

260 industry-sponsored lunches: Frederick Sierles et al., "Medical Students' Exposure
to and Attitudes About Drug Company Interactions: A National Survey," *JAMA*
294, no. 9 (2005): 1034–42, doi: 10.1001/jama.294.9.1034, as cited in Austad,
Avorn, and Kesselheim, "Medical Students' Exposure."

260 "virtually unfettered access to young doctors": Angell, "Big Pharma."

260 think more critically: F. Sierles et al., "A National Survey," as cited in Austad,
Avorn, and Kesselheim, "Medical Students' Exposure."

260 believe they're entitled: F. Sierles et al., "A National Survey," as cited in Austad, Avorn, and Kesselheim, "Medical Students' Exposure."

261 Some wrongly believe: F. Sierles et al., "A National Survey," as cited in Austad, Avorn, and Kesselheim, "Medical Students' Exposure."

261 Even seasoned doctors: F. Sierles et al., "A National Survey," as cited in Austad, Avorn, and Kesselheim, "Medical Students' Exposure."

261 when otherwise they wouldn't have: Elaine K. Howley, "Do Drug Company Payments to Doctors Influence Which Drugs They Prescribe?," *US News & World Report*, August 31, 2018, https://health.usnews.com/health-care/patient-advice /articles/2018-08-31/do-drug-company-payments-to-doctors-influence-which -drugs-they-prescribe.

261 upped their prescriptions for branded drugs: Colette DeJong et al., "Pharmaceutical Industry–Sponsored Meals and Physician Prescribing Patterns for Medicare Beneficiaries," *JAMA Internal Medicine* 176, no. 8 (2016): 1114–22, doi: 10.1001 /jamainternmed.2016.2765, as cited in Michelle Llamas, "Selling Side Effects: Big Pharma's Marketing Machine," *DrugWatch*, May 24, 2019, https://www .drugwatch.com/featured/big-pharma-marketing/.

261 believe that only "completely safe" drugs are allowed: Pew Charitable Trust, "Persuading the Prescribers: Pharmaceutical Industry Marketing and Its Influence on Physicians and Patients," November 11, 2013, https://www.pewtrusts.org /en/research-and-analysis/fact-sheets/2013/11/11/persuading-the-prescribers -pharmaceutical-industry-marketing-and-its-influence-on-physicians-and-patients, as cited in Llamas, "Selling Side Effects."

261 another 10 percent entirely false: Adrienne E. Faerber and David H. Kreling, "Content Analysis of False and Misleading Claims in Television Advertising for Prescription and Nonprescription Drugs," *Journal of General Internal Medicie* 29, no. 1 (2014): 110–18, doi: 10.1007/s11606-013-2604-0; Llamas, "Selling Side Effects."

261 direct-to-consumer (DTC) marketing: Llamas, "Selling Side Effects."

261 ads often promote more expensive options: "Can You Trust Drug Ads on TV?," *Consumer Reports*, January 11, 2015, https://www.consumerreports.org/cro/news /2015/01/can-you-trust-drug-ads-on-tv/index.htm, as cited in Llamas, "Selling Side Effects."

261 voted to ban DTC marketing: Llamas, "Selling Side Effects."

262 asked by patients for inappropriate drugs: Pamela Hallquist Viale and Deanna Sanchez Yamamoto, "The Attitudes and Beliefs of Oncology Nurse Practitioners Regarding Direct-to-Consumer Advertising of Prescription Medications," *Oncology Nursing Forum* 31, no. 4 (July 1, 2004): 777–83, doi: 10.1188/04.ONF.777 -783, as cited in Llamas, "Selling Side Effects."

262 succumb to the pressure: Llamas, "Selling Side Effects."

262 insisted that the university researchers tweak the data: Philip J. Hilts, "Company Tried to Block Report That Its H.I.V. Vaccine Failed," *New York Times*, November 1, 2000, https://www.nytimes.com/2000/11/01/us/company-tried-to-block -report-that-its-hiv-vaccine-failed.html.

262   "I would think I have certain rights": Douglas M. Birch and Gary Cohn, "Standing Up to Industry," *Baltimore Sun*, June 26, 2001, https://www.baltimoresun.com /bal-te.research26jun26-story.html.

CHAPTER 14: PULSE

263   "turned residencies into another profitable business": Elisabeth Rosenthal, *An American Sickness: How Healthcare Became Big Business and How You Can Take It Back* (New York: Penguin Press, 2017), 42–43.

263   Residents work grueling hours: Rosenthal, *An American Sickness*, 43.

263   $171,000 annually per resident: U.S. Government Accountability Office, *Physician Workforce: Caps on Medicare-Funded Graduate Medical Education at Teaching Hospitals*, May 2021, 8, https://www.gao.gov/assets/gao-21-391.pdf.

263   worked 100 and even 120 hours per week: Ryan Park, "Why So Many Young Doctors Work Such Awful Hours," *The Atlantic*, February 21, 2017, https://www.the atlantic.com/business/archive/2017/02/doctors-long-hours-schedules/516639/.

264   average of 80 per week: Park, "Why So Many."

264   "same amount of work in less time": Park, "Why So Many."

264   work more hours than permitted: Park, "Why So Many."

264   submit false reports: Kyle M. Fargen and Charles L. Rosen, "Are Duty Hour Regulations Promoting a Culture of Dishonesty Among Resident Physicians?," *Journal of Graduate Medical Education* 5, no. 4 (2013): 553–55, doi: 10.4300/JGME -D-13-00220.1.

264   hourly restrictions pertain only: Park, "Why So Many."

264   five hours or fewer per night: DeWitt C. Baldwin Jr. and Steven R. Daugherty, "Sleep Deprivation and Fatigue in Residency Training: Results of a National Survey of First- and Second-Year Residents," *Sleep* 27, no. 2 (March 2004): 217–23, doi: 10.1093/sleep/27.2.217.

264   significant medical errors: Baldwin and Daugherty, "Sleep Deprivation."

264   half what American residents: Park, "Why So Many."

264   hourly wage of the hospital janitors: Catherine Rampell, "Solving the Shortage in Primary Care Doctors," *New York Times*, December 14, 2013, https://www .nytimes.com/2013/12/15/business/solving-the-shortage-in-primary-care -doctors.html?_r=0.

264   "better than break-even deal": Rosenthal, *An American Sickness*, 43.

265   bullying: Amar R. Chadaga, Dana Villines, and Armand Kridorian, "Bullying in the American Graduate Medical Education System: A National Cross-Sectional Survey," *PLoS One* 11, no. 3 (2016): e0150246, doi: 10.1371/journal.pone.0150246.

265   "pecking order of seniority": Elizabeth Paice et al., "Bullying Among Doctors in Training: Cross Sectional Questionnaire Survey," *British Medical Journal* 329, no. 7467 (2004): 658–59, doi: 10.1136/bmj.38133.502569.AE, as cited in Heather B. Leisy and Meleha Ahmad, "Altering Workplace Attitudes for Resident Education (A.W.A.R.E.): Discovering Solutions for Medical Resident Bullying Through

Literature Review," *BMC Medical Education* 16 (April 27, 2016): 127, doi: 10.1186 /s12909-016-0639-8.

265   Abuse took several forms: Chadaga, Villines, and Kridorian, "Bullying in the American."

265   BIPOC and female trainees: Chadaga, Villines, and Kridorian, "Bullying in the American."

265   had considered suicide: Judith Graham, "Why Are Doctors Plagued by Depression and Suicide? A Crisis Comes into Focus," *Stat*, July 21, 2016, https://www .statnews.com/2016/07/21/depression-suicide-physicians/.

265   "I definitely graduated med school with PTSD": Pamela Wible, "Why Doctors Kill Themselves," TEDMED, 2015, https://www.tedmed.com/talks/show?id=528918.

265   "little tolerance for": Graham, "Why Are Doctors Plagued."

266   "owed something for your suffering": Marilyn R. Peterson, *At Personal Risk: Boundary Violations in Professional-Client Relationships* (New York: W. W. Norton, 1992), 173.

266   how they wield their power: Peterson, *At Personal Risk*, 174.

266   narrative medicine: Rita Charon, "What to Do with Stories: The Sciences of Narrative Medicine," *Canadian Family Physician* 53, no. 8 (2007): 1265–67, https:// www.ncbi.nlm.nih.gov/pmc/articles/PMC1949238/.

266   "quails before any more gladiatorial encounters": Alice James, *The Death and Letters of Alice James: Selected Correspondence*, ed. Ruth Bernard Yeazell (Berkeley: University of California Press, 1981), 112, as cited in Jean Strouse, *Alice James: A Biography* (Cambridge: Harvard University Press, 1999), 236.

267   caused by "anxiety & strain": James, *The Death*, 123, as cited in Strouse, *Alice James*, 237.

267   all he could offer her: James, *The Death*, 123–24.

267   "one of the most *potent* creations": Strouse, *Alice James*, 267.

267   "even I felt suicidal": Wible, "Why Doctors Kill Themselves."

267   300 to 400 suicide deaths annually: Graham, "Why Are Doctors Plagued."

267   "overextended and overworked": Physicians Foundation, *2018 Survey of America's Physicians: Practice Patterns and Perspectives*, https://physiciansfoundation.org/wp -content/uploads/2018/09/physicians-survey-results-final-2018.pdf.

267   "empathy burnout": Pamela Wible, interview by Jamie Passaro, "Pamela Wible on What's Missing from Healthcare Reform," *The Sun*, November 2009, https:// thesunmagazine.org/issues/407/who-will-heal-the-healers.

267   working an average of 51 hours a week: Physicians Foundation, *2018 Survey*.

268   burnout often or all the time: Physicians Foundation, *2018 Survey*.

268   was the job: Carol Peckham, "Medscape National Physician Burnout and Depression Report 2018," *Medscape*, January 17, 2018, https://www.medscape.com /slideshow/2018-lifestyle-burnout-depression-6009235.

268   would not choose the medical profession: Physicians Foundation, *2018 Survey*.

268   "patient-physician relationship": Pamela Wible, interview with Passaro, "Pamela Wible."

268 loss of clinical autonomy: Physicians Foundation, *2018 Survey*.

268 "pawn[s] in a moneymaking game": Meghan O'Rourke, "Doctors Tell All—and It's Bad," *The Atlantic*, November 2014, https://www.theatlantic.com/magazine /archive/2014/11/doctors-tell-all-and-its-bad/380785/.

268 "moral injury": Wendy Dean, Austin Charles Dean, and Simon G. Talbot, "Why 'Burnout' Is the Wrong Term for Physician Suffering," *Medscape*, July 23, 2019, https://www.medscape.com/viewarticle/915097_1.

269 resulting administrative burdens: Alex Patten, "Before COVID-19, Health-care Worker Burnout Was Rampant. The Pandemic Has Only Made It Worse," *Webshrink*, July 25, 2020, https://www.webshrink.com/general/general-news /before-covid-19-healthcare-worker-burnout-was-rampant-the-pandemic-has -only-made-it-worse; Emily Gee and Topher Spiro, "Excess Administrative Costs Burden the U.S. Healthcare System," Center for American Progress, April 8, 2019, https://webshrink.com/general/general-news/pandemic-worsens-doctor-burnout.

269 number of healthcare administrators: Patten, "Before COVID-19."

269 whose job it is to deny treatment: Patten, "Before COVID-19."

269 increase the risk of medical error: Leisy and Ahmad, "Altering Workplace Attitudes."

269 no federal laws requiring hospitals: Martin Makary and Michael Daniel, "Medical Error—The Third Leading Cause of Death in the US," *BMJ* 353 (2016): i2139, doi: 10.1136/bmj.i2139.

269 unnecessary deaths: Institute of Medicine, "To Err Is Human: Building a Safer Health System," November 1999, https://nap.nationalacademies.org/resource /9728/To-Err-is-Human-1999--report-brief.pdf.

269 medical error: Alan Dumoff, "Where the Danger Lies: Misplaced Concerns, Mis-drawn Standards of Informed Consent," *Alternative and Complementary Therapies* 9, no. 5 (2003): 268–73, doi: 10.1089/107628003322490724.

269 third leading cause of death: Makary and Daniel, "Medical Error."

269 account only for hospital deaths: Makary and Daniel, "Medical Error."

270 "number of errors is not small at all": Danielle Ofri, *When We Do Harm: A Doctor Confronts Medical Error* (Boston: Beacon Press, 2020), 2.

270 dismissive healthcare providers: Tressie McMillan Cottom, "I Was Pregnant and in Crisis. All the Doctors and Nurses Saw Was an Incompetent Black Woman," *Time*, January 8, 2019, https://time.com/5494404/tressie-mcmillan-cottom-thick -pregnancy-competent/.

270 inadequately trained to treat the chronically ill: Jonathan D. Darer et al., "More Training Needed in Chronic Care: A Survey of US Physicians," *Academic Medicine* 79, no. 6 (2004): 541–48, doi: 10.1097/00001888-200406000-00009, as discussed in Meghan O'Rourke, "What's Wrong with Me?," *New Yorker*, August 26, 2013, 32–37, https://www.newyorker.com/magazine/2013/08/26/whats-wrong-with-me.

270 fail to include anything about ME/CFS: T. Mark Peterson et al., "Coverage of CFS Within U.S. Medical Schools," *Universal Journal of Public Health* 1, no. 4 (2013): 177–79, doi: 10.13189/ujph.2013.010404, as cited in Committee on the Diagnostic Criteria for Myalgic Encephalomyelitis/Chronic Fatigue Syndrome,

Board on the Health of Select Populations, Institute of Medicine, *Beyond Myalgic Encephalomyelitis/Chronic Fatigue Syndrome: Redefining an Illness* (Washington, DC: National Academies Press, 2015), https://www.ncbi.nlm.nih.gov/books /NBK274235/, as cited in Meghan O'Rourke, "A New Name, and Wider Recognition, for Chronic Fatigue Syndrome," *New Yorker*, February 27, 2015, https:// www.newyorker.com/tech/annals-of-technology/chronic-fatigue-syndrome-iom -report.

270　scant mention in just 40 percent of textbooks: Leonard A. Jason et al., "Frequency and Content Analysis of Chronic Fatigue Syndrome in Medical Text Books," *Australian Journal of Primary Health* 16, no. 2 (2010): 174–78, doi: 10.1071/PY09023.

271　illnesses caused by toxic chemicals: Stephen G. Pelletier, "Experts See Growing Importance of Adding Environmental Health Content to Medical School Curricula," *AAMCNews*, September 27, 2016, https://news.aamc.org/medical-education /article/experts-importance-environmental-health-content/.

271　"inadequate" instruction in environmental health: Pelletier, "Experts See Growing Importance."

271　little training in nutrition: Pamela Wible, interview with Passaro, "Pamela Wible."

271　"on the lookout for hysterical females": Maya Dusenbery, "Is Medicine's Gender Bias Killing Young Women?," *Pacific Standard*, March 23, 2015, http://www.psmag .com/health-and-behavior/is-medicines-gender-bias-killing-young-women.

271　gout, rheumatism, and digestive issues: Strouse, *Alice James*, 273.

271　"too stimulating for jangled nerves": Strouse, *Alice James*, 274.

271　commonplace book: Strouse, *Alice James*, 268.

272　Katharine was called back: Strouse, *Alice James*, 274.

272　"that infinite sky": Strouse, *Alice James*, 269.

272　"began to keep a diary": Strouse, *Alice James*, 272.

272　"so here goes, my first Journal!": Strouse, *Alice James*, 25.

272　"How sick one gets of being 'good'": Alice James, *The Diary of Alice James*, ed. Leon Edel (Boston: Northeastern University Press, 1999), 64.

273　"can't say *damn*!'": James, *Diary*, 66, as cited in Strouse, *Alice James*, 261.

273　"shape the formless mass within": James, *Diary*, 113, as cited in Strouse, *Alice James*, 292.

273　lack the time to be empathic: Empathetics, "Proven," 2016, http://empathetics .com/.

273　antidote to burnout: Sandra G. Boodman, "How to Teach Doctors Empathy," *The Atlantic*, March 15, 2015, https://www.theatlantic.com/health/archive/2015/03 /how-to-teach-doctors-empathy/387784/.

273　empathy declines during medical training: Helen Riess et al., "Empathy Training for Resident Physicians: A Randomized Controlled Trial of a Neuroscience-Informed Curriculum," *Journal of General Internal Medicine* 27, no. 10 (2012): 1280–86, doi: 10.1007/s11606-012-2063-z.

273　*that* is a buffer against burnout: L. Carol Ritchie, "Does Taking Time for Compassion Make Doctors Better at Their Jobs?," National Public Radio, April 26, 2019, https://www.npr.org/sections/health-shots/2019/04/26/717272708/does-taking-time-for-compassion-make-doctors-better-at-their-jobs.

274   Empathic communication skills are critical: Riess et al., "Empathy Training"; Ritchie, "Does Taking Time."

274   fewer malpractice claims: Riess et al., "Empathy Training."

274   provide online Empathetics® education courses: https://empathetics.com/press-release-march-2022/.

274   empathy can be learned: Riess et al., "Empathy Training."

274   "churning patients through": Pamela Wible, interview with Passaro, "Pamela Wible."

274   prescribing drugs are the logical shortcuts: Elizabeth Klodas, "One Cardiologist's Mission to Reduce Statin Use for Cholesterol," CNN Health, January 14, 2019, https://www.cnn.com/2019/01/08/health/cardiologist-statin-cholesterol-mission.

274   "doctors on the assembly line": Pamela Wible, interview with Passaro, "Pamela Wible."

275   community forums: Pamela Wible, interview with Passaro, "Pamela Wible."

275   in partnership with her patients: Pamela Wible, "The Community-Focused Family Medicine Clinic: A 'New Model' in Oregon," *Journal of Family Practice* 54, no. 8 (2005): 704–705, https://www.mdedge.com/familymedicine/article/60387/practice-management/community-focused-family-medicine-clinic-new-model.

275   "by humanizing the experience": Pamela Wible, interview with Passaro, "Pamela Wible."

276   "altogether wretched": Strouse, *Alice James*, 296.

276   a "consoling answer": James, *Diary*, 135.

276   to nurse her: Strouse, *Alice James*, 297.

276   "you will die or *recover!*": James, *Diary*, 142.

276   "the ignorant asininity of the medical profession": James, *Diary*, 150.

276   "The Healer's Art": "Healer's Art Overview," Institute for the Study of Health & Illness, 2021, http://www.rishiprograms.org/healers-art/.

277   more med schools have added this course: Rachel Remen, "The Healer's Art—Inspiring Medical Students Nationwide and Abroad," *Rachel's Blog*, November 2012, http://www.rachelremen.com/wordpress/wp-content/uploads/2012/11/BarChart9-2012.pdf.

277   each era can be defined by certain emblematic diseases: David B. Morris, *Illness and Culture in the Postmodern Age* (Berkeley: University of California Press, 1998), 51.

278   "Postmodern illness": Morris, *Illness and Culture*, 58.

278   "interpenetrated by culture": Morris, *Illness and Culture*, 70–71.

278   introduced the biopsychosocial perspective: George L. Engel, "The Need for a New Medical Model: A Challenge for Biomedicine," *Science* 196, no. 4286 (1977): 129–36, doi: 10.1126/science.847460.

278   most effectively viewed through a biopsychosocial lens: Morris, *Illness and Culture*, 248.

278   "claimed the body of its patient as its territory": Arthur W. Frank, *The Wounded*

Storyteller: Body, Illness, and Ethics, 2nd ed. (Chicago: University of Chicago Press, 2013), 10.

278 "The story told by the physician": Frank, *The Wounded Storyteller*, 5.

278 "the colonization was judged worth the cure": Frank, *The Wounded Storyteller*, 11.

279 "too untidy for laboratory analysis": Morris, *Illness and Culture*, 245.

279 "medicine's reduction of their suffering to its general unifying view": Frank, *The Wounded Storyteller*, 11.

279 "a fragmentary narrative": Morris, *Illness and Culture*, 277–78.

279 "than the medical story can tell": Frank, *The Wounded Storyteller*, 24.

279 "return to normal obligations of work and family": Frank, *The Wounded Storyteller*, 82.

279 "an 'it' to be cured": Frank, *The Wounded Storyteller*, 85.

279 "The body is the means and medium of my life": Arthur Frank, *At the Will of the Body: Reflections on Illness* (Boston, New York: A Mariner Book, Houghton Mifflin Company, 2002), 10.

280 "attempts to curtail storytelling by patients": Frank, *The Wounded Storyteller*, 58.

280 "medical monologue": Morris, *Illness and Culture*, 264.

280 initiating at least half of the interruptions: Howard B. Beckman and Richard B. Frankel, "The Effect of Physician Behavior on the Collection of Data," *Annals of Internal Medicine* 318, no. 1 (1988): 692–96, doi: 10.7326/0003-4819-101-5-692, as cited in Morris, *Illness and Culture*, 264.

280 "narrative surrender": Frank, *The Wounded Storyteller*, 16.

280 defined heroism by *doing* rather than, say, persevering: Frank, *The Wounded Storyteller*, 134.

281 Program in Narrative Medicine at Columbia University: Charon, "What to Do with Stories."

281 Narrative medicine curricula: Charon, "What to Do with Stories."

282 "Restitution stories": Frank, *The Wounded Storyteller*, 115.

282 "more to buy, whatever needs fixing will be fixed": Frank, *The Wounded Storyteller*, 86.

282 "only outcome Parsons considers as acceptable": Frank, *The Wounded Storyteller*, 82–83.

282 "pit of narrative wreckage": Frank, *The Wounded Storyteller*, 110.

282 "only denies what is being experienced": Frank, *The Wounded Storyteller*, 110.

282 quest story: Frank, *The Wounded Storyteller*, 115–36.

282 transforming that suffering into testimony: Frank, *The Wounded Storyteller*, 18.

282 "to guide others who will follow them": Frank, *The Wounded Storyteller*, 17.

283 *The Hero with a Thousand Faces*: Frank, *The Wounded Storyteller*, 411.

283 *Star Wars*: Bill Moyers, *Joseph Campbell and the Power of Myth*, 1988, https://billmoyers.com/series/joseph-campbell-and-the-power-of-myth-1988/.

283 "Woman as Temptress," for instance: Joseph Campbell, *The Hero with a Thousand Faces*, 2nd ed. (Princeton, NJ: Princeton University Press, 1968), 120.

283 "she is become the queen of sin": Campbell, *The Hero*, 123.

284 Stephen Straus betrayed his bias: Stephen E. Straus, "Chronic Fatigue Syndrome," *British Medical Journal* 313 (1996): 831–32, doi: 10.1136/bmj.313.7061.831, as cited in Mary Dimmock and Matthew Lazell-Fairman, *Thirty Years of Disdain: How HHS and a Group of Psychiatrists Buried Myalgic Encephalitis*, December 2015, https://www.dropbox.com/s/bycueauxmh49z4l/Thirty%20Years%20of%20 Disdain%20-%20Background.pdf?dl=0, 38.

285 "cultural causes and contexts of illness": Morris, *Illness and Culture*, 276–77.

CHAPTER 15: TREASURE HOUSE

286 *neurasthenia* in my Merriam-Webster's dictionary: "Neurasthenia," in *Merriam-Webster's Collegiate Dictionary*, 10th ed., 1993, http://merriam-webstercollegiate. com/dictionary/neurasthenia; Neurasthenia is defined as "nervous debility and exhaustion occurring in the absence of objective causes or lesions; nervous exhaustion," "Neurasthenia" in Dictionary.com, 2012, https://www.dictionary.com /browse/neurasthenia.

286 "a physical not a mental state": George M. Beard, *American Nervousness: Its Causes and Consequences* (New York: G. P. Putnam's Sons, 1881), 17, as cited in Charles E. Rosenberg, "The Place of George M. Beard in Nineteenth-Century Psychiatry," *Bulletin of the History of Medicine* 36 (1962): 245–59, 349, https://pubmed.ncbi .nlm.nih.gov/14037559/.

286 mind and body as intrinsically interconnected: Rosenberg, "The Place," 247; Suzanne Poirier, "The Weir Mitchell Rest Cure: Doctors and Patients," *Women's Studies* 10 (1983): 16.

286 "inhibiting the normal flow of life": William James, "The Hidden Self," https:// en.wikisource.org/wiki/The_Hidden_Self.

287 "even the scientific sect": William James, *The Varieties of Religious Experience* (New York: Longmans, Green, and Co., 1902), 95, https://csrs.nd.edu/assets/59930 /williams_1902.pdf.

287 "keys for unlocking the world's treasure-house": James, *The Varieties*, 95.

287 Robert Ader made a serendipitous discovery: Stephen Pincock, "Robert Ader," *The Lancet* 379, no. 9813 (2012): P308, doi: 10.1016/S0140-6736(12)60134-2.

287 conditioning the immunosuppressive effects: Pincock, "Robert Ader."

287 contradicting the long-held belief: Robert Ader and Nicholas Cohen, "Behaviorally Conditioned Immunosuppression," *Psychosomatic Medicine* 37, no. 4 (1975): 333–40, doi: 10.1097/00006842-197507000-00007.

288 first indications of neuroimmune interaction: John M. Williams and David L. Felten, "Sympathetic Innervation of Murine Thymus and Spleen: A Comparative Histofluorescence Study," *The Anatomical Record* 199, no. 4 (1981): 531–42, doi: 10.1002/ar.1091990409.

288 groundbreaking findings in the March 1973 issue of *Science*: Candace B. Pert and Solomon H. Snyder, "Opiate Receptor: Demonstration in Nervous Tissue," *Science* 179, no. 4077 (1973): 1011–14, doi: 10.1126/science.179.4077.1011.

288   "the new interdisciplinary field of neuroscience": Candace Pert, *Molecules of Emotion: Why You Feel the Way You Feel* (New York: Scribner, 1997), 34.

288   as well as the rest of the body: Pert, *Molecules of Emotion,* 21.

289   ligands: Pert, *Molecules of Emotion,* 23.

289   more fluid and poetic: Pert, *Molecules of Emotion,* 84.

289   "wiggle, shimmy, and even hum": Pert, *Molecules of Emotion,* 22.

289   "from the Latin *ligare,* 'that which binds,'": Pert, *Molecules of Emotion,* 24.

289   morphine made by the body itself: Pert, *Molecules of Emotion,* 63.

289   would permeate every field of medicine: Pert, *Molecules of Emotion,* 30.

289   Pert and her team went on to find: Pert, *Molecules of Emotion,* 80.

289   regulating virtually all life processes: Pert, *Molecules of Emotion,* 25.

289   Peptides are produced in many parts of the body: Pert, *Molecules of Emotion,* 70.

290   located peptide receptors in all parts of the brain: Pert, *Molecules of Emotion,* 86.

290   communicate back and forth through their peptide messengers: Pert, *Molecules of Emotion,* 163–64.

290   interpret those sensations as emotions: "William James, "What Is an Emotion?," *Mind* 9, no. 34 (1884): 188–205, doi: 10.1093/mind/os-IX.34.188, as discussed in Pert, *Molecules of Emotion,* 135–37.

290   said emotions come first: Pert, *Molecules of Emotion,* 135–37.

290   communication goes both ways: Pert, *Molecules of Emotion,* 135–37.

290   "play as an integrated entity": *Molecules of Emotion,* Pert, 148.

290   "biochemical substrate of emotion": Candace B. Pert et al., "Neuropeptides and Their Receptors: A Psychosomatic Network," *Journal of Immunology* 135, no. 2 (1985), http://candacepert.com/wp-content/uploads/2014/05/Psychosomatic-network-peptides-receptors-Pert-JI85-Pert-820-6.pdf, as cited in Pert, *Molecules of Emotion,* 179.

290   "intelligently orchestrated symphony of life": Pert, *Molecules of Emotion,* 185.

292   "he told her that women don't need to *make* the journey": Maureen Murdock, *The Heroine's Journey: Woman's Quest for Wholeness* (Boston: Shambhala, 1990), 2.

292   "an exercise in exploring the shadow": Sarah Ramey, *The Lady's Handbook for Her Mysterious Illness: A Memoir* (New York: Doubleday, 2020), 221.

292   "the heroine's journey is a journey *in*": Ramey, *The Lady's Handbook,* 219.

292   "most untraveled corners of used-book stores": Ramey, *The Lady's Handbook,* 227.

293   "cyclically, with everything else": Ramey, *The Lady's Handbook,* 227, 230.

293   an "*ecological* initiation": Ramey, *The Lady's Handbook,* 230.

293   can fall anywhere on the spectrum of masculinity and femininity: Ramey, *The Lady's Handbook,* 255.

293   mythic heroine is the protector of the interior: Ramey, *The Lady's Handbook,* 235.

293   need the feminine to balance the masculine: Ramey, *The Lady's Handbook,* 224.

293   "a fluency with darkness": Ramey, *The Lady's Handbook,* 238.

293   traits seen as masculine rank higher: Ramey, *The Lady's Handbook,* 239–40.

294   "strongest medicine there is on Earth": Ramey, *The Lady's Handbook,* 396.

294   "This is wisdom, not weakness": Ramey, *The Lady's Handbook,* 249.

295 always striving for more: Ramey, *The Lady's Handbook*, 248.

295 "to slay dragons": Ramey, *The Lady's Handbook*, 251.

295 "is missing its other half": Ramey, *The Lady's Handbook*, 250.

295 "with the fertile void": Ramey, *The Lady's Handbook*, 232.

295 "the need for the feminine corrective": Ramey, *The Lady's Handbook*, 253.

296 "the missing medicine in Medicine": Ramey, *The Lady's Handbook*, 260.

296 functional medicine provides the balanced approach: Ramey, *The Lady's Handbook*, 260–62.

296 the scan revealed: Ramey, *The Lady's Handbook*, 385–87.

296 "because I am a woman": Ramey, *The Lady's Handbook*, 388.

297 emotions are a critical element: Antonio Damasio, *Descartes' Error: Emotion, Reason, and the Human Brain* (New York: Penguin, 1994), 170–72.

297 make decisions with the help of the sensations in our bodies: Damasio, *Descartes' Error*, 179.

297 increases the efficiency of the decision-making: Damasio, *Descartes' Error*, 173.

297 helps us project into the future: Damasio, *Descartes' Error*, 175.

298 not psychosomatic but "neurosomatic": Jay Goldstein, *Betrayal by the Brain: The Neurologic Basis of Chronic Fatigue Syndrome, Fibromyalgia Syndrome, and Related Neural Network Disorders* (New York: Haworth Medical Press, 1996), 6.

298 "biochemical neural network of dysfunction": Goldstein, *Betrayal by the Brain*, 2.

298 limbic hypothesis: Jay Goldstein, "CFS: Limbic Encephalopathy in a Dysfunctional Neuroimmune Network," in eds. Byron M. Hyde, Jay Goldstein, and Paul Levine, *The Clinical and Scientific Basis of Myalgic Encephalomyelitis/Chronic Fatigue Syndrome* (Ogdensburg, NY: Nightingale Research Foundation Press, 1992), 400–406, as cited in Erica F. Verrillo and Lauren M. Gellman, *Chronic Fatigue Syndrome: A Treatment Guide* (St. Louis, MO: Quality Medical Publishing, 1998), 75.

298 kindling: Iris R. Bell, Claudia S. Miller, and Gary E. Schwartz, "An Olfactory-Limbic Model of Multiple Chemical Sensitivity Syndrome: Possible Relationships to Kindling and Affective Spectrum Disorders," *Biological Psychiatry* 32, no. 3 (1992): 218–42, doi: 10.1016/0006-3223(92)901045-9.

299 eventually nonetheless provoked convulsions: Graham V. Goddard, "Development of Epileptic Seizures Through Brain Stimulation at Low Intensity," *Nature* 214, no. 5092 (1967): 1020–21, doi: 10.1038/2141020a0, as cited in Niki Gratrix, "Limbic Kindling: Hard Wiring the Brain for Hypersensitivity and Chronic Fatigue Syndrome," *HealthRising* (blog), May 17, 2014, https://www.healthrising.org/blog/2014/05/17/limbic-kindling-hard-wiring-brain-hypersensitives-chronic-fatigue-syndrome/.

299 induce kindling through chemical stimulation: Goddard, "Development of Epileptic Seizures," as cited in Gratrix, "Limbic Kindling."

299 intermittent nature of low-level chemical exposures: Bell, Miller, and Schwartz, "An Olfactory-Limbic Model."

299 limbic kindling may play a role in ME/CFS: Leonard Jason et al., "Kindling and

Oxidative Stress as Contributors to Myalgic Encephalomyalitis/Chronic Fatigue Syndrome," *Journal of Behavioral and Neuroscience Research* 7, no. 2 (2009): 1–17, https://www.researchgate.net/publication/49772972_Kindling_and_Oxidative_Stress_as_Contributors_to_Myalgic_EncephalomyelitisChronic_Fatigue_Syndrome/citation/download.

300   leads to impaired immune response: Ashok Gupta, "Unconscious Amygdalar Fear Conditioning in a Subset of Chronic Fatigue Syndrome Patients," *Medical Hypotheses* 59, no. 6 (2001): 727–35, doi: 1.1016/s0306-9877(02)00321-3, as cited in Jason et al., "Kindling and Oxidative Stress."

300   integrative biopsychosocial theory: Benjamin N. Goertzel et al., "Combinations of Single Nucleotide Polymorphisms in Neuroendocrine Effector and Receptor Genes Predict Chronic Fatigue Syndrome," *Pharmacogenomics* 7, no. 3 (2006): 475–83, doi: 10.2217/14622416.7.3.475, as cited in Vegard B. Wyller, Hege R. Eriksen, and Kirsti Malterud, "Can Sustained Arousal Explain the Chronic Fatigue Syndrome?," *Behavioral and Brain Functions* 5, no. 10 (2009), doi: 10.1186/1744-9081-5-10.

300   "a unifying theoretical framework": Wyller, Eriksen, and Malterud, "Can Sustained Arousal Explain."

300   "the butterfly effect": James Gleick, *Chaos: Making a New Science* (New York: Penguin, 1987), 322 (notes). Gleick suggests that the term may have emerged from Lorenz's 1972 paper, "Predictability: Does the Flap of a Butterfly's Wings in Brazil Set Off a Tornado in Texas?" presented at the annual meeting of the American Association for the Advancement of Science.

301   "Chaos and the Limits of Modern Medicine": James S. Goodwin, "A Piece of My Mind. Chaos, and the Limits of Modern Medicine," *JAMA* 278, no. 17 (1997): 1399–400, https://www.researchgate.net/publication/13873560_A_piece_of_my_mind_Chaos_and_the_limits_of_modern_medicine.

302   "solver of puzzles": Gleick, *Chaos,* 37.

303   "has an interdisciplinary character": Gleick, *Chaos,* 37.

303   Chaos theory helped to connect: Gleick, *Chaos,* 114.

303   Max Planck: Max Planck, *Scientific Autobiography, and Other Papers,* trans. F. Gaynor (New York: Greenwood Press, 1968), 18–19.

303   "A new scientific truth": Planck, *Scientific Autobiography,* as cited in Bernard Barber, "Resistance by Scientists to Scientific Discovery," *Science* 134, no. 3479 (1961): 596–97, https://science.sciencemag.org/content/134/3479/596.

303   a long lag: Daniel Niven, "Closing the 17-Year Gap Between Scientific Evidence and Patient Care," *University Affairs,* January 17, 2017, https://www.universityaffairs.ca/opinion/in-my-opinion/closing-17-year-gap-scientific-evidence-patient-care/.

304   an outlier: Benoit B. Mandelbrot, *The Fractalist: Memoir of a Scientific Maverick* (New York: Pantheon, 2012), 228.

304   could discern a pattern that no one else had seen: Mandelbrot, *The Fractalist,* 216–19.

304 "it was a naturalist's approach": Gleick, *Chaos*, 110.

305 "mountains are not cones": Jacob Goldstein, "Clouds Are Not Spheres, Mountains Are Not Cones," *Planet Money*, October 18, 2010, https://www.npr.org/sections /money/2010/10/18/130643155/-clouds-are-not-spheres-mountains-are-not -cones.

305 "for which there was no geometry": Benoit Mandelbrot, "Fractals and the Art of Roughness," TED, https://www.ted.com/talks/benoit_mandelbrot_fractals_and _the_art_of_roughness.

305 many other systems in the body also bear fractal elements: Gleick, *Chaos*, 108–10.

305 a pair of human lungs, spread out: Gleick, *Chaos*, 109.

305 breathing patterns are fractal: Mark Ward, *Beyond Chaos: The Underlying Theory Behind Life, the Universe, and Everything* (New York: St. Martin's Press, 2001), 145.

306 follow fractal laws: Ward, *Beyond Chaos*, 145.

306 "critical point": Ward, *Beyond Chaos*, 140–41. Ward writes about the critical state, aka critical point (54), and writes about it in terms of the body (146).

306 would wear out more quickly: Ward, *Beyond Chaos*, 140.

306 don't follow fractal patterns: *Beyond Chaos*, Ward, 143.

306 "not as creative": Ward, *Beyond Chaos*, 146.

306 "Systems disordered in the right way are highly adaptable": Crystal Ives, "Human Beings as Chaotic Systems," 2004, http://fractal.org/Life-Science-Technology /Publications/Human-beings-as-fractal-systems.pdf.

306 applied to research: Kathy A. Svitil and Dan Winters, "Fire in the Brain," *Discover Magazine* 23, no. 5 (May 2002): 50.

307 predict the early course of the COVID-19 pandemic: Sylvain Mangiarotti et al., "Chaos Theory Applied to the Outbreak of COVID-19: An Ancillary Approach to Decision Making in Pandemic Context," *Epidemiology and Infection* 148 (2020): e95, doi: 10.1017/S0950268820000990.

307 "harmonious arrangement of order and disorder": Gleick, *Chaos*, 117.

307 "essentially hostile to wild nature": Gleick, *Chaos*, 117.

308 systems that pulse: William E. Odum, Eugene P. Odum, and Howard T. Odum, "Nature's Pulsing Paradigm," *Estuaries* 18, no. 4 (1995): 552, doi: 10.2307/1352375.

308 earth's ecosystem, like a beating heart: Carolyn Merchant, *The Columbia Guide to American Environmental History* (New York: Columbia University Press, 2002), 190.

PART V: RECOVERY

309 Ursula Le Guin: Ursula Le Guin (speech, National Book Awards, November 19, 2014), https://www.poetryfoundation.org/harriet/2014/11/change-begins-in-art -ursula-k-le-guins-amazing-nba-acceptance-speech.

309 Rebecca Solnit, *Hope in the Dark*: Rebecca Solnit, *Hope in the Dark: Untold Histories, Wild Possibilities*, 3rd ed. (Chicago: Haymarket Books, 2016), xxvi.

310 great human orchestra: Sandra Steingraber, as quoted in Robert Shetterly's book

of portraits *Americans Who Tell the Truth* (New York: Dutton Books for Young Readers, 2005). Reprinted with permission.

CHAPTER 16: REWIRING

312 *Wired for Healing*: Annie Hopper, *Wired for Healing: Remapping the Brain to Recover from Chronic and Mysterious Illnesses* (Victoria, BC: The Dynamic Neural Reprogramming System, 2014), 5.

312 broken-down houseboat: Hopper, *Wired for Healing*, 8–9.

313 "longing for *action*, relentlessly denied": Alice James, *The Diary of Alice James*, ed. Leon Edel (Boston: Northeastern University Press, 1999), 151.

313 her "restricted career": Jean Strouse, *Alice James: A Biography* (Cambridge: Harvard University Press, 1999), 276.

313 "little rubbish-heap": James, *Diary*, 78, as cited in Strouse, *Alice James*, 276.

313 "proportionate to the excess of weakness": Strouse, *Alice James*, 276.

313 "the varying degrees of discomfort": *Alice James: Her Life in Letters*, ed. Linda Anderson (Bristol, England: Thoemmes Press, 1996), 263.

313 Italianate townhouse: Strouse, *Alice James*, 297–98.

314 homeostasis: Sapolsky, *Why Zebras*, 9.

314 absence of disease: Sung W. Lee, "A Copernican Approach to Brain Advancement: The Paradigm of Allostatic Orchestration," *Frontiers in Human Neuroscience* 13 (2019): 129, doi: 10.3389/fnhum.2019.00129.

314 a postmodern paradigm: allostasis: Peter Sterling and Joseph Eyer, "Allostasis: A New Paradigm to Explain Arousal Pathology," *Handbook of Life Stress, Cognition and Health*, eds. Shirley Fisher and James Reason (New York: John Wiley & Sons, 1988), 629–49.

314 "measurements of the internal milieu": Sterling and Eyer, "Allostasis," 631.

314 compensatory changes: Sterling and Eyer, "Allostasis," 645–46.

314 anticipatory changes: Lee, "A Copernican Approach."

314 body as a complex ecosystem: Lee, "A Copernican Approach."

315 set point is likely to be regulated cooperatively: Robert M. Sapolsky, *Why Zebras Don't Get Ulcers*, 3rd ed. (New York: Times Books, 2004), 9.

315 "optimal anticipatory oscillation": Lee, "A Copernican Approach."

316 brain is in fact surprisingly malleable: Norman Doidge, *The Brain That Changes Itself: Stories of Personal Triumph from the Frontiers of Brain Science* (New York: Viking, 2007), xviii.

316 "cascading stress response": Hopper, *Wired for Healing*, xx.

316 "an *acquired brain injury* that affects many systems": Hopper, *Wired for Healing*, 12.

316 "excessive stress inhibits synaptic function and neuronal growth": Hopper, *Wired for Healing*, 31.

316 impair detoxification processes: Hopper, *Wired for Healing*, 48.

316 "neurons that fire together wire together": Doidge, *The Brain That Changes*, 63.

317 "allostatic impairment": Lee, "A Copernican Approach."

317   persistent assaults on the brain can impact all of the systems: Lee, "A Copernican Approach."

317   repair of the social fabric: Lee, "A Copernican Approach."

318   constraint-induced movement therapy: Doidge, *The Brain That Changes*, 134, 136.

318   CIMT restores reduced neuronal brain maps: Doidge, *The Brain That Changes*, 149.

318   motor functions substantially improved: J. Liepert et al., "Motor Cortex Plasticity During Constraint-Induced Movement Therapy in Stroke Patients," *Neuroscience Letters* 250, no. 1 (1998): 5–8, doi: 10.1016/s0304-3940(98)00386-3, as cited in Doidge, *The Brain That Changes*, 149.

318   neuroplastic changes can reach across brain hemispheres: Bruno Kopp et al., "Plasticity in the Motor System Related to Therapy-Induced Improvement of Movement After Stroke," *NeuroReport* 10, no. 4 (1999): 807–10, doi: 10.1097/00001756 -199903170-00026, as cited in Doidge, *The Brain That Changes*, 149.

318   "going downhill at a steady trot": James, *Diary*, 207.

318   "out of the formless void": James, *Diary*, 207.

318   As she exulted in her diary: James, *Diary*, 206, as cited in Strouse, *Alice James*, 301.

318   "hyperaesthesia": James, *Diary*, 207.

319   "a certain value as an indestructible quantity": James, *Diary*, 207, as cited in Strouse, *Alice James*, 301.

319   "whisperings of release in the air": James, *Diary*, 194, as cited in Strouse, *Alice James*, 304.

319   "I have always had a significance for myself": James, *Diary*, 195, as cited in Strouse, *Alice James*, 305.

319   morphine that had worked for a time: Strouse, *Alice James*, 308.

319   an article by a nearby doctor about hypnosis: Strouse, *Alice James*, 309.

319   "deep sea of divine *cessation*": James, *Diary*, 232, as cited in Strouse, *Alice James*, 312.

319   began regularly hypnotizing her: Strouse, *Alice James*, 309.

320   "vast field of therapeutic possibilities": Strouse, *Alice James*, 222.

320   "modern complicated mechanism": James, *Diary*, 223, as cited in Strouse, *Alice James*, 309.

321   showed similar brain map changes: Alvaro Pascual-Leone et al., "Modulation of Muscle Responses Evoked by Transcranial Magnetic Stimulation During the Acquisition of New Fine Motor Skills," *Journal of Neurophysiology* 74, no. 3 (1995): 1037–45, doi: 10.1152/jn.1995.74.3.1037, as cited in Doidge, *The Brain That Changes*, 201.

321   her limbic system calmed: Hopper, *Wired for Healing*, 80–81.

322   vulnerable to fascism: William I. Robinson, "Global Capitalist Crisis and Twenty-First Century Fascism: Beyond the Trump Hype," *Science & Society* 83, no. 2 (2019): 481–509, https://doi.org/10.1521/siso.2019.83.2.155; "Fascism on the Rise: Where Does It Come From, and How to Stop It, with a Common European Response," European Economic and Social Committee, October 30, 2018, https:// www.eesc.europa.eu/en/news-media/news/fascism-rise-where-does-it-come -and-how-stop-it-common-european-response.

322 "mechanistic view of change": Solnit, *Hope in the Dark*, 60.

322 social change starts in the imagination: Solnit, *Hope in the Dark*, 26.

323 legislator chose to do his mother's bidding: Solnit, *Hope in the Dark*, xx.

323 photo essay by Thilde Jensen: Thilde Jensen, "Everything Makes Them Sick," *New York Times*, September 17, 2011, https://archive.nytimes.com/www.nytimes.com /interactive/2011/09/18/opinion/sunday/20110918_OPINION_ALLERGY GOBIG.html?ref=opinion#1.

324 author of the paper: Ashok Gupta, "Unconscious Amygdalar Fear Conditioning in a Subset of Chronic Fatigue Syndrome Patients," *Medical Hypotheses* 59, no. 6 (2001): 727–35, doi: 1.1016/s0306-9877(02)00321-3.

327 "would love you to believe that it's hopeless": Solnit, *Hope in the Dark*, xi.

327 "both excuse themselves from acting": Solnit, *Hope in the Dark*, xiv.

327 Confederate statues fell: Jaia Clingham-David, "5 Key Achievements of Black Lives Matter Movement in 2020, So Far," *One Green Planet*, 2020, https://www .onegreenplanet.org/human-interest/5-key-achievements-of-black-lives-matter -movement-in-2020-so-far/.

327 jury pronounced Chauvin guilty: Janelle Griffith, "Derek Chauvin Sentenced to 22.5 Years for the Murder of George Floyd," NBC News, June 25, 2021, https:// www.nbcnews.com/news/us-news/derek-chauvin-be-sentenced-murder-death -george-floyd-n1272332.

328 Passamaquoddy Nation recently reacquired: Colin Woodard, "Passamaquoddy Tribe Reacquires Island Stolen More Than 150 Years Ago," *Portland Press Herald*, May 17, 2021, https://www.pressherald.com/2021/05/17/passamaquoddy-tribe -reacquires-island-stolen-more-than-150-years-ago/.

328 Johnson & Johnson began removing known and probable carcinogens: Jane Kay, "Johnson & Johnson Removes Some Chemicals from Baby Shampoo, Other Products," *Scientific American*, May 6, 2013, https://www.scientificamerican.com /article/johnson-and-johnson-removes-some-chemicals-from-baby-shampoo -other-products/.

328 ordinance recognizing the rights of nature: Ben Price, personal communication, December 5, 2020.

328 into its constitution: Ben Price, personal communication, December 5, 2020.

328 "litanies or recitations or monuments": Solnit, *Hope in the Dark*, xxi.

329 even a forced smile: Elizabeth Millard, "Forcing a Smile May Improve Your Mood, Study Suggests," *verywellmind*, August 31, 2020, https://www.verywellmind .com/news-science-shows-smiling-really-does-make-us-feel-better-5075811 #citation-2.

330 "invisible except through storytelling": Solnit, *Hope in the Dark*, 71.

332 to start on the margins: Solnit, *Hope in the Dark*, 28–29.

333 finally when women spoke out, people listened: "#MeToo: A Timeline of Events," *Chicago Tribune*, February 4, 1021, https://www.chicagotribune.com/lifestyles/ct -me-too-timeline-20171208-htmlstory.html.

333 doesn't make this: Ashley Fetters Maloy and Paul Farhi, "Five Years On, What

Happened to the Men of #MeToo?," *Washington Post*, October 16, 2022, https://www.washingtonpost.com/lifestyle/2022/10/16/metoo-men-what-happened.

333 "not a finished Utopia": Bertrand Russell, *Political Ideals* (New York: The Century Co., 1917), chapter 1, as cited in Rutger Bregman, *Utopia for Realists: How We Can Build the Ideal World* (New York: Little, Brown, 2017), 21.

333 Energy-saving lightbulbs: Sophie Lewis, "Trump Rolls Back Obama-Era Regulations on Energy-Efficient Light Bulbs," CBS News, September 4, 2019, https://www.cbsnews.com/news/trump-rolls-back-obama-era-regulations-on-energy-efficient-light-bulbs/.

334 to lower smokestack emissions: Diane Bacher, "Devices Used to Remove Pollutants from Smoke Stacks," *Sciencing*, November 22, 2019, https://sciencing.com/about-5568843-devices-remove-pollutants-smoke-stacks.html.

334 The internet: Mariana Mazzucato, *The Entrepreneurial State: Debunking Public vs. Private Sector Myths* (New York: Penguin, 2013), https://marianamazzucato.com/books/the-entrepreneurial-state.

334 begin with the word *public*: Charles C. W. Cooke, "Notes on a Ridiculous Meme," *National Review*, October 19, 2015, https://www.nationalreview.com/2015/10/socialism-united-states-meme/.

334 first ever study: Dale Guenter, "DNRS Research Results at NAPCRG Conference," December 17, 2019, https://www.youtube.com/watch?v=KgQ1IN0b2J0.

335 average healthy Canadian generally scores: Dale Guenter et al., "Neuroplasticity-Based Treatment for Fibromyalgia, Chronic Fatigue and Multiple Chemical Sensitivity: Feasibility and Outcomes," 2019, https://retrainingthebrain.com/research/.

335 "it lasts": Guenter, "DNRS Research Results."

335 also significantly reduced: Guenter et al., "Neuroplasticity-Based Treatment."

335 randomized controlled trial of a brain retraining program: Alex Bratty, "A Pilot Study Published in the Journal of Clinical Medicine," the Gupta Program, 2022, https://www.guptaprogram.com/fibrostudy/.

335 measured the effects of the Gupta Program: Juan P. Sanabria-Mazo et al., "Mindfulness-Based Program Plus Amygdala and Insula Retraining (MAIR) for the Treatment of Women with Fibromyalgia: A Pilot Randomized Controlled Trial," *Journal of Clinical Medicine* 9, no. 10 (2020): 3246, doi: 10.3390/jcm9103246, https://www.guptaprogram.com/wp-content/uploads/2020/10/jcm-09-03246.pdf.

336 comfort the afflicted and afflict the comfortable: Robert Deis, "Comfort the Afflicted, and Afflict the Comfortable," *This Day in Quotes*, July 30, 2020, http://www.thisdayinquotes.com/2020/07/comfort-afflicted-and-afflict.html?m=1.

337 "until the vanishing point is reached": James, *Diary*, 229–30.

337 "the poor, shabby old thing": James, *Diary*, 230, as cited in Strouse, *Alice James*, 189.

337 "Alice was making sentences": James, *Diary*, 232–33, as cited in Strouse, *Alice James*, 313.

338 "did not succumb": Strouse, *Alice James*, 315.

338 "anything but a failure": Strouse, *Alice James*, 315.

338 laborers belonged to unions: Howard Zinn, *A People's History of the United States,* 35th anniversary edition (New York: HarperPerennial, 2015), 328.

338 Industrial Workers of the World: Zinn, *A People's History,* 329.

338 rallied strikers all over the country: Zinn, *A People's History,* 329, 331.

339 risen to four thousand: Zinn, *A People's History,* 339.

339 just twenty-five work stoppages: Bureau of Labor Statistics, "Annual Work Stoppages Involving 1,000 or More Workers, 1947–Present," February 23, 2022, https://www.bls.gov/web/wkstp/annual-listing.htm.

339 Social Democratic Party: Zinn, *A People's History,* 340.

340 largest women's march in history up until that time: Zinn, *A People's History,* 344.

340 protesting Trump's inauguration in 2017: Tim Wallace and Alicia Parlapiano, "Crowd Scientists Say Women's March in Washington Had 3 Times as Many People as Trump's Inauguration," *New York Times,* January 22, 2017, https://www.nytimes.com/interactive/2017/01/22/us/politics/womens-march-trump-crowd-estimates.html.

340 largest single-day protest in U.S. history: Matt Broomfield, "Women's March Against Donald Trump Is the Largest Day of Protests in US History, Say Political Scientists," *Independent,* January 23, 2017, https://www.independent.co.uk/news/world/americas/womens-march-anti-donald-trump-womens-rights-largest-protest-demonstration-us-history-political-scientists-a7541081.html.

340 prevent women of color from voting: Anna North, "The 19th Amendment Didn't Give Women the Right to Vote," *Vox,* August 18, 2020, https://www.vox.com/2020/8/18/21358913/19th-amendment-ratified-anniversary-women-suffrage-vote.

341 plug-in air fresheners: Toxic Free Future, "Top 10 Tips to Go Toxic-Free on the Cheap," https://toxicfreefuture.org/healthy-choices/10-tips-to-go-toxic-free-on-the-cheap/.

341 Shell alone emitted: Seth Wynes and Kimberly A. Nicholas, "The Climate Mitigation Gap: Education and Government Recommendations Miss the Most Effective Individual Actions," *Environmental Research Letters* 12, no. 7 (2017): e074024, doi: 10.1088/1748-9326/aa7541; Cassandra Roxburgh, "Individuals Are Not to Blame for the Climate Crisis," *Yes!* January 31, 2022, https://www.yesmagazine.org/environment/2022/01/31/climate-change-fossil-fuel-industry-individual-responsibility.

341 "industry-funded 'deflection campaigns'": Michael E. Mann, "Lifestyle Changes Aren't Enough to Save the Planet. Here's What Could," *Time,* September 12, 2019, https://time.com/5669071/lifestyle-changes-climate-change/.

341 cannot be achieved: Morten Fibieger Byskov, "Focusing on How Individuals Can Stop Climate Change Is Very Convenient for Corporations," Fast Company, January 11, 2019, https://www.fastcompany.com/90290795/focusing-on-how-individuals-can-stop-climate-change-is-very-convenient-for-corporations.

341 diversion from actual political action: Wesley Morris and Jenna Wortham, "Circular(s): Why Conscious Consumption Isn't Enough to Combat Climate

Change," Still Processing, *New York Times*, March 14, 2019, https://www.nytimes.com/2019/03/14/podcasts/still-processing-circulars-climate-change.html.

342 Frank R. Lautenberg Chemical Safety for the 21st Century Act: Noah M. Sachs, "Will the New Toxic Chemical Safety Law Protect Us?," *The Conversation*, June 16, 2016, https://theconversation.com/will-the-new-toxic-chemical-safety-law-protect-us-60769.

343 ban chain store pharmacies from their state: Stacy Mitchell, Interview by Tracy Frisch, "Unfair Advantage: Stacy Mitchell on How Amazon Undermines Local Economies," *The Sun*, November 2018.

343 city's investments out of corporations: Mitchell, Interview by Frisch, "Unfair Advantage."

CHAPTER 17: WEB

344 latent in my system: Jonathan R. Kerr, "Epstein-Barr Virus (EBV) Reactivation and Therapeutic Inhibitors," *Journal of Clinical Pathology* 72 (2019): 651–58, https://doi.org/10.1136/jclinpath-2019-205822, as cited in Mike McRae, "A New Therapy Attacking a Common Virus Shows Huge Promise for Multiple Sclerosis," *ScienceAlert*, April 13, 2022, https://www.sciencealert.com/experimental-therapy-targeting-epstein-barr-infections-shows-promise-as-ms-treatment.

344 MTHFR: Stephanie Eckelkamp, "What Exactly Is Methylation & Why Is It So Essential to Overall Health?," *mindbodygreen*, March 23, 2022, https://www.mindbodygreen.com/articles/what-is-methylation.

344 COMT gene: Tchiki Davis, "What Is the COMT Gene? And How Does It Affect Your Health?," *Psychology Today* (blog), January 15, 2020, https://www.psychologytoday.com/us/blog/click-here-happiness/202001/what-is-the-comt-gene-and-how-does-it-affect-your-health.

345 "fear conditioning in the amygdala": Ashok Gupta, "Unconscious Amygdalar Fear Conditioning in a Subset of Chronic Fatigue Syndrome Patients," *Medical Hypotheses* 59, no. 6 (2001): 727–35, doi: 1.1016/s0306-9877(02)00321-3.

347 critical hours of connection: Kathryn Landon-Malone, PhD, RN, CPNP-R, personal communication, November 17–30, 2020. Landon-Malone's PhD is in clinical psychology with a concentration in somatic psychology, and for her dissertation on second pregnancies she used existing research in early trauma, pre- and perinatal psychology, and somatic psychology to make assertions that traumatic early experiences shared with mother and baby could lead to definable psychological effects in the mother's and child's futures.

347 "trauma in infancy appears to lead to supersensitization": Norman Doidge, *The Brain That Changes Itself: Stories of Personal Triumph from the Frontiers of Brain Science* (New York: Viking, 2007), 240.

347 more easily stressed for the rest of their lives: Doidge, *The Brain That Changes*, 387 (notes).

347 critical imprinting time: Landon-Malone, personal communication, November 17–30, 2020.

348 "it's a shared experience": Landon-Malone, personal communication, November 17–30, 2020.

349 Adverse Childhood Experiences (ACE) score: Christine Heim et al., "Early Adverse Experience and Risk for Chronic Fatigue Syndrome," *Archives of General Psychiatry* 63, no. 11 (2006): 1258–66, doi: 10.1001/archpsyc.63.11.1258; Christine Heim et al., "Childhood Trauma and Risk for Chronic Fatigue Syndrome: Association with Neuroendocrine Dysfunction," *Archives of General Psychiatry* 66, no. 1 (2009): 72–80, doi: 10.1001/archgenpsychiatry.2008.508.

349 believed stress played a role: Alison Clements et al., "Chronic Fatigue Syndrome: A Qualitative Investigation of Patients' Beliefs About the Illness," *Journal of Psychosomatic Research* 42, no. 6 (1997): 615–24, doi: 10.1016/S0022-3999(97)00087-1.

349 Limbic system impairment could be: Annie Hopper, *Wired for Healing: Remapping the Brain to Recovery from Chronic and Mysterious Illnesses* (Victoria, BC: The Dynamic Neural Reprogramming System, 2014), xix; Vegard B. Wyller, Hege R. Eriksen, and Kirsti Malterud, "Can Sustained Arousal Explain the Chronic Fatigue Syndrome?," *Behavioral and Brain Functions* 5, no. 10 (2009), doi: 10.1186/1744 -9081-5-10.

349 including long COVID: "COVID Long-Haulers Treatment: Neuroplasticity-Based Approach Showing Promising Results," Dynamic Neural Retraining System, https://retrainingthebrain.com/long-haulers-treatment-covid/.

350 TED Talk: Jennifer Brea, "What Happens When You Have a Disease Doctors Can't Diagnose," TEDSummit, January 7, 2017, https://www.ted.com/talks/jennifer _brea_what_happens_when_you_have_a_disease_doctors_can_t_diagnose ?language=en.

350 fully in her body for the first time: Jennifer Brea, personal communication, January 28, 2021.

350 no longer met the criteria for ME/CFS: Jennifer Brea, "CCI + Tethered Cord Series," *Medium,* March 26, 2019, https://jenbrea.medium.com/cci-tethered-cord -series-e1e098b5edf.

351 "People are looking for one answer": Jennifer Brea, personal communication, January 28, 2021.

351 experienced significant improvements from: Jacob Teitelbaum, "Other People with ME/CFS Have Experienced Significant Improvements from: IVIG—Intravenous Gamma Globulin Therapy for Chronic Fatigue Syndrome (ME/CFS), Fibromyalgia and POTS," Health Rising, 2017, https://www.healthrising.org/treating-chronic-fatigue-syndrome/drugs/ivig-intravenous-gamma-globulin-therapy/; Selim Akarsu et al., "The Efficacy of Hyperbaric Oxygen Therapy in the Management of Chronic Fatigue Syndrome," *Undersea and Hyperbaric Medicine* 40, no. 2 (2013): 197–200, https://pubmed.ncbi.nlm.nih.gov/23682549/; Robert Phair, "Metabolic Traps in ME/CFS," Open Medicine Foundation, October 2, 2019, https://www.youtube.com/watch?v=d9oVHDh8rjk.

351 "once the fire has been put out": Jennifer Brea, @jenbrea, "I think of brain retraining as something that might help some people turn off the alarms once

the fire has been put out," Twitter, January 29, 2021, https://twitter.com/jenbrea/status/1355227868125483008.

351 "not an intellectual process": Hopper, *Wired for Healing*, 108.

352 like the polluted air had a *texture*: Jennifer Brea, personal communication, January 28, 2021.

353 from a homeostatic perspective: Jessica Del Pozo, interview with Kevin Gallagher, "Emergent Resilience for Health, Community, and Our Climate: Building Community, Resilience, and Reconnecting to Our Natural Environments," *Psychology Today* (blog), February 16, 2020, https://www.psychologytoday.com/us/blog/being-awake-better/202002/emergent-resilience-health-community-and-our-climate-0.

353 "in an ongoing conversation with that world": Del Pozo, interview with Kevin Gallagher, "Emergent Resilience."

355 wanted her diary posthumously published: Alice James, *The Diary of Alice James*, ed. Leon Edel (Boston: Northeastern University Press, 1999), xxix, as cited in Strouse, *Alice James*, 320.

355 "leaf in the family laurel crown": Jean Strouse, *Alice James: A Biography* (Cambridge: Harvard University Press, 1999), 319.

356 Oyster Bay Nation: Tasmania Parks and Wildlife Service, "Maria Island National Park," https://parks.tas.gov.au/explore-our-parks/maria-island-national-park.

357 debunking the Darwinian notion: David Korten, Interview by Arnie Cooper, "Everybody Wants to Rule the World: David Korten on Putting an End to Global Competition," *The Sun*, September 2007, https://www.thesunmagazine.org/issues/381/everybody-wants-to-rule-the-world.

357 because we were more socially oriented: Rutger Bregman, *Humankind: A Hopeful History*, trans. Elizabeth Manton and Erica Moore (New York: Little, Brown, 2020), 59–60, 68–72.

357 a leg up on the other hominins: Bregman, *Humankind*, 68–72.

357 "cells come together in this extraordinary cooperative enterprise": Korten, Interview by Cooper, "Everybody Wants to Rule the World."

EPILOGUE

365 died from COVID-19: Hannah Ritchie et al., "Coronavirus (COVID-19) Deaths," Our World in Data, August 25, 2022, https://ourworldindata.org/covid-deaths; "How Many Died in the American Civil War?," History Channel, January 6, 2022, https://www.history.com/news/american-civil-war-deaths.

365 long COVID: Destin Groff et al., "Short-Term and Long-Term Rates of Postacute Sequelae of SARS-CoV-2 Infection: A Systematic Review," *JAMA Network Open* 4, no. 10 (2021): e2128568, doi: 10.1001/jamanetworkopen.2021.28568.

365 similarities between long COVID and ME/CFS: Timothy L. Wong and Danielle J. Weitzer, "Long COVID and Myalgic Encephalomyelitis/Chronic Fatigue Syndrome (ME/CFS)—a Systemic Review and Comparison of Clinical

Presentation and Symptomology," *Medicina* 57, no. 5 (May 2021): 418, doi: 10.3390/medicina57050418.

365   wind up with long COVID: Pam Belluck, "Many 'Long Covid' Patients Had No Symptoms from Their Initial Infection," *New York Times*, March 8, 2021, https://www.nytimes.com/2021/03/08/health/long-covid-asymptomatic.html?search ResultPosition=2.

365   rate of long COVID among fully vaccinated: Katelyn Jetelina, "How Vaccines Reduce Long Covid," *Your Local Epidemiologist*, November 17, 2021, https://your localepidemiologist.substack.com/p/how-vaccines-reduce-long-covid.

EPIGRAPH

367   "Window on the Body": from *Walking Words* by Eduardo Galeano, translated by Mark Fried. Copyright © 1993 by Eduardo Galeano. Translation copyright © 1995 by Mark Fried. Used by permission of the author and W. W. Norton & Company, Inc.

APPENDIX

373   charter revocation laws: Joel Bakan, *The Corporation: The Pathological Pursuit of Profit and Power* (New York: Free Press, 2004), 157.

374   can freely vote their consciences: Katrina vanden Heuvel, "Ranked-Choice Voting Is Already Changing Politics for the Better," *Washington Post*, May 4, 2021, https://www.washingtonpost.com/opinions/2021/05/04/ranked-choice-voting-is -already-changing-politics-better/.